Virtual Reality Technologies for Health and Clinical Applications

Series Editor

Paul Sharkey

For further volumes:
http://www.springer.com/series/13399

Patrice L. (Tamar) Weiss • Emily A. Keshner
Mindy F. Levin
Editors

Virtual Reality for Physical and Motor Rehabilitation

Springer

Editors
Patrice L. (Tamar) Weiss
Department of Occupational Therapy
University of Haifa
Mount Carmel
Haifa, Israel

Emily A. Keshner
Department of Physical Therapy and Department of Electrical and Computer Engineering, Temple University
Philadelphia, PA, USA

Mindy F. Levin
School of Physical and Occupational Therapy, McGill University
Montreal, QC, Canada

ISBN 978-1-4939-0967-4 ISBN 978-1-4939-0968-1 (eBook)
DOI 10.1007/978-1-4939-0968-1
Springer New York Heidelberg Dordrecht London

Library of Congress Control Number: 2014942842

Printed on acid-free paper

Springer is part of Springer Science+Business Media (www.springer.com)

Contents

Contributors

Sergei V. Adamovich, Ph.D. Department of Biomedical Engineering, New Jersey Institue of Technology, Newark, NJ, USA
sergei.adamovich@njit.edu

Eric R. Anson, P.T. Department of Kinesiology, University of Maryland, College Park, MD, USA
eanson1@umd.edu

Lara A. Boyd, P.T., Ph.D. Department of Physical Therapy, University of British Columbia, Vancouver, BC, Canada
lara.boyd@ubc.ca

Nicoleta Bugnariu, P.T., Ph.D. Physical Therapy Program, University of North Texas Health Science Center, Fort Worth, TX, USA
nicoleta.bugnariu@unthsc.edu

Katharine L. Cheung, M.Sc. Department of Physical Therapy, University of British Columbia, Vancouver, BC, Canada
katharine.cheung@alumni.ubc.ca

Sarah H. Creem-Regehr, Ph.D. Department of Psychology, University of Utah, Salt Lake City, UT, USA
sarah.creem@psych.utah.edu

Judith E. Deutsch, P.T., Ph.D. RiVERS Lab, Department of Rehabilitation and Movement Science, Rutgers University, Newark, NJ, USA
deutsch@shrp.rutgers.edu

Stephen R. Ellis, Ph.D. Human Systems Integrations Division, Advanced Controls and Displays Laboratory, NASA Ames Research Center, Moffet Field, CA, USA
stephen.r.ellis@nasa.gov

Gerard G. Fluet Department of Rehabilitation and Movement Science, Rutgers University, Newark, NJ, USA
fluet179@comcast.net

Joyce Fung, P.T., Ph.D. School of Physical and Occupational Therapy, McGill University, Montréal, QC, Canada
joyce.fung@mcgill.ca

Dido Green, O.T., Ph.D. Centre for Rehabilitation, Faculty of Health and Life Sciences, Oxford Brookes University, Oxford, UK
dido.green@brookes.ac.uk

Jeffrey M. Hausdorff, Ph.D. Movement Disorders Unit, Department of Neurology, Tel-Aviv Sourasky Medical Center, Tel-Aviv, Israel
jhausdor@tlvmc.gov.il

John Jeka, Ph.D. Department of Kinesiology, Temple University, Philadelphia, PA, USA
jjeka@temple.edu

Michal Kafri, P.T., Ph.D. Department of Physical Therapy, Faculty of Social Welfare & Health Sciences, University of Haifa, Mount Carmel, Haifa, Israel
kafri.michal@gmail.com

Robert V. Kenyon, P.T., Ph.D. Department of Computer Science, University of Illinois at Chicago, Chicago, IL, USA
Kenyon@uic.edu

Emily A. Keshner, P.T., Ph.D. Department of Physical Therapy and Department of Electrical and Computer Engineering, Temple University, Philadelphia, PA, USA
ekeshner@temple.edu

Anouk Lamontagne, P.T., Ph.D. School of Physical and Occupational Therapy, McGill University, Montréal, QC, Canada
anouk.lamontagne@mcgill.ca

Daneille E. Levac, P.T., Ph.D. School of Rehabilitation Sciences, Faculty of Health Sciences, University of Ottawa, Ottawa, ON, Canada
dlevа2@uottawa.ca

Mindy F. Levin, P.T., Ph.D. School of Physical and Occupational Therapy, McGill University, Montreal, QC, Canada
mindy.levin@mcgill.ca

Dario G. Liebermann, Ph.D. Physical Therapy Department, The Stanley Steyer School of Health Professions, Sackler Faculty of Medicine, Tel Aviv University, Tel Aviv, Israel
dlieberm@post.tau.ac.il

Alma S. Merians P.T., Ph.D. Department of Rehabilitation and Movement Science, Rutgers University, Newark, NJ, USA
alma.merians@shrp.rutgers.edu

Anat Mirelman, P.T., Ph.D. Movement Disorders Unit, Department of Neurology, Tel-Aviv Sourasky Medical Center, Tel-Aviv, Israel
anatmi@tlvmc.gov.il

Heidi Sveistrup, Ph.D. School of Rehabilitation Sciences, Faculty of Health Sciences, University of Ottawa, Ottawa, ON, Canada
hsveist@uottawa.ca

Eugene Tunik, P.T., Ph.D. Department of Rehabilitation & Movement Science, UMDNJ, Newark, NJ, USA
eugene.tunik@rutgers.edu

William H. Warren, Ph.D. Department of Cognitive, Linguistic, and Psychological Sciences, Brown University, Providence, RI, USA
bill_warren@brown.edu

Patrice L. (Tamar) Weiss, O.T., Ph.D. Department of Occupational Therapy, Faculty of Social Welfare and Health Sciences, University of Haifa, Mount Carmel, Haifa, Israel
tamar@research.haifa.ac.il

Peter Wilson, Ph.D. School of Psychology, Australian Catholic University, Melbourne, VIC, Australia
peterh.wilson@acu.edu.au

W. Geoffrey Wright, Ph.D. Departments of Physical Therapy and Biomedical Engineering, Temple University, Philadelphia, PA, USA
wrightw@temple.edu

Chapter 1
Volume Introduction and Overview

Patrice L. (Tamar) Weiss, Emily A. Keshner, and Mindy F. Levin

Objective To introduce the reader to the scope and content of the volume.

The development of technologies that can be applied to rehabilitation offers tremendous promise for enhancing functional capacity by eliminating or minimizing the functional limitations imposed by disability. As new rehabilitation technologies emerge, it is our responsibility as scientists and clinicians to determine how these can best be used to support and modify human behavior. This requires that we understand both how technology development interfaces with human performance and how therapeutic interventions can be adapted to employ the technology effectively. Technologies based on virtual reality (VR) provide multiple levels at which this interface may occur, ranging from the most basic sensorimotor mechanisms to the more complex learning and psychosocial aspects of human behavior.

P.L. (Tamar) Weiss (✉)
Department of Occupational Therapy, Faculty of Social Welfare and Health Sciences,
University of Haifa, Mount Carmel, Haifa 3498838, Israel
e-mail: tamar@research.haifa.ac.il

E.A. Keshner
Department of Physical Therapy and Department of Electrical and Computer Engineering,
Temple University, 3307 N. Broad ST, Philadelphia, PA 19140, USA
e-mail: ekeshner@temple.edu

M.F. Levin
School of Physical and occupational Therapy, McGill University,
3654 Promenade Sir William Osler, Montreal, QC, Canada, H3G 1Y5
e-mail: mindy.levin@mcgill.ca

P.L. (Tamar) Weiss et al. (eds.), *Virtual Reality for Physical and Motor Rehabilitation*, Virtual Reality Technologies for Health and Clinical Applications,
DOI 10.1007/978-1-4939-0968-1_1,

This first volume of the Virtual Reality Technologies for Health and Clinical Applications series aims to provide a comprehensive overview of how VR technologies are applied to motor rehabilitation. The first part of this volume identifies the characteristics of VR that affect the mechanisms underlying the motor control processes that support motor relearning. The second part of the volume consists of critical overviews of VR applications that address (1) different therapeutic objectives (e.g., increasing muscle strength, improving sitting balance) and (2) user (client) goals including their relationship to the environment (e.g., participation in work, study, recreation). Chapter authors focus on the latest research findings on the clinical application of VR technology for remediation of motor disorders due to specific physical disabilities (e.g., stroke, traumatic brain injury, Parkinson's syndromes, cerebral palsy, degenerative conditions such as amyotrophic lateral sclerosis and multiple sclerosis). In this first chapter we provide a short summary of each of the subsequent chapters.

Chapter 2 by Katharine L. Cheung, Eugene Tunik, Sergei V. Adamovich, and Lara A. Boyd presents the key aspects of neuroplasticity and how VR technology can capitalize on and influence this phenomenon to promote motor rehabilitation. The nature of neuroplasticity and the physiological mechanisms involved in the induction of both short- and long-term changes in the brain that enable us to store and retrieve motor memories for later use is discussed. The ways in which neuroplastic changes can be classified using the biological principles related to neuroplasticity and the underlying tenets of learning are reviewed. The fundamental elements of experience-dependent neuroplasticity and clinical interventions, including VR technology, which have the potential to induce and affect neuroplasticity are considered. The empirical evidence of the effects of VR on neuroplastic changes in the brain is summarized.

Chapter 3 by Danielle E. Levac and Heidi Sveistrup presents four fundamental variables influencing client motor learning and describe how attributes of VR technologies provide opportunities to target these variables. It summarizes the rationale and evidence for attributes of VR technology that target the motor learning variables of practice, augmented feedback, motivation, and observational learning. The potential for motor learning achieved with VR-based therapy to transfer and generalize to the tasks in the physical environment is discussed. Recommendations are provided for clinicians interested in emphasizing motor learning using VR-based therapy.

Chapter 4 by Robert V. Kenyon and Stephen R. Ellis examines aspects of the technology that are needed to transfer visual information in the physical world to the virtual world by presenting how characteristics of human vision and human perception interface with a virtual environment. The advantages of VR systems for coincident viewing of physical and virtual objects and control of vision are presented. Perception of self-motion and visual perception including vection, vergence, stereovision, size-constancy, and rehabilitation in VR are reviewed.

Chapter 5 by W. Geoffrey Wright, Sarah H. Creem-Regehr, William H. Warren, Eric R. Anson, John Jeka, and Emily A. Keshner deals with the issue of resolving ambiguity between motion of objects in the world and self-motion that reflects interdependence between multimodal signals. A growing body of evidence suggests that visual, vestibular, non-visual, and non-vestibular aspects of virtual world immersion play an important role in perception of self-motion. In this chapter, five experts from the fields of postural and locomotor control present the work they have engaged in to understand how the brain uses multiple pathways of sensory feedback to organize motor behavior. Each discusses their work showing how VR may help us understand or engage the mechanisms underlying sensorimotor integration.

Chapter 6 by Mindy F. Levin, Judith E. Deutsch, Michal Kafri, and Dario G. Liebermann describes the quality of different types of VR environments and their influence on the production of movement. The chapter summarizes the current evidence on the validity of upper and lower limb movements made in different 2D and 3D VR environments. Movement patterns are considered directly as kinematic performance (e.g., endpoint trajectories) and motor quality measures (e.g., joint rotations), or indirectly, as surrogate measures of performance (e.g., heart rate).

Chapter 7 by Alma S. Merians and Gerard G. Fluet describes current clinical evidence for the effectiveness of VR applications on upper limb recovery in individuals who have had a stroke. The chapter summarizes outcomes of upper limb rehabilitation studies using the International Classification of Functioning, Disability, and Health model as a framework and describes motor learning approaches that have been used in VR simulations and interventions for upper limb recovery after stroke. The chapter includes a case study that explores how to effectively use VR/robotic technology for an individualized treatment intervention based on motor learning principles.

Chapter 8 by Anat Mirelman, Judith E. Deutsch, and Jeffrey M. Hausdorff presents a review of VR augmented training for improving walking and reducing fall risk in patients with neurodegenerative disease. It describes the common impairments in gait that are fundamental to neurodegenerative diseases and provides examples from studies on aging, Parkinson's disease and multiple sclerosis. Factors that contribute to problems in mobility are discussed along with current treatment approaches. The review of these topics leads to the rationale and potential advantages of VR-based methods for improving walking and mobility in patients with neurodegenerative disease.

Chapter 9 by Anouk Lamontagne, Emily A. Keshner, Nicoleta Bugnariu, and Joyce Fung reviews how VR can be used to investigate normal and disturbed mechanisms of balance and locomotor control. Loss of upright balance control resulting in falls is a major health problem for older adults and stroke survivors. Balance and mobility deficits arise not only from motor or sensory impairments but also from the inability to select and reweight pertinent sensory information. In particular, the role of the vestibular system and effects of age and stroke on the ability of the central nervous system to resolve sensory conflicts is emphasized, as well as the potential for rehabilitation protocols that include training in virtual environments to improve balance.

Chapter 10 by Dido Green and Peter Wilson provides an overview of the evolution of VR technologies across domains of childhood disability that focuses on the evidence base for applications in research, clinical and community settings in order to optimize outcomes for the child and family. It explores how changing patterns of childhood participation and engagement provide opportunities for using VR technologies for children with disabilities. The International Classification of Functioning, Disability, and Health—Children and Youth version is used as a framework to consider the role of VR technologies in evaluation and intervention across body structures and body function, activity performance and participation across different contexts. Benefits of VR are viewed through the lens of current theory and research to consider broader aspects of the potential impact on brain–behavior relationships.

Chapter 11 by Patrice L. (Tamar) Weiss, Emily A. Keshner, and Mindy F. Levin presents an overview of the evidence for effectiveness of VR for motor rehabilitation and a review of the major technology "breakthroughs" (1986–1995; 1996–2005; 2006–present) that have led to the use of VR for motor rehabilitation. A "Force Field" analysis is presented that looks to the future regarding developments anticipated to occur over the next 5–10 years. Forces that appear to be key factors in helping VR technology have a positive impact on motor rehabilitation have been identified from the information reported in the chapters of this volume, In addition, the forces that currently limit positive progress and, in some cases, prevent advancement towards the goal of effective use of VR technology for motor rehabilitation have been identified.

In conclusion, this volume focuses on the current state-of-the-art in the field of applications of VR for motor rehabilitation. The content has been purposely limited to motor applications in order to critically highlight both the advances that have been made over the past two decades and those that are anticipated in the coming years. At the same time, we recognize the importance of interpreting activity of the motor system within the context of various psychological and cognitive phenomena, as presented in Volume 2 of this series (Psychological and Neurocognitive Interventions edited by Albert A. "Skip" Rizzo and Stéphane Bouchard). We are also aware that technology-based motor rehabilitation must take into account many exciting developments in the world of gaming as presented in Volume 3 of this series (edited by Eva Petersson Brooks and David Brown). Finally, improved motor applications will greatly benefit from the material presented in Volume 4 of this series (Design, Technologies, Tools, Methodologies & Analysis edited by Sue Cobb and Belinda Lange). Thus, to assist the reader, when appropriate, references are made to other chapters in this volume as well as to the three companion volumes in this book series.

Chapter 2
Neuroplasticity and Virtual Reality

Katharine L. Cheung, Eugene Tunik, Sergei V. Adamovich, and Lara A. Boyd

Objective To present the key aspects of neuroplasticity and how VR technology can capitalise on and influence this phenomenon to promote motor rehabilitation.

2.1 Definition of Neuroplasticity

In this chapter we discuss neuroplasticity and consider how VR technology may be used to promote motor learning and rehabilitation. First, we discuss the nature of neuroplasticity and the physiological mechanisms involved in the induction of both short- and long-term changes that enable us to store and retrieve memories for later use. Second, we review how neuroplastic changes can be indexed using biological principles and the underlying tenets of learning. Third, we consider the fundamental

K.L. Cheung, MSc (✉) • L.A. Boyd
Department of Physical Therapy, University of British Columbia,
212-2177 Wesbrook Mall, Vancouver,
BC, Canada, V6T 1Z3
e-mail: katharine.cheung@alumni.ubc.ca; lara.boyd@ubc.ca

E. Tunik, P.T., Ph.D.
Department of Rehabilitation & Movement Science, UMDNJ,
323 M. L. King Blvd., University Heights, Newark, NJ 07102, USA
e-mail: eugene.tunik@rutgers.edu

S.V. Adamovich, Ph. D.
Department of Biomedical Engineering,
New Jersey Institute of Technology, Newark, NJ, USA
e-mail: sergei.adamovich@njit.edu

P.L. (Tamar) Weiss et al. (eds.), *Virtual Reality for Physical and Motor Rehabilitation*, Virtual Reality Technologies for Health and Clinical Applications,
DOI 10.1007/978-1-4939-0968-1_2, © Springer Science+Business Media New York 2014

elements of experience-dependent neuroplasticity and clinical interventions that have the potential to induce and affect neuroplasticity. Finally, we consider empirical evidence of the effects of VR on neuroplastic changes in the brain.

The incidence of brain trauma is significant across the globe, and the resultant brain damage of such traumas often carries significant social, economic and human (personal) implications. Fortunately, the brain is highly capable, even beyond its developmental years, to exhibit physiological, functional and structural changes over time; this is likely the substrate for recovery of lost function following an injury (Nudo, 2006). The ability of the nervous system to undergo physiological changes as a result of genetic, behavioural and environmental changes is referred to as neuroplasticity. The processes of development, ageing, learning, memory and neural response to trauma all involve the critical concept of neuroplasticity. (N.B. We will often discuss the concepts of this chapter in terms of the brain following insult or injury—oftentimes it is easier to demonstrate normal brain function by comparing and contrasting with pathological brain states.)

2.1.1 Short-Term Versus Long-Term Changes

Neuroplasticity can occur on multiple levels, meaning the nature and extent of neuroplasticity can vary. Relatively short-term cellular changes can occur as a result of a temporary alteration in excitability of a population of neurons whereas relatively long-term structural changes can occur following long-term practice of a skill or an insult to the brain such as a stroke (Johansen-Berg et al., 2002). For example, short-term neural excitability changes (on the scale of seconds to hours) can be observed by inducing voltage changes in cortical regions of the brain via single-pulsed transcranial magnetic stimulation (TMS); a technique that has been shown to induce only short-term transient effects on the excitability of the brain (Barker, 1999). An example of a longer-term change in the brain can be observed in individuals who have become proficient at certain tasks. For example, empirical evidence of expanded areas of the motor cortex associated with finger movement has been shown in pianists (e.g. Pascual-Leone, Cammarota, Wassermann, Brasil-Neto, Cohen & Hallett, 1993); this is a clear demonstration of how behaviour can result in a long-term physical change in brain regions over time. Long-lasting changes in the brain (on the scale of years to decades) can also be readily observed following insults to the brain such as stroke, which can cause significant tissue damage (Hallet, 2001). Given appropriate rehabilitation however, neuroplastic changes may occur over time that allow for full or partial recovery of any lost function after the insult. Indeed, the neuroplastic nature of the brain allows for it to restructure over time with training and practice. Later in this chapter we discuss ways in which the properties of brain plasticity can be exploited to create long-lasting changes in the brain using technology such as VR.

2.1.2 *Changes in Neuronal Traffic*

2.1.2.1 Synaptic Pruning and Hebbian Mechanisms

Individual connections between neurons in the brain are continuously being altered depending on environmental and behavioural stimulation and responses to bodily injury. A key component of the theory of neuroplasticity is this dynamic change in neural connectivity, which involves the interplay of two phenomena: synaptic pruning and Hebbian neural interactions. Although synaptic pruning was initially characterised in the visual system (for review, Tessier and Broadie, 2009), pruning can be considered more generally as a genetically programmed reduction in the number of physical synapses between neurons in all sensory–motor systems in the nervous system. This process of pruning is strongly influenced by stimulation from the environment and interactions between neurons during learning—a process termed Hebbian interaction (Hebb, 1949). For example, pairs of neurons that are often excited together will likely exhibit less pruning and perhaps strengthened mutual connectivity, whereas the connections of two neurons that fire independently of one another will become either pruned or weakened. This principle is known colloquially as: "neurons that fire together wire together; neurons that fire apart wire apart" (Bliss & Lomo, 1973). If connections between neurons are no longer being used, their level of connectivity may be reduced or eliminated to allow more room and resources for active connections to be strengthened. Effectively, the connections between neurons are constantly being altered and redefined. An understanding of the principles of synaptic pruning and Hebbian interactions is helpful when considering the design and implementation of technology geared towards altering the connectivity between neurons during the processes of learning and rehabilitation.

2.1.2.2 LTP and LTD Hypothesis of Learning and Memory

While much remains to be elucidated about the nature of learning and memory, the theory of long-term potentiation (LTP) is well documented and a strong candidate as a cellular correlate for learning and memory. LTP is defined as a long-lasting enhancement in signal transmission between neurons that occurs when two neurons are stimulated simultaneously (Bliss & Lomo, 1973); it is one of the ways by which chemical synapses are able to alter in strength. The counterpart of LTP, long-term depression (LTD), occurs when the postsynaptic effects of a given neuron on another are weakened. LTP and LTD are activity-dependent processes that result in an accentuation or a reduction, respectively, in the efficacy of synaptic transmission either through changes in the number of connections between neurons, the modulation of neurotransmitter exchange between neurons, or both (Mulkey & Malenka, 1992).

2.1.3 Gross Anatomical Changes

2.1.3.1 Changes in Connectivity

Changes in synaptic dynamics through pruning and Hebbian interactions are evidenced on a macroscopic brain level as connections between different brain regions that are strengthened or weakened over time and by experience. Importantly, the brain has the ability to form new functional connections after it has experienced an injury or perturbation (for review see Calautti & Baron, 2003). Clear evidence of this has been demonstrated in the human motor system. For example, work from Nudo and Milliken (1996) has shown that after a focal stroke in the area of motor cortex responsible for hand function, neurons adjacent to the stroke lesion take over some of the lost motor function. These data and others demonstrate that changes in connectivity within the brain underlie the ability of an individual to recover some of their lost motor function after injury. Despite potential benefits, however, changes in connectivity can also result in pathological consequences. For example, repeated consumption of an addictive substance may result in neural connectivity changes that lead to an increased desire to continue to seek the substance (for review, Alcantra et al., 2011; Thomas, Kalivas, & Shaham, 2008).

2.1.3.2 Changes in Brain Activity Patterns Over Time

There are many current methods that may be used to assess changes in brain activity over time. Although we provide an overview of functional magnetic resonance imaging (fMRI) as an assay tool in more detail below, it is helpful to introduce it here as one way in which global changes in brain activity have been measured. fMRI measures the blood-oxygen-level-dependent (BOLD) signal and, because of its high spatial resolution, is particularly well-suited to investigate whether shifts in brain activity patterns occur over time. Changes in both the location and level of the BOLD signal can reveal evidence of neuroplasticity. Motor learning, for instance, has been shown to change BOLD patterns across distributed brain circuits in both healthy and patient populations. For example, BOLD patterns in different brain regions were examined before and after participants learned a novel motor sequence task (Meehan et al., 2011). Learning the new task changed patterns of brain network activity in both healthy and stroke-damaged brains. Importantly, these data show that individuals after a stroke may compensate by relying on different brain regions than matched healthy controls (e.g. dorsolateral prefrontal cortex instead of dorsal premotor cortex) to support some forms of motor learning (Fig. 2.1).

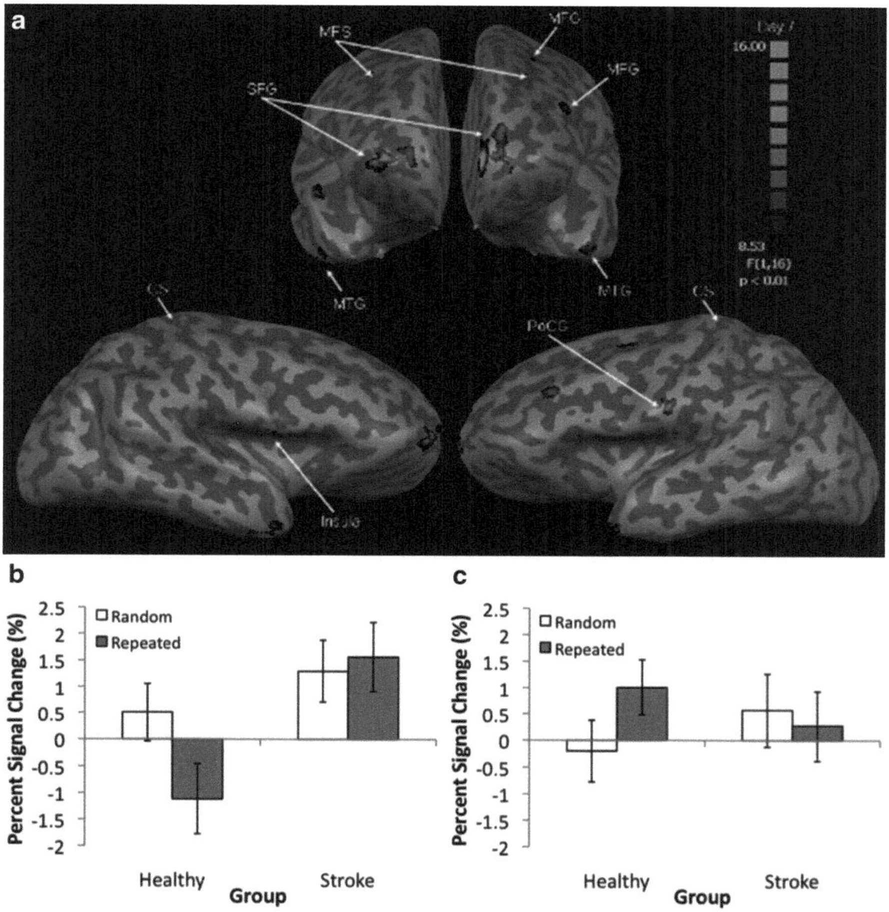

Fig. 2.1 (**a**) Sample fMRI showing the contrast in neural activity between individuals with stroke and matched healthy controls. Importantly, individuals with stroke rely on dorsolateral prefrontal cortex during motor sequence learning (**b**) while matched controls activate the premotor cortex to perform repeated sequences at a delayed retention test (**c**). Adapted from Meehan et al., 2011

2.2 How Can We Index Neuroplasticity?

There are several established methods of measuring neuroplastic changes in the nervous system. Here we discuss methods used to measure changes in excitability of different brain regions, methods to measure changes in metabolic demands in the brain, and methods of evaluating behaviour associated with neural changes.

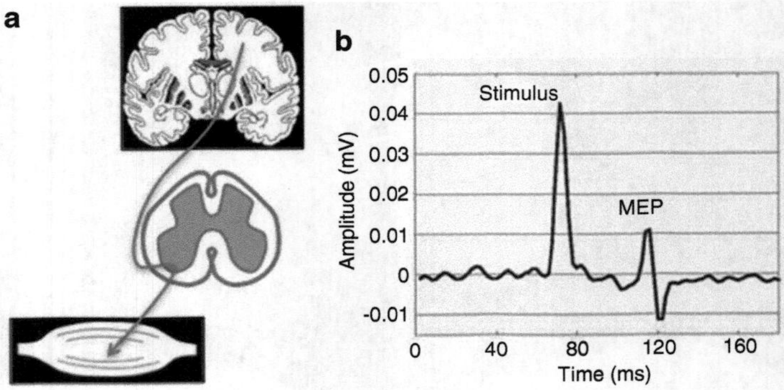

Fig. 2.2 Example of transcranial magnetic stimulation induced motor evoked potential. Stimulation over primary motor cortex induces depolarisation of pyramidal cells (**a**) and leads to an induced muscle response in the periphery (**b**)

2.2.1 Measuring Changes in Excitability of Brain Regions

2.2.1.1 Evoked Potentials

One common method of measuring changes in brain excitability is by presenting a stimulus to the nervous system and recording the electric potential that is evoked. This is called an evoked potential or response (Rothwell, 1997). Signals are typically recorded from the cerebral cortex, brainstem, spinal cord or peripheral nerves. For example, motor-evoked potentials (MEPs) can be recorded by stimulating the motor cortex of a subject and recording the electrical potential evoked in the muscle corresponding to the cortical area being stimulated (Pascual-Leone et al., 2002) (Fig. 2.2). The value of this technique is that differences in cortical excitability associated with disease, recovery or clinical intervention can be examined over time within the same individual. For example, measures of neural excitability could be obtained prior to, and following, a clinical intervention in order to examine the efficacy of the intervention (e.g. the effect of TMS applied to the motor cortex on general cortical excitability). While this technique provides a direct measure of the excitability state of the motor neurons in the brain and spinal cord, it is limited in its ability to assay the excitability of other brain regions, which do not have descending projections to muscles. For assessing more global brain areas, other measures are more appropriate.

2.2.1.2 Electroencephalography (EEG)

Electroencephalography (EEG) is used to measure electrical activity of the brain over time. More specifically, it measures the fluctuation of voltage between different areas in the brain as a result of changes in net ion flow across neuronal membranes during synaptic transmission (Huang et al., 2007). EEG can be used as a diagnostic tool in clinical settings, for example, for the assessment of neural activity during epilepsy, encephalopathies and coma. Although EEG measures electrical activity across the entire surface of the head, the ability to pinpoint the source of the electrical signal using EEG methodology is limited (though more sophisticated source localisation algorithms are emerging (e.g. Koessler et al., 2007)). The main advantage of EEG arises from its outstanding temporal resolution that allows characterisation of changes in brain activity at the millisecond time scale.

2.2.1.3 Magnetoencephalography (MEG)

Magnetoencephalography (MEG) is a technique used to examine magnetic fields produced by electrical currents in the brain. Like EEG, MEG signals are generated by net ion flow throughout neurons in the brain. The advantage of MEG is that it also offers millisecond scale temporal resolution as well as improved spatial resolution over EEG. Some source localisation algorithms show promise in identifying sub-cortical activity in addition to cortical activity (Hämäläinen et al., 1993). These acuity advantages arise because magnetic fields are less susceptible to distortion by the skull and scalp than are the electrical fields measured by EEG. However, MEG is only sensitive to tangential current sources (i.e. those which are parallel to the scalp), allowing it to mainly identify sources coming from depressions in the surface of the brain (sulci) while EEG is sensitive to both radial (directed towards or away from the scalp) and tangential sources (Huang et al., 2007), allowing it to be sensitive to both sulcal sources *and* sources from ridges surrounding the sulci (e.g. gyri). In this regard, MEG and EEG provide supplementary information concerning different parts of the brain and may be used in conjunction with each other to capture multiple physiological processes (Hämäläinen et al., 1993).

2.2.2 Measuring BOLD Contrast and Metabolic Changes

2.2.2.1 Functional Magnetic Resonance Imaging (fMRI)

Functional magnetic resonance imaging (fMRI) is a non-invasive, indirect method of localising and measuring neural activity in the brain based on the relationship between neural activity and the metabolic demands associated with the increased neural activity. As stated earlier in this chapter, most fMRI experiments measure a blood-oxygen-level-dependent (BOLD) response. Changes in the BOLD signal result from changes in the blood deoxyhaemoglobin level in the brain. An increase in neuronal activity results in an increase in oxygen consumption, regional cerebral blood volume and regional cerebral blood flow, increasing the concentration of deoxyhaemoglobin and decreasing the concentration of oxyhaemoglobin (for review see Logothetis & Wandell, 2003; Norris, 2003). By comparing the BOLD response across two or more test conditions (e.g. before and after learning a task), activation in a given brain area can be considered as increased or decreased relative to the control condition. Magnetic resonance imaging (MRI) is also used to acquire an anatomical scan of the brain prior to imaging with fMRI so that the location of any changes in the BOLD signal can be readily identified on a subject-specific basis.

The advantage of using fMRI lies in its unsurpassed spatial resolution (as much as 1 mm accuracy) and its ability to index the connectivity between functionally activated brain regions. This means that one is able to study how different brain areas interact with each other during certain tasks, or how brain activity in different areas changes following an insult to the brain. Studies have demonstrated that while neurological and behavioural tests may not be able to detect changes in brain function following traumatic brain injuries such as concussion, there is increasing evidence that advanced neuroimaging methods can provide more sensitive indications of the underlying brain pathology (e.g. Johnson et al., 2012). These findings suggest that fMRI may show promise as a prognostic tool to evaluate the neurological status of asymptomatic individuals who are suspected of injury (e.g. military personnel who are suspected of developing post-traumatic stress disorder). However, a significant limiting factor of fMRI is the relatively sluggish haemodynamics of blood flow, thus markedly limiting the temporal resolution of this approach. For example, while EEG and MEG allow one to characterise neural response at the millisecond time scale, fMRI operates on a multi-second time scale. Along the same vein, fMRI is only an indirect inference of neural activity (through changes in blood flow) while the other approaches measure neural activity more directly. Recently, new techniques have allowed for the measurement of brain activity via fMRI during interactions with virtual environments (VEs), thereby enabling one to examine whether or not exposure to VEs can influence a damaged brain's activity patterns and levels (e.g. Slobounov et al., 2010; Saleh et al., 2013).

2.2.2.2 Magnetic Resonance Spectroscopy (MRS)

Magnetic resonance spectroscopy (MRS) is a non-invasive imaging technique that uses the nuclear magnetic resonance properties of hydrogen to quantify brain metabolites in vivo. It can be used to study metabolic changes in neuropathies such as brain tumours, strokes and seizure disorders (Cirstea et al., 2011; Federico et al., 1998; Marino, Ciurleo, Bramanti, Federico, & De Stefano, 2011). The neurometabolites detectable by MRS often fluctuate in response to neuronal injury, hypoxia, cellular energy metabolism and membrane turnover (Brooks et al., 2001). These include: N-acetyl aspartate (a marker for neuronal integrity), lactate (a by-product of anaerobic metabolism during periods of hypoxia), creatine (related to the energy potential available in brain tissue), choline (an indicator of cell density and cell wall turnover), myo-inositol (an astrocytic marker and possibly a indicator of intracellular osmotic integrity) and glutamate (the main excitatory neurotransmitter in the central nervous system).

2.2.3 *Measuring Changes in Behaviour*

The neuroplastic nature of the brain enables the process of learning and re-learning to occur. Because the process of learning is supported by neuroplasticity, change in an individual's behaviour over time is an important index of cortical reorganisation. Indeed, all procedural and episodic learning, and relearning after injury to the brain, is supported by neuroplastic change. Motor learning is an ideal example to illustrate this concept. Motor learning is defined as the acquisition of a new behaviour through skilled practice and results in a relatively permanent change in the ability of an individual to perform a movement (Salmoni et al., 1984; Schmidt and Lee, 2011). Once a skilled movement is learned, the ability to perform the skill is robust and stable. Experience, practice or change in behaviour stimulates the brain to reorganise. Neuroplasticity, in the context of motor learning, refers to changes in neural organisation associated with skilled practice or modifications of movement patterns (Berlucchi and Buchtel, 2009). When a skill is repeatedly practised, neural changes occur as a result of functional reorganisation across many brain regions (Karni et al., 1998). As we will discuss later on (and in Chap. 3), technology such as virtual reality, which has the ability to enforce stereotyped, repeated practice of skills is an excellent method by which to promote learning and rehabilitation (e.g. by using sophisticated forms of feedback, practice schedules, engaging and rewarding practice environments, and the possibility of mass practice) to reinforce and perhaps even bolster neuroplasticity.

2.3 Experience-Dependent Neuroplasticity

2.3.1 *Motor Learning and New Technology*

Overall, learning and practising new motor skills is critical for inducing neuroplastic change and functional recovery after an insult to the nervous system. There is ample evidence to suggest that plasticity of the brain is dependent on use and that intensity, frequency and duration of practice are all important factors in determining the extent of neural reorganisation (for review see Adamovich, Fluet, Tunik, & Merians, 2009). Given the central role of practice for experience-dependent plasticity there is now acute interest in the development of new techniques, such as virtual reality interfaces, that enable the user to control or modify the task parameters to foster motor learning. These technologies may allow training to occur in a life-like enriching yet controlled environment, integrated into the clinical setting, and tailored to the specific needs of each individual.

2.3.2 Neuroplasticity in the Context of Motor Learning

Importantly, experience appears to be one of the main drivers of neuroplastic change. In fact, substantial short-term changes in the rate of both changes in skill and functional organisation can be observed even within a single training session. In the context of motor learning, "fast learning" (Doyon and Benali, 2005) is the rapid change often seen early in practice; however, this does not necessarily translate to sustained improvements in motor skill. With practice over multiple training sessions, improvement commonly plateaus and the slope of change associated with learning lessens (Karni et al., 1998). This characterises the "slow learning" phase (Doyon and Benali, 2005), which can continue for long periods of time. In addition, following the conclusion of a practice session, motor memories may be strengthened or enhanced by an offline process known as consolidation, which allows memories to stabilise and be available to be recalled at a later date (Brashers-Krug et al., 1996). A key question centres on why the speed of change associated with motor skill acquisition varies within and across practice sessions. Neurophysiology provides the answer. Rapid changes in the amount and location of neurotransmitters, within and between the neurons of the brain support fast learning (Nudo, 2006); while the structural modifications enabling new contacts between neurons underpin slow learning (Kleim et al., 2004). Because altering neuron structure requires more time than does reallocating neurotransmitters, rates of change in behaviour associated with learning vary between early and late learning (Karni et al., 1998).

Overall, an understanding of the mechanisms of neuroplasticity in the context of motor learning is important in designing and implementing tools to promote neuroplastic change. Notably, these properties can be particularly well exploited by technology such as VR to provide user experiences that promote the processes of both fast and slow learning.

2.4 What Is the Role of Virtual Reality in Neuroplasticity?

Generally, following damage to the brain an individual's ability to interact with the physical environment is diminished (Rose, Brooks, & Rizzo, 2005). New technology, such as VR, may potentially help reduce the burden of such physical limitations by providing an alternative, favourable environment in which to practice motor skills. VR can be defined as "an approach to user-computer interface that involves real-time simulation of an environment, scenario or activity that allows for user interaction via multiple sensory channels" (Adamovich, Fluet, et al., 2009).

New VR training approaches capitalise on recent technological advances including improved robotic design, the development of haptic interfaces and the advent of human–machine interactions in virtual reality (Merians, Poizner, Boian, Burdea, & Adamovich, 2006). There are many VR applications currently in use. For example, VR has been used in clinical settings as a training tool for surgeons and as a tool to deliver cognitive, post-traumatic stress disorder and pain therapy (Adamovich,

Fluet, et al., 2009; Bohil, Alicea, & Biocca, 2011). It also has the potential to aid in studying processes such as the dynamics of neurodevelopment and neuro-connectivity (Bohil et al., 2011) and to study the neural circuitry underlying certain animal behaviours (Dombeck & Reiser, 2012). VR allows for the possibility of delivering patient-specific opportunities for interaction with the environment via technology such as head-mounted displays or screens which require less set-up and effort than would be needed to provide a patient with an opportunity to interact with the real environment (Rose et al., 2005). It is this naturalistic environment allowing for interactive behaviour while being monitored and recorded that is the primary advantage of implementing VR technology (Bohil et al., 2011). This means VR technology can be used to deliver meaningful and relevant stimulation to an individual's nervous system and thereby capitalise on the plasticity of the brain to promote motor learning and rehabilitation (see Chap. 3).

2.4.1 VR Practice

As discussed above, learning and performing new skills is critical for inducing neuroplastic change and functional recovery after an insult to the nervous system. Virtual reality simulations are particularly effective tools that allow for monitoring of behaviour in three-dimensional space. VR set-ups allow for thorough analysis of the user's actions and the ability to provide guidelines and precise real-time feedback to promote the desired behavioural result. Research has shown, for example, that virtual-reality augmented robotically-facilitated repetitive movement training may potentially aid in improving motor control in patients with moderate to severe upper extremity impairment (who have difficulty performing unassisted movements) (Merians et al., 2006).

The majority of empirical data using VR paradigms has involved persons with chronic stroke or children with cerebral palsy (Chaps. 7 and 10). Virtual reality gaming and task simulations are becoming increasingly popular as a means of providing repetitive intensive practice to chronic stroke patients. This is posited to be a particularly effective form of rehabilitation due to its potential to promote increased interest of participants by virtue of task novelty. This may in turn lead to greater programme compliance, which may ultimately facilitate better clinical outcomes compared to traditional rehabilitation programmes (Adamovich, Fluet, et al., 2009; Merians et al., 2006; You et al., 2005).

2.4.2 Categorisation of VR Technology

Virtual environments (VEs) can be used to present complex, interactive multimodal sensory information to the user (Bohil et al., 2011). In fact, a major development in the use and clinical outcome efficacy of VR came with the addition of tactile information and interaction forces into the visual experience of VR (Merians, Fluet, Qiu, Lafond, & Adamovich, 2011). This is important as the more relavant and realistic the training programme, the more easily it may be transferred into daily life. Further, fMRI data show that motor training that is specific to the task being learned induces larger neuroplastic change as compared to simply increasing arm use after stroke (Boyd, Randhawa, Vidoni, & Wessel, 2010). In general, VR systems are typically classified by the visual presentations they provide to a participant, the presence or absence of somatosensory feedback and the modality used to collect data from the participant (Chap. 5, Adamovich, Fluet, et al., 2009). In addition to providing visual–motor feedback, haptic technology allows virtual environments to provide force feedback. This refers to force and touch feedback provided to the user by the computer through specialised interfaces, which can simulate interactions with objects (Merians et al., 2006). This ability to provide visual–motor and somatosensory feedback to the user is paramount; the more relevant and realistic the input presented to the brain during training, the more valuable the training and the more likely this sensory information will be integrated and used to help re-organise the brain in a favourable manner.

2.4.3 Effects of VR on Neural Circuits

Embarking on a discussion of the potential neural processes that may be affected through VR interaction beckons a brief digression to the role that visual input has on the brain (see Chap. 4). Visual information can provide a potent signal for reorganisation of sensorimotor circuits. For example, visual errors can influence motor cortical areas during motor learning (Bray, Shimojo, & O'Doherty, 2007; Hadipour-Niktarash et al., 2007; Muellbacher et al., 2001, 2002; Richardson et al., 2006). Active and rewarded practice by which one learns to use feedback to reduce errors in movement shapes neural activity in motor and premotor areas (Bray et al., 2007; Wise et al., 1998). Moreover, repeated and intentional observation of actions can facilitate the magnitude of MEPs and influence cortico-cortical interactions (both intracortical facilitation and inhibition) in the motor and premotor areas (Leonard & Tremblay, 2007; Patuzzo, Fiaschi, & Manganotti, 2003; Stefan et al., 2005; Strafella & Paus, 2000). From retrograde tracer studies, it is also known that rich intra-hemispheric cortico-cortical connections link the occipital, parietal and frontal cortices which process visual, somatic and motor information (Dum & Strick, 2005; Fang, Stepniewska, & Kass, 2005; Lewis et al., 2005; Lewis & Van Essen, 2000a, 2000b; Mitchell & Cauller, 2001; Stepniewska, Fang, & Kaas, 2005). Likewise, single unit data show that a substantial number of neurons in motor, premotor and parietal areas are modulated by visual information (Graziano, 1999; Graziano & Gandhi, 2000; Graziano & Gross, 1998a, 1998b; Kakei, Hoffman, & Strick, 2003) thus providing direct modification of movement by visual information. Moreover, unlike proprioception, which is obligatorily coupled to active and/or passive limb movement, visual feedback of movement can be provided independent of the movement itself through illusory manipulations. For example, patients with severe paresis or absence of volitional control can be asked to make an intention to move (or imagine movement) and this motor effort can be coupled with biological limb motion displayed through the VR interface (see Adamovich, August, Merians, & Tunik, 2009). Thus visual feedback offers a means to modulate the motor system without requiring overt movement. Indeed, the visual system is robust in that its influence over the brain often overrides other afferent modalities, such as proprioception, when a sensory conflict is introduced (Snijders, Holmes, & Spence, 2007). Finally, by virtue of the relatively distant location between the motor and visual systems and their largely separate vascular supply, the visual regions of the brain can often remain intact despite lesions to the motor system. These features of the visual brain position VR as a highly desirable tool to provide visual feedback to optimise motor learning in neurologically impaired individuals.

VR can provide sophisticated sensory information to users and elicit a feeling of real presence or immersion in the ongoing task (Riva, 1998; Riva, Castelnuovo, & Mantovani, 2006). Perhaps one of the strongest attributes of VR is that it enables sensory manipulations that are not possible in the real world (i.e. colour/brightness, location, form, auditory input, temporal/spatial distortions, presenting feedback in different vantage points, allow the user to playback movements for feedback or to freeze motion on the screen). Indeed these properties might maximise chances for feedback-induced neural reorganisation. For example, the clinician can control various parameters that cannot be controlled in the natural world—such as "freezing" motion of one of the virtual hands, or parts of a hand, to focus attention to salient aspects of feedback, or to augment the quality of movement observed in VR. Early evidence suggests that skills acquired after VR-based training may transfer to real-world functions (Chap. 6, Adamovich et al., 2004; Deutsch et al., 2004; Holden, 2005; Kenyon & Afenya, 1995; Merians et al., 2002; Merians et al., 2006). For example, training in virtual environments has been shown to lead to clinical and kinematic improvements that are attributed to mitigation of impairment rather than compensatory strategies (Subramanian, Lourenço, Chilingaryan, Sveistrup, & Levin, 2013). In two studies, functional improvements were paralleled by a shift from a predominantly contralesional sensorimotor activation pre-therapy to a predominantly ipsilesional activation post-therapy (Jang et al., 2005; You et al., 2005). Similar shifts in hemispheric lateralisation are observed after therapy performed in the real world (Carey et al., 2002, 2006; Small et al., 2002), which suggests that training an affected limb in VR with high-fidelity feedback may tap into similar neural reorganisation changes (e.g. neuroplastic changes) observed after training in the real world.

More recently, research has explored specific ways in which distortions can be introduced in VR to invoke neural plasticity. In this case, the neuroplastic change is generally measured as an increase or decrease in the excitability of the motor cortex. For example, in a study by Adamovich, et al. (Adamovich, Fluet, et al., 2009), healthy subjects and patients with chronic stroke performed a simple finger flexion task while observing their movement as a virtual reality doppleganger representation on an LCD display. The display was positioned over their hand such that the

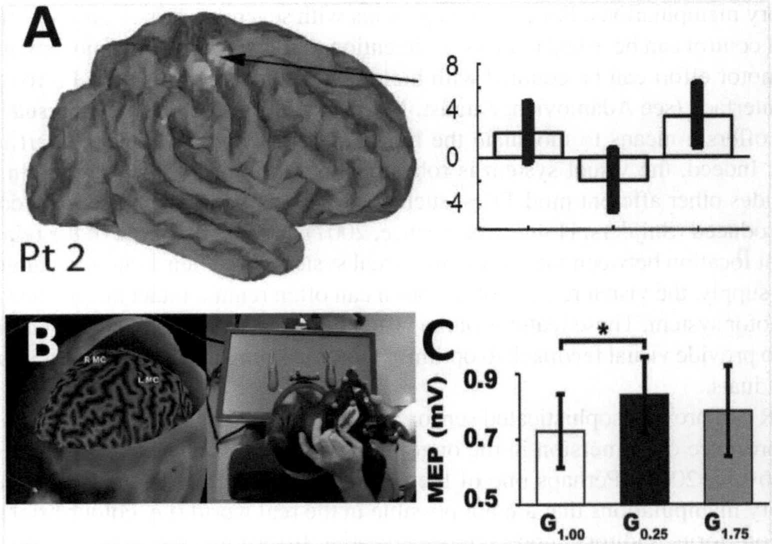

Fig. 2.3 (**a**) Adapted from Saleh, Adamovich, & Tunik, 2012. Significant activation in a chronic stroke subject performing a targeted finger flexion task with the affected hand. Feedback was presented in VR as either veridical (G1.00), scaled down (G0.25) or scaled up (G1.75) movement of a virtual hand model. The ipsilesional sensorimotor areas were significantly more activated in the G.25 and G1.75 conditions, compared to the veridical condition (betas for each condition shown in the right panel, error bars indicate 90 % confidence intervals). (**b, c**) Adapted from Bagce et al., 2012. The role of the corticospinal system in processing the gain discordance was tested with TMS. The task was as described above. Group mean MEPs were significantly increased in the G0.25 condition relative to the veridical condition

virtual hand was overlaid on the subject's actual hand. The VR hand model was actuated in real-time by the subjects' actual hand movement (recorded using a data glove). During the experiments, brain activity was assayed using fMRI and TMS measures. VR was used to manipulate the relationship between what the subjects did and what the subjects saw by scaling the amplitude of the VR hand motion (relative to their own movement) or by having subjects observe the virtual hand move without actually moving themselves. This work revealed a distributed parieto-frontal network involved in observation of movements performed by the virtual hand (Adamovich, Fluet, et al., 2009). Interestingly, the primary motor cortex (M1) seems particularly important for reconciling discrepancy between intended actions and discordant visual feedback ("visuomotor discordance") (Bagce, Saleh, Adamovich, & Tunik, 2011, 2012; Saleh et al., 2011, 2012).

Our preliminary data in healthy individuals (manuscript in preparation), reveal that activity of M1 can be facilitated by as much as 50 % after subjects had the opportunity to adapt to the discordant feedback and only by 12 % if subjects had not adapted. Figure 2.3 shows preliminary data for stroke patients who were exposed to similar gain discordance conditions. The observation that excitability can be increased (even partially) in the affected motor cortex in individuals with stroke suggests that neuroplasticity may be harnessed in patients through VR-based interactions. In other words, what these findings suggest is that visual manipulations presented through VR may invoke similar responses, at least at the level of M1, in stroke and healthy subjects alike. However, what remains unclear is whether cumulative exposure to such visuomotor discordance, as typically occurs in learning paradigms, would translate to the same neural changes in the two groups. Given the unique advantages of VR that have been discussed (such as delivery of mass-practice and sophisticated feedback), this technology may be an important tool for clinicians to drive neuroplastic changes. The long-term clinical and neuroplastic outcome of VR training is currently under investigation. Nonetheless, these data illustrate how virtual reality manipulations may be used as a probe of neural function on the one hand, and as a training tool on the other.

2.4.4 Limitations of VR

While virtual reality environments offer many unique advantages to other approaches, limitations to their efficacy and practicality exist (Chap. 6). Firstly, larger clinical studies are required to establish the efficacy of using VR in sensorimotor rehabilitation in different clinical populations. Additionally, to date there is little information on the generalisability of the training effects of VR to the corresponding physical environment in general, and the VR training parameters associated with optimal transfer to real-world functional improvements remain yet to be elucidated. Furthermore, it is unclear whether advantages of VR over real-world training exist, and if so, precisely what these advantages are. It is important to investigate whether there is something unique to VR that can be exploited that cannot be with other types of therapies, or whether any benefits of VR can be attributed to the gaming platforms associated with VR themselves (i.e. are VR therapies only more effective therapeutics because they are more entertaining and therefore keep subjects more engaged and motivated throughout their training session? Is greater intervention adherence alone the cause of any discrepancies in VR treatments versus alternative ones?). While limitations in VR technology exist, the potential for favourable neuroplastic change afforded by such technology undoubtedly warrant further investigation.

2.5 Conclusion

Virtual reality allows for the observation of neural activity during realistic simulations using sensorimotor input. While much remains to be elucidated in the realm of VR and its clinical applications, the unique aspects of VR, which are not present in other therapies, have shown great potential in the field of rehabilitation therapy. A key component of the theory of neuroplasticity is the dynamic nature of change in neural connectivity, and motor rehabilitation therapy implementing VR technology that can be tailored based on the specific needs of a particular subject may be particularly effective. The use of virtual reality technology in rehabilitation for brain damage in particular is becoming more prevalent in clinical settings. There is sufficient evidence demonstrating its efficacy to suggest it may become an integral part of cognitive assessment and rehabilitation treatments in the future. Given the unique elements virtual reality technology carries with it, significant effort into studying and refining rehabilitation approaches implementing virtual reality technology is well justified.

References

Adamovich, S. V., August, K., Merians, A., & Tunik, E. (2009). A virtual reality-based system integrated with fmri to study neural mechanisms of action observation-execution: A proof of concept study. *Restorative Neurology and Neuroscience, 27*(3), 209–223.

Adamovich, S. V., Fluet, G. G., Tunik, E., & Merians, A. S. (2009). Sensorimotor training in virtual reality: A review. *NeuroRehabilitation, 25*, 29–44.

Adamovich, S. V., Merians, A. S., Boian, R., Tremaine, M., Burdea, G. S., Recce, M., et al. (2004). A virtual reality based exercise system for hand rehabilitation post-stroke: Transfer to function. *Conference Proceedings - IEEE Engineering in Medicine and Biology Society, 7*, 4936–4939.

Alcantra, A. A., Lim, H. Y., Floyd, C. E., Garces, J., Mendenhall, J., Lyons, C. L., et al. (2011). Cocaine- and morphine-induced synaptic plasticity in the nucleus accumbens. *Synapse, 65*, 309–320.

Bagce, H. F., Saleh, S., Adamovich, S. V., & Tunik, E. (2011). Visuomotor discordance in virtual reality: Effects on online motor control. *Conference Proceedings - IEEE Engineering in Medicine and Biology Society, 2011*, 7262–7265.

Bagce, H. F., Saleh, S., Adamovich, S. V., & Tunik, E. (2012). Visuomotor gain discordance alters online motor performance and enhances primary motor cortex excitability in patients with stroke. *Neuromodulation, 15*(4), 361–366.

Barker, A.T. (1999). The history and basic principles of magnetic nerve stimulation. *Electroencephalography and Clinical Neurophysiology, 51*(Suppl), 3–21.

Berlucchi, G., & Buchtel, H.A. (2009). Neuronal plasticity: historical roots and evolution of meaning. *Experimental Brain Research, 192*(3), 307–319.

Bliss, T. V., & Lomo, T. (1973). Long-lasting potentiation of synaptic transmission in the dentate area of the anaesthetized rabbit following stimulation of the perforant path. *Journal of Physiology, 232*, 331–356.

Bohil, C. J., Alicea, B., & Biocca, F. A. (2011). Virtual reality in neuroscience research and therapy. *Nature Reviews. Neuroscience, 12*, 752–762.

Boyd, L. A., Randhawa, B., Vidoni, E. D., & Wessel, B. D. (2010). Motor learning after stroke: Is skill acquisition a prerequisite for contralesional neuroplastic change? *Neuroscience Letters, 482*, 21–25.

Brashers-Krug, T., Shadmehr, R., & Bizzi, E. (1996). Consolidation in human motor memory. *Nature, 382*, 252–255.

Bray, S., Shimojo, S., & O'Doherty, J. P. (2007). Direct instrumental conditioning of neural activity using functional magnetic resonance imaging-derived reward feedback. *Journal of Neuroscience, 27*(28), 7498–7507.

Brooks, J.C.W., Roberts, N., Kemp, G.J., Gosney, M.A., Lye, M., & Whitehouse, G.H. (2001). A proton magnetic resonance spectroscopy study of age-related changes in frontal lobe metabolite concentrations. *Cerebral Cortex, 11*(7), 598–605.

Calautti, J. C., & Baron, J. C. (2003). Functional neuroimaging studies of motor recovery after stroke in adults: A review. *Stroke, 34*, 1553–1566.

Carey, L. M., Abbott, D. F., Puce, A., Jackson, G. D., Syngeniotis, A., & Donnan, G. A. (2002). Reemergence of activation with poststroke somatosensory recovery: A serial fMRI case study. *Neurology, 59*(5), 749–752.

Carey, L. M., Abbott, D. F., Egan, G. F., O'Keefe, G. J., Jackson, G. D., Bernhardt, J., et al. (2006). Evolution of brain activation with good and poor motor recovery after stroke. *Neurorehabilitation and Neural Repair, 20*(1), 24–41.

Cirstea, C. M., Brooks, W. M., Craciunas, S. C., Popescu, E. A., Choi, I. Y., Lee, P., et al. (2011). Primary motor cortex in stroke: A functional MRI-guided proton MR spectroscopic study. *Stroke, 42*(4), 1004–1009.

Deutsch, J. E., Merians, A. S., Adamovich, S., Poizner, H., & Budrea, G. C. (2004). Development and application of virtual reality technology to improve hand use and gait of individuals post-stroke. *Restorative Neurology Neuroscience, 22*(3–5), 371–386.

Dombeck, D. A., & Reiser, M. B. (2012). Real neuroscience in virtual worlds. *Current Opinion in Neurobiology, 22*, 3–10.

Doyon, J., & Benali, H. (2005). Reorganization and plasticity in the adult brain during learning of motor skills. *Current Opinion in Neurobiology, 15*(2), 161–167.

Dum, R. P., & Strick, P. L. (2005). Frontal lobe inputs to the digit representations of the motor areas on the lateral surface of the hemisphere. *Journal of Neuroscience, 25*(6), 1375–1386.

Fang, P. C., Stepniewska, I., & Kass, J. H. (2005). Ipsilateral cortical connections of motor, premotor, frontal eye, and posterior parietal fields in a prosimian primate, *Otolemur garnetti. The Journal of Comparative Neuroscience, 490*(3), 305–333.

Federico, F., Simone, I. L., Lucivero, V., Giannini, P., Laddomada, G., Mezzapesa, D. M., et al. (1998). Prognostic value of proton magnetic resonance spectroscopy in ischemic stroke. *Archives of Neurology, 55*(4), 489–494.

Graziano, M. S. (1999). Where is my arm? The relative role of vision and proprioception in the neuronal representation of limb position. *Proceedings of the National Academy of Science, 96*(18), 10418–10421.

Graziano, M. S., & Gandhi, S. (2000). Location of the polysensory zone in the precentral gyrus of anesthetized monkeys. *Experimental Brain Research, 135*(2), 259–266.

Graziano, M. S., & Gross, C. G. (1998a). Spatial maps for the control of movement. *Current Opinion in Neurobiology, 8*(2), 195–201.

Graziano, M. S., & Gross, C. G. (1998b). Visual responses with and without fixation: Neurons in premotor cortex encode spatial locations independently of eye position. *Experimental Brain Research, 118*(3), 373–380.

Hadipour-Niktarash, A., et al. (2007). Impairment of retention but not acquisition of a visuomotor skill through time-dependent disruption of primary motor cortex. *Journal of Neuroscience, 27*(49), 13413–13419.

Hallet, M. (2001). Plasticity of the human motor cortex and recovery from stroke. *Brain Research Reviews, 36*, 169–174.

Hämäläinen, M., Hari, R., Ilmoniemi, R., Knuutila, J., & Lounasmaa, O. V. (1993). Magnetoencephalography – Theory, instrumentation, and applications to noninvasive studies of signal processing in the human brain. *Reviews of Modern Physics, 65*(2), 413–497.

Hebb, D. O. (1949). *The organization of behavior*. New York, NY: Wiley and Sons.

Holden, M. K. (2005). Virtual environments for motor rehabilitation: Review. *Cyberpsychology, Behavior and Social Networking, 8*(3), 187–211.

Huang, M., Song, T., Hagler, D., Podgorny, I., Jousmaki, V., Cui, L., et al. (2007). A novel integrated MEG and EEG analysis method for dipolar sources. *NeuroImage, 37*(3), 731–748.

Jang, S. H., You, S. H., Hallett, M., Cho, Y. W., Park, C., Cho, S., et al. (2005). Cortical reorganization and associated functional motor recovery after virtual reality in patients with chronic stroke: An experimenter-blind preliminary study. *Archives of Physical Medicine and Rehabilitation, 86*(11), 2218–2223.

Johansen-Berg, H., Dawes, H., Guy, C., Smith, S. M., Wade, D. T., & Matthews, P. M. (2002). Correlation between motor improvements and altered fMRI activity after rehabilitative therapy. *Brain, 125*, 2731–2742.

Johnson, B., Zhang, K., Gay, M., Horovitz, S., Hallett, M., Sebastianelli, W., et al. (2012). Alteration of brain default network in subacute phase of injury in concussed individuals: Resting-state fMRI study. *NeuroImage, 59*(1), 511–518.

Kakei, S., Hoffman, D. S., & Strick, P. L. (2003). Sensorimotor transformations in cortical motor areas. *Neuroscience Research, 46*(1), 1–10.

Karni, A., Meyer, G., Rey-Hipolito, C., Jezzard, P., Adams, M. M., Turner, R., et al. (1998). The acquisition of skilled motor performance: Fast and slow experience-driven changes in primary motor cortex. *Proceedings of the National Academy of Science, 95*, 861–868.

Kenyon, R. V., & Afenya, M. B. (1995). Training in virtual and real environments. *Annals of Biomedical Engineering, 23*(4), 445–455.

Kleim, J.A., Hogg, T.M., VandenBerg, P.M., Cooper, N.R., Bruneau, R., & Remple, M. (2004). Cortical synaptogenesis and motor map reorganization occur during late, but not early, phase of motor skill learning. *The Journal of Neuroscience, 24*(3), 628–633.

Koessler, L., Maillard, L., Benhadid, A., Vignal, J. P., Braun, M., & Vespignani, H. (2007). Spatial localization of EEG electrodes. *Clinical Neurophysiology, 37*, 97–102.

Leonard, G., & Tremblay, F. (2007). Corticomotor facilitation associated with observation, imagery and imitation of hand actions: A comparative study in young and old adults. *Experimental Brain Research, 177*(2), 167–175.

Lewis, J. W., & Van Essen, D. C. (2000a). Corticocortical connections of visual, sensorimotor, and multimodal processing areas in the parietal lobe of the macaque monkey. *The Journal of Comparative Neurology, 428*(1), 112–137.

Lewis, J. W., & Van Essen, D. C. (2000b). Mapping of architectonic subdivisions in the macaque monkey, with emphasis on parieto-occipital cortex. *The Journal of Comparative Neurology, 428*(1), 79–111.

Lewis, S. J. G., Slabosz, A., Robbins, T. W., Barker, R. A., & Owen, A. M. (2005). Dopaminergic basis for deficits in working memory but not attentioanl set-shifting in Parkinson's disease. *Neuropsychologia, 43*(6), 823–832.

Logothetis, N.K., & Wandell, B.A. (2003). Interpreting the BOLD signal. *Annual Review of Physiology, 66*, 735–769.

Marino, S., Ciurleo, R., Bramanti, P., Federico, A., & De Stefano, N. (2011). 1H-MR spectroscopy in traumatic brain injury. *Neurocritical Care, 14*(1), 127–133.

Meehan, S.K., Randhawa, B., Wessel, B., & Boyd, L.A. (2011). Implicit sequence-specific motor learning after subcortical stroke is associated with increased prefrontal brain activations: an fMRI study. *Human Brain Mapping, 32*(2), 290–303.

Merians, A. S., Fluet, G. G., Qiu, Q., Lafond, I., & Adamovich, S. V. (2011). Learning in a virtual environment using haptic systems for movement re-education: Can this medium be used from remodeling other behaviors and actions? *Journal of Diabetes Science and Technology, 5*(2), 301–308.

Merians, A. S., Poizner, H., Boian, R., Burdea, G., & Adamovich, S. (2006). Sensorimotor training in a virtual reality environment: Does it improve functional recovery poststroke. *Neurorehabilitation and Neural Repair, 20*(2), 252–267.

Merians, A. S., Jack, D., Boian, R., Tremaine, M., Burdea, G. C., Adamovich, S. V., et al. (2002). Virtual reality-augmented rehabilitation for patients following stroke. *Physical Therapy, 82*(9), 898–915.

Mitchell, B. D., & Cauller, L. J. (2001). Corticocortical and thalamocortical projection to layer I of the frontal neocortex in rats. *Brain Research, 921*(1–2), 68–77.

Muellbacher, W., Ziemann, U., Boroojerdi, B., Cohen, L., & Hallett, M. (2001). Role of the human cortex in rapid motor learning. *Experimental Brain Research, 136*(4), 431–438.

Muellbacher, W., Ziemann, U., Wissel, J., Dang, N., Kofler, M., Facchini, S., et al. (2002). Early consolidation in human primary motor cortex. *Nature, 415*(6872), 640–644.

Mulkey, R. M., & Malenka, R. C. (1992). Mechanisms underlying induction of homosynaptic long-term depression in area CA1 of the hippocampus. *Neuron, 9*, 967–975.
Norris, D. G. (2003). High field human imaging. *Journal of Magnetic Resonance Imaging, 18*(5), 519–529.
Nudo, R. J. (2006). Plasticity. *NeuroRx: The Journal of the American Society for Experimental NeuroTherapeutics, 3*, 420–427.
Nudo, R. J., & Milliken, G. W. (1996). Reorganization of movement representations in primary motor cortex following focal ischemic infarcts in adult squirrel monkeys. *Journal of Neurophysiology, 75*(5), 2144–2149.
Pascual-Leone, A., Cammarota, A., Wassermann, E.M., Brasil-Neto, J.P., Cohen, L.G., & Hallett, M. (1993). Modulation of motor cortical outputs to the reading hand of braille readers. *Annals of Neurology, 34*(1), 33–37.
Patuzzo, S., Fiaschi, A., & Manganotti, P. (2003). Modulation of motor cortex excitability in the left hemisphere during action observation: A single- and paired-pulse transcranial magnetic stimulation study of self- and non-self-action observation. *Neuropsychologia, 41*(9), 1272–1278.
Richardson, A. G., Overduin, S. A., Valero-Cabré, A., Padoa-Schioppa, C., Pascual-Leone, A., Bizzi, E., et al. (2006). Disruption of primary motor cortex before learning impairs memory of movement dynamics. *Journal of Neuroscience, 26*(48), 12466–12470.
Riva, G. (1998). Virtual environments in neuroscience. *IEEE Transactions of Information Technology of Biomedicine, 2*(4), 275–281.
Riva, G., Castelnuovo, G., & Mantovani, F. (2006). Transformation of flow in rehabilitation: The role of advanced communication technologies. *Behavioural Research Methods, 38*(2), 237–244.
Rose, F. D., Brooks, B. M., & Rizzo, A. A. (2005). Virtual reality in brain damage rehabilitation: Review. *CyberPsychology and Behaviour, 8*, 241–271.
Rothwell, J. C. (1997). Techniques and mechanisms of action of transcranial stimulation of the human motor cortex. *Journal of Neuroscience Methods, 74*, 113–122.
Saleh, S., Adamovich, S., & Tunik, E. (2012). Resting state functional connectivity and task-related effective connectivity changes after upper extremity rehabilitation: A pilot study. *Conference Proceedings - IEEE Engineering in Medicine and Biology Society, 2012*, 4559–4562.
Saleh, S., Adamovich, S.V., & Tunik, E. (2013). Visual feedback discordance mediates changes in brain activity and effective connectivity: A stroke fMRI dynamic causal modeling study. *Advances in Biomedical Engineering (ICAMBE), 2nd International Conference*, 85–88.
Saleh, S., Bagce, H., Qiu, Q., Fluet, G., Merians, A., Adamovich, S., et al. (2011). Mechanisms of neural reorganization in chronic stroke subjects after virtual reality training. *Conference Proceedings - IEEE Engineering in Medicine and Biology Society, 2011*, 8118–8121.
Salmoni, A.W., Schmidt, R.A., & Walter, C.B. (1984). Knowledge of results and motor learning: A review and critical reappraisal. *Psychological Bulletin, 95*(3), 355–386.
Schmidt, R. A., & Lee, T.D. (2011). *Motor control and learning: A behavioral emphasis*, 5th ed. (Champaign, IL: Human Kinetics).
Slobounov, S. M., Zhang, K., Pennell, D., Ray, W., Johnson, B., & Sebastianelli, W. (2010). Functional abnormalities in normally appearing athletes following mild traumatic brain injury: A functional MRI study. *Experimental Brain Research, 202*(2), 341–354.
Small, S. L., Hlustik, P., Noll, D. C., Genovese, C., & Solodkin, A. (2002). Cerebellar hemispheric activation ipsilateral to the paretic hand correlated with functional recovery after stroke. *Brain, 125*(7), 1544–1557.
Snijders, H. J., Holmes, N. P., & Spence, C. (2007). Direction-dependent integration of vision and proprioception in reaching under the influence of the mirror illusion. *Neuropsychologia, 45*(3), 496–505.
Stefan, K., Cohen, L. G., Duque, J., Mazzocchio, R., Celnik, P., Sawaki, L., et al. (2005). Formation of a motor memory by action observation. *Journal of Neuroscience, 25*(41), 9339–9346.

Stepniewska, I., Fang, P. C., & Kaas, J. H. (2005). Microstimulation reveals specialized subregions for different complex movements in posterior parietal cortex of prosimian galagos. *Proceedings of the National Academy of Sciences, 102*(13), 4878–4883.

Strafella, A. P., & Paus, T. (2000). Modulation of cortical excitability during action observation: A transcranial magnetic stimulation study. *Neuroreport, 11*(10), 2289–2292.

Subramanian, S. K., Lourenço, C. B., Chilingaryan, G., Sveistrup, H., & Levin, M. F. (2013). Arm motor recovery using a virtual reality intervention in chronic stroke: Randomized control trial. *Neurorehabilitation and Neural Repair, 27*(1), 13–23.

Thomas, M. J., Kalivas, P. W., & Shaham, Y. (2008). Neuroplasticity in the mesolimbic dopamine system and cocaine addiction. *British Journal of Pharmacology, 154*, 327–342.

Tessier, C.R. & Broadie, K. (2009). Activity-dependent modulation of neural circuit synaptic connectivity. *Frontiers in Molecular Neuroscience, 2*, 8.

Wise, S. P., Moody, S. L., Blomstrom, K. J., & Mitz, A. R. (1998). Changes in motor cortical activity during visuomotor adaptation. *Experimental Brain Research, 121*(3), 285–299.

You, S. H., Jang, S. H., Kim, Y. H., Hallet, M., Ahn, S. H., Kwon, Y. H., et al. (2005). Virtual reality-induced cortical reorganization and associated locomotor recovery in chronic stroke-An experimenter-blind randomized study. *Stroke, 36*, 1166–1171.

Chapter 3
Motor Learning and Virtual Reality

Danielle E. Levac and Heidi Sveistrup

Objective To present four fundamental variables influencing client motor learning and describe how attributes of VR technologies provide opportunities to target these variables. To discuss how clinicians can harness these attributes to help clients transfer and generalize the learning achieved in VR-based therapy to better performance in the physical environment.

3.1 Introduction

The primary goal of physical rehabilitation is to help the individual return to functional performance of daily life activities through acquisition of new motor skills and recovery or compensation of lost motor skills. To do so, clinicians seek to promote *motor learning*, defined as "a set of internal processes associated with practice or experience leading to relatively permanent changes in the capability for a motor skill" (Schmidt & Lee, 2011, p. 327). Motor learning is emphasized when clinicians organize practice conditions in ways that promote long-term retention, transfer, and generalization of the skills learned in therapy to their implementation within real-world activities (Wishart, Lee, Ezekiel, Marley, & Lehto, 2000). Decisions about

D.E. Levac (✉)
School of Rehabilitation Sciences, Faculty of Health Sciences, University of Ottawa,
200 Lees Ave (Room A120), Ottawa, ON, Canada, K1N 6N5
e-mail: dleva2@uottawa.ca

H. Sveistrup
School of Rehabilitation Sciences, Faculty of Health Sciences, University of Ottawa,
451 Smyth (Room 3028), Ottawa, ON, Canada, K1H 8M5
e-mail: hsveist@uottawa.ca

P.L. (Tamar) Weiss et al. (eds.), *Virtual Reality for Physical and Motor Rehabilitation*, Virtual Reality Technologies for Health and Clinical Applications,
DOI 10.1007/978-1-4939-0968-1_3, © Springer Science+Business Media New York 2014

Table 3.1 Summary of attributes of virtual reality that align with motor learning variables

Motor learning variable	Attributes
Observational learning	Users can view their own image interacting with virtual objects in the VE
	Users can view an avatar mirroring their movements
	Users can view a virtual teacher demonstrating optimal movement patterns
	VEs can facilitate mental practice or motor imagery
Practice: amount, task specificity, and meaning	Potential for abundant repetition of practice trials
	Ecologically valid VEs enhance task specificity of practice
	Train movements that are identical to those required in real-life tasks
	Options to individualize to different challenge levels
	Enriched environment
	Goal-oriented tasks
	Familiarity of commercially available VR gaming systems
Augmented Feedback	Precise and consistent
	Auditory, visual, or tactile
	Knowledge of performance
	Knowledge of results
	Positive motivational feedback
Motivation	Novelty of VR technology
	Gaming features
	Feedback
	Goal-oriented tasks
	Capacity to individualize treatment options
	Users can select tasks
	Competition against other players
	Match between cognitive and physical effort

the way practice conditions are organized within therapy sessions involve motor learning variables: for example; the type of task to be practiced, the order in which the tasks are practiced, and the type of feedback provided (Levac, Missiuna, Wishart, DeMatteo, & Wright, 2011). Consideration of these motor learning variables is recommended within rehabilitation (Wishart et al., 2000; Zwicker & Harris, 2009; Schmidt 1991) and is supported by the link between motor learning and neuroplasticity (see Chap. 2) (Kleim & Jones, 2008; Krakauer, 2006; Ploughman, 2002).

The scientific rationale for use of virtual reality (VR) technology within rehabilitation can be found in the field of motor learning (Holden, 2005). Therapeutic interventions using VR systems and delivered in virtual environments (VEs) are attractive rehabilitation options because the motor learning variables underlying experience-dependent neuroplasticity are inherent attributes of VR systems (Levin, 2011). The primary objective of this chapter is to summarize the attributes of VR technology that align with four fundamental motor learning variables: practice, augmented feedback, motivation, and observational learning (Table 3.1). We discuss the potential for training in VEs to promote transfer and generalization of learning to the physical environment and describe the features of VR technologies that may impede motor learning processes in clients recovering from central nervous system (CNS) injury.

Secondly, we focus on clinical implications of VR tool implementation in rehabilitation by providing recommendations for clinicians interested in emphasizing motor learning within VR-based therapy (Levac & Galvin, 2013). Finally, the chapter highlights directions for research to further evaluate how learning in VR-based therapy can transfer and generalize to actions performed in the physical environment.

3.2 Motor Learning Variables

3.2.1 Practice

Animal and human studies provide substantial evidence of the importance of abundant, intensive, salient practice for motor learning and neuroplastic change (Adamovich, August, Merians, & Tunik, 2009; Adamovich, Fluet, Tunik, & Merians, 2009; Schmidt & Lee, 2011). The use of VR technologies enables clinicians to provide these practice conditions to individuals undergoing rehabilitation (Adamovich, August, et al., 2009; Adamovich, Fluet, et al., 2009; Levin, 2011). In particular, VR allows for plentiful, task-specific, and meaningful practice opportunities.

3.2.1.1 Amount of Practice

Amount of practice is a fundamental factor supporting motor learning. A greater number of practice trials will improve learning, although the law of practice states that this effect is most evident in early stages of learning and decreases over time (Schmidt & Lee, 2011). Intensity of practice is another key factor driving neuroplastic change in rehabilitation (Kleim & Jones, 2008). Evidence from animal models shows that abundant, intensive practice is needed in the early stages of recovery from a brain injury (Krakauer, Carmichael, Corbett, & Wittenberg, 2012). Indeed, individuals recovering from stroke require a greater number of repetitions as compared to healthy individuals in order to achieve improvements in movement outcomes (Cirstea, Ptito, & Levin, 2003). The flexibility of many VR applications implies that training in meaningful, enriched environments can be provided earlier in recovery from CNS injury than conventional exercises, maximizing the potential to target neuroplastic processes and providing the cortical stimulation needed to prevent functional deterioration of affected structures (Adamovich, August, et al., 2009; Adamovich, Fluet, et al., 2009; Kleim & Jones, 2008).

Compared to training in a physical environment (PE), training in a VE can offer the potential for massed repetition of practice trials (Adamovich, August, et al., 2009; Adamovich, Fluet, et al., 2009; Lange et al., 2012; Weiss & Katz, 2004). The automaticity of many systems implies ease of consistent task repetition, and VEs may motivate users to engage in more repetitions or longer practice durations as compared to conventional exercises (Holden, 2005). However, there is variation in

VR intervention studies regarding the length of training time and the number of movement repetitions completed during VR training. Specifically, the body of evidence comparing the amount of training time or number of repetitions performed in a VE to that in a PE is small. Mirelman, Patritti, Bonato, and Deutsch (2010) trained individuals recovering from stroke in a robot coupled with a VE and compared this condition to training with the robot alone, finding that the group who had trained with the addition of the VE had a significantly greater average training time, required fewer rests, and reported less fatigue as compared to the robot-alone group. However, the number of repetitions performed throughout the training was not significantly different between the two groups (Mirelman et al., 2010). Bryanton et al. (2006) compared ankle exercises undertaken in a VE to conventional home exercises in a group of children with cerebral palsy (CP). They found that children completed more repetitions of the conventional exercise during the specified training time, although the quality of movement was poor as compared to the VE practice condition. However, despite fewer repetitions being recorded in the VE condition, the children in this group achieved and maintained the desired training position for longer periods of time, indicating additional benefits of practice in the VE.

3.2.1.2 Task-Specific Practice

The *specificity of learning hypothesis* posits that motor learning is promoted when the practice conditions of skill acquisition are as similar as possible to those expected for performance of the task in the physical environment (Barnett, Ross, Schmidt, & Todd, 1973; Schmidt & Lee, 2011). VEs may exhibit varying degrees of task specificity. Highly immersive VEs that are *ecologically valid* are the most task-specific. Ecologically valid VEs are designed to recreate conditions of the physical environment and include manipulation of real-world constraints, challenges, or environmental obstacles (Rizzo & Kim, 2005). Many such VEs enable users to practice tasks that may not yet be feasible to accomplish in the real world, such as using a motorized wheelchair, driving a car, or crossing the street. Kizony, Levin, Hughey, Perez, and Fung (2010) developed a VE mimicking a grocery aisle that combined walking on a treadmill with the cognitive task of following shopping instructions. Task-specific VEs that replicate realistic, difficult or dangerous real-life skills can provide safe testing and training rehabilitation environments (Rizzo & Kim, 2005).

VEs are lower on the continuum of task specificity when they are less immersive and do not include the haptic feedback involved in an interaction as experienced in the physical world. However, many can still be considered somewhat task-specific because they provide practice conditions in which the user accomplishes tasks using body movements that are similar to those required when undertaking the task in the PE. Examples include moving boxes from one conveyor belt to another [GestureTek's Interactive Rehabilitation Exercise System (IREX)], responding to obstacles in a VE while standing on an moving force platform (Motek Medical Computer Assisted Rehabilitation Enivornment [CAREN]), being a goalie in a soccer game [IREX], playing table tennis [Microsoft's Kinect], or skiing down a mountain [Nintendo Wii]. Interfaces with the VE may also enhance task specificity; for example, a sensor glove can be used to train finger and hand movements (Golomb et al., 2010) and additions mimicking real-life objects, such as a tennis racquet or a golf club, can be attached to a handheld remote control. The body of literature evaluating whether movement kinematics of upper extremity pointing, reaching, and grasping tasks are in fact similar in physical and virtual environments is reviewed in Chap. 5.

VEs lowest on the task-specificity continuum are those that include fantasy-based games, such as GestureTek's "Sharkbait" where the task to be accomplished has no real-world equivalent. Moreover, some VEs may include attributes that refute task specificity in favor of providing practice conditions that are *enhanced* as compared to those available in the real world: for example; more abundant augmented feedback, greater opportunities for consistent task repetition, and optimal control over parameterization of practice challenge levels.

3.2.1.3 Meaningful Practice

Learning is optimized when learners are engaged in meaningful tasks that are optimally challenging (Kleim & Jones, 2008). Repetition alone is not sufficient for learning; rather, practice must be done in the context of skill acquisition and must provide opportunities for learners to find the solution to the movement task (Lee, Swinnen, & Serrien, 1994; Lehto et al., 2001). There should be an optimal intersection between the cognitive effort required for the client to engage in problem-solving activities during movement repetitions and the challenging nature of the task (Lee et al., 1994).

VR offers an enriched environment that contributes to task meaning and salience. Individuals undergoing rehabilitation may benefit from this increased interaction with an enriched environment (Rose et al., 2000; Sveistrup, 2004). Studies using animal models demonstrate that environmental enrichment of housing conditions enhances cognitive processing abilities through neuroplastic change in the cerebral cortex, and improves learning, problem solving, and cognitive performance after brain damage (Nithianantharajah & Hannan, 2006; Rose, Attree, Brooks, & Johnson, 1998). However, patients do not always receive substantial amounts of time in therapy activities during inpatient stays (Bernhardt, Dewey, Thrift, & Donnan, 2004). The use of VR can be one option to make environmentally enriched practice conditions more accessible to people with sensory or motor impairments (Rose et al., 1998).

The goal-oriented nature of many tasks in VEs may enhance cognitive engagement with the task and thus their salience (Walker et al., 2010). VR games typically have goals to attain that can be progressed in terms of difficulty (Weiss, Kizony, Feintuch, Rand, & Katz, 2006). Working to achieve a goal may enhance attention and concentration in therapy, potentially increasing the efficacy of rehabilitation interventions (Eng et al., 2007; Holden, 2005). Working towards a goal of achieving a high score in a game, for example, may enhance children's enjoyment of therapy (Gordon & Okita, 2010).

The familiarity of commercially available video games may enhance their meaning and salience for rehabilitation clients. Mouawad, Doust, Max, and McNulty (2011) suggest that the familiarity of participants in their study with the Nintendo Wii system is a factor that may have enhanced motivation and motor learning. In a qualitative study of physical therapists using the Wii with children and youth with acquired brain injury, the therapists remarked that they felt the familiarity of the games encouraged children to move and to participate in therapy (Levac, Miller, & Missiuna, 2011).

VR simulations have been added to other types of therapy such as body weight support treadmill training (BWSTT) and constraint induced movement therapy (CIMT) to enhance the salience of the repetitive practice required in these interventions. In BWSTT, a VE with which the user interacts while walking on a treadmill can add motivation to practice of a repetitive walking task through the experience of being part of an activity such as walking down a street (Walker et al., 2010). The Nintendo Wii games have also been used during CIMT programs for children with the rationale that they may increase engagement of task practice given the long hours of training required by the protocol (Gordon & Okita, 2010).

3.2.2 Augmented Feedback

Augmented feedback—information provided about an action that is supplemental to the inherent feedback typically received from the sensory system—is a major factor supporting motor learning (Schmidt & Lee, 2011). Much research investigates the most effective methods of providing augmented feedback to learners, including its nature, timing, and frequency (Molier, Van Asseldonk, Hermens, & Jannink, 2010). Feedback nature can be classified as knowledge of performance (KP)—information about how a person performed a movement—or knowledge of results (KR)—information about whether the movement produced the desired goal (Schmidt & Lee, 2011). Feedback can be provided either during the practice trial (concurrent) or after its completion (terminal), and can be provided at a set frequency, either as a summary after a certain number of trials, or less frequently as learning evolves (faded) (Molier et al., 2010). Molier et al. (2010) conducted a systematic review of studies evaluating the role of feedback in motor relearning of the hemiparetic arm following stroke. They concluded that "…augmented feedback in general has an added value for stroke rehabilitation" (Molier et al., 2010 p. 1799). Because of the variety of studies included in the review, the authors could not determine which combinations of types and schedules of feedback were most beneficial.

VEs offer auditory, visual, and/or tactile feedback that is intuitive, interpretable, provided in real time, and enhanced in precision and consistency as compared to what is available in the real world (Holden, 2005; Subramanian, 2010). Given that many VR systems provide abundant feedback in all these forms, clinicians have opportunities to select the type of feedback that would be most beneficial for learning in the context of an individual's particular impairments (Deutsch et al., 2011).

VR technologies can provide KP feedback representing movement kinematics, muscle activity, or force generation. They can provide KR through visual feedback of the game score or number of successful versus unsuccessful attempts, auditory feedback reflecting whether the movement resulted in a successful outcome, or by a collection of summary information to convey knowledge of results to the user (Mumford & Wilson, 2009). VEs can also provide simple positive feedback linked to success that may enhance motivation and engagement (Deutsch et al., 2011).

Proprioceptive feedback about the contact of a body part with a virtual object is provided by haptic feedback in many VR systems (Feintuch et al., 2006). This type of feedback can increase realism of the interaction and may be important for activation of sensory–motor networks (Robertson & Roby-Brami, 2010). Adamovich et al. (Adamovich, August, et al., 2009; Adamovich, Fluet, et al., 2009) suggest that the tactile feedback provided by a robotic interface to the VE enhances the sensory experience and provides forces that better mimic interaction with objects in the real world. Indeed, haptic feedback is likely essential for accurate grasp in VEs (Hibbard & Bradshaw, 2003). Studies have compared kinematics of upper extremity reach and grasp in VEs using haptic feedback from gloves to identical movements made in physical environments. For example, Magdalon, Michaelson, Quevedo, and Levin (2011) found that movement trajectories and reach to grasp coordination were similar in both environments in healthy individuals (see Chap. 5).

What is the evidence for the impact of feedback provided in a VE on motor learning outcomes in rehabilitation clients? A recent systematic review evaluating whether extrinsic feedback improves motor learning in the upper limb in people who have had a stroke calls for more research to explore whether the enhanced feedback provided by VEs results in improved motor learning as compared to training in a PE (Subramanian, 2010). However, two studies have specifically addressed this question. Mirelman, Bonato, and Deutsch (2009) compared training of ankle movements post-stroke in a robot and a VE to a robot alone, with both groups supervised by a clinician. They suggest that feedback from the VE improved the clinician's efficiency because the clinician could direct the user's attention to the most relevant aspects of the VE's feedback (see Chap. 5). More recently, Subramanian, Lourenço, Chilingaryan, Sveistrup, and Levin (2013) completed a randomized control trial comparing training of upper extremity function in people with stroke in a three-dimensional VE to a PE. The authors suggest that the KP feedback provided by the VE contributed to the demonstrated improvements, possibly because subjects undertook greater cognitive effort and motor planning to achieve the movement pattern required for success at the task.

3.2.3 *Observational Learning*

The "mirror neuron" or "action observation" system in the primary motor cortex is one neurophysiological mechanism underlying learning by imitation or observational learning (Petrosini et al., 2003). Observation of goal-oriented movements provides sensory feedback about movement patterns and outcomes which may contribute to motor learning (Krakauer, 2006). Observing these goal-oriented movements activates neurons that pick up on essential components of the activity that are similar across repetitions, allowing for an image to develop upon which to base movement (Buccino, Solodkin, & Small, 2006).

The mirror neuron system may be engaged in VEs in four ways: (1) Through motion capture VR technology in which the user views his/her own image interacting with virtual objects, allowing for observation of movement accuracy (Weiss, Rand, Katz, & Kizony, 2004) and provision of visual feedback about body position in space (Flynn, Palma, & Bender, 2007); (2) Through VEs in which an avatar mirrors the user's movements; (3) Through VEs in which a virtual teacher demonstrates optimal movement patterns for users to mimic, in the same spatial frame of reference as the users' own movements (Eng et al., 2007; Holden, 2005); or (4) Through VR applications that facilitate mental practice or motor imagery.

With respect to evidence, there is conflicting information as to whether observation in a VE activates the same mirror neuron network as observation in a PE. Adamovich et al. (Adamovich, August, et al., 2009; Adamovich, Fluet, et al., 2009) developed a VR system compatible with functional magnetic resonance imaging (fMRI) and asked healthy subjects to observe preprogrammed movement sequences of a virtual hand as well as movement sequences of a virtual hand controlled in real time by their own hand movements. In both conditions, the same neural networks as those activated by physical world observation were recruited. Cameirao, Badia, Oller, and Verschure (2010) developed the Rehabilitation Gaming System, in which the user controls the movement of two virtual limbs to train finger and arm movements using a first person perspective. They postulated that this first person perspective should facilitate activation of the mirror neuron network. Holden, Todorov, Callahan, and Bizzi (1999) created a VE displayed on a desktop computer showing a "teacher" repeatedly performing the correct movement, allowing the user to match his movement to that of the teacher for training in real time. The authors conclude that subjects could transfer improved performance of reaching movements to the physical environment because they were imitating the teacher within the same frame of reference, negating the need for spatial transformation and allowing subjects to more quickly identify their movement errors.

With respect to evidence in rehabilitation clients, Tunik, Saleh, Bagce, Merians, and Adamovich (2011) found that observing movements of a virtual hand activated the sensorimotor cortex corresponding to the paretic hand in people with chronic stroke, suggesting that this could be a mechanism to train neural reorganization. Researchers investigating the use of GestureTek's IREX in adults with stroke and children with cerebral palsy have also credited activation of the mirror neuron system with the improvements seen after training (Jang, You, & Hallett, 2005; You et al., 2005).

In contrast, evidence exists to suggest that observation in a VE does not in fact recruit the same neural pathways as observation in a PE. The extent to which VEs can target the processes involved in action observation may be dependent on their similarity to the physical world (Adamovich, August, et al., 2009; Adamovich,

Fluet, et al., 2009). Some evidence suggests that observation of virtual effectors may recruit fewer neural circuits than observation of real-world actions. For example, Perani et al. (2001) asked healthy young adults to observe a virtual hand performing a reaching task and a real hand performing the same task, finding less activation in relevant brain areas on fMRI for the virtual observation. Despite including two levels of VR simulations, there was no difference according to the degree of realism of the VR hand. They concluded that observation in a VE did not activate existing action representation maps.

Mental practice or motor imagery could be another mechanism to target observational learning. Gaggioli, Meneghini, Morganti, Alcaniz, and Riva (2006) created a VR system to facilitate mental practice of the affected limb, evaluating it in a case study of an individual following stroke, and demonstrating improvement in arm function after an 8-week training program. However, they could not isolate whether these benefits were due to the mental practice or to the observation of the virtual limb. A brain–computer interface in which subjects wear electroencephalogram (EEG) sensors allows researchers to measure activity patterns in the primary and secondary motor areas of the brain during action observation and imitation of VR tasks (Bermudez, Badia, Samaha, Garcia Morgade, & Verschure, 2011). The developers postulated that the virtual avatar could be controlled via sensory motor rhythms picked up by the EEGs and that an immobile patient could train the motor cortex by controlling the virtual avatar through motor imagery.

VR may also augment the effects of learning by observation by "distorting reality" to highlight movement errors. This can be done by augmenting movement trajectories, exaggerating movement features (Gordon & Okita, 2010; Robertson & Roby-Brami, 2010) and adding more movement replays (Adamovich, August, et al., 2009; Adamovich, Fluet, et al., 2009). However, evidence is required to determine whether these augmentations offer motor learning benefits.

3.2.4 *Motivation*

Learners must be motivated to engage in practice (Schmidt & Lee, 2011). Expectations that rehabilitation should include the large number of repetitions required to regain lost skills after injury can be enhanced if individuals are motivated to participate in the therapy task (Holden, 2005). While this applies to all patient populations, it may be particularly relevant for children for whom engagement in the task may facilitate the maintenance of attention and participation in rehabilitation (Gordon & Magill, 2011; Laufer & Weiss, 2011).

Several hypotheses exist as to why training in a VE might provide motivating practice for clients in rehabilitation. Users may be motivated to participate because of the novelty of these interventions (Lewis & Rosie, 2012). The gaming features of many VR systems, including commercially available interactive video games, may increase motivation (Deutsch, Borbely, Filler, Huhn, & Guarrera-Bowlby, 2008; Jack et al., 2001; Rizzo & Kim, 2005). For example, Mouawad et al. (2011) suggest that the Nintendo Wii games motivate players through the visual and auditory cues that provide commentary, rewards, and feedback related to progress. The motivation provided by the goal-oriented nature of VR applications was also supported in a study where a parent of a child with CP who had participated in a VR gaming intervention commented on the motivation provided by the scoring system (Bryanton et al., 2006). Other studies have suggested that viewing movement trajectories or performance results may motivate users to improve their movement (Gordon & Okita, 2010) and that the unpredictable challenge and variation of stimulus presentation within many VR games motivates children to maintain attention and participation (Harris & Reid, 2005).

VR systems can provide clinicians with a significant capacity to individualize treatment options through manipulating levels of task difficulty and stimulus presentation (Rizzo & Kim, 2005), which may also be a mechanism to achieve and enhance motivation by progressing practice challenge (Golomb et al., 2011; Holden, 2005, Lange et al., 2012; Wang & Reid, 2011). Cameirao et al. (2010) discussed how their Rehabilitation Gaming System adapts the task on a trial by trial basis so that the user averages approximately 70 % correct trials, with the goal of preventing boredom and frustration. VEs may also facilitate task simplification, which may motivate the learning process as the user no longer needs to distinguish the most important elements of the task (Holden, 2005). The capacity to individualize may also enhance motivation by allowing the user to select his or her own practice tasks and schedule (Deutsch et al., 2008; Huber et al., 2008; Miller & Reid, 2003). Overall, many VR systems allow for stimulus control and consistency in terms of individualization and manipulation of treatment parameters to create optimal learning conditions (Rizzo & Kim, 2005).

Competition, either against another player or against a virtual opponent, may also enhance motivation (Deutsch et al., 2008; Harris & Reid, 2005). In the VEs associated with the Lokomat robotic gait trainer, the virtual opponent can be set to walk faster than the user, potentially motivating him or her to participate more actively (Brutsch et al., 2011; Koenig et al., 2008). Ballester, Bermudez, Badia, and Verschure (2011) found that subjects performed a greater amplitude of upper extremity reaching movements when they played competitively against other players as compared to when they played alone, suggested the multiplayer social gaming interaction motivated users to improve their performance.

The body of evidence evaluating these hypotheses, exploring motivation from users' perspectives, or specifically investigating the relationship between motivation and outcomes is small. Motivation typically is assessed through qualitative responses and using a wide variety of standardized and non-standardized outcome measures whose psychometric properties may not be established.

Reviews of the pediatric VR literature conclude that VR interventions motivate children to participate in the repetitive activities needed to gain skills (Laufer & Weiss, 2011; Parsons, Rizzo, Rogers, & York, 2009; Snider, Majnemer, & Darsaklis, 2010). Schuler, Brutsch, Muller, van Hedel, and Meyer-Heim (2011) assessed electromyographic (EMG) activity in lower limb muscles in children with CP and typically developing children walking within a VE as compared to those walking in normal overground conditions on a treadmill. The authors found that EMG activity in both groups of children was significantly higher during walking in the VR scenario and suggest that this provides evidence that the VE contributes to children's motivation and engagement to participate in walking tasks. A narrative review has summarized themes from studies investigating users' responses to VR game use in rehabilitation, distilling comments from users about different aspects that motivated them to participate in the VR interventions (Lewis & Rosie, 2012). Qualitative studies have explored the motivational appeal of VR from the perspective of both clinicians and clients. Levac et al. (2011) asked a small group of physical therapists about their use of the Nintendo Wii with pediatric neurological populations. Therapists described their perceptions that the Wii enhances children's motivation to participate in therapy and to practice movements that they would otherwise be reluctant to try. Lewis, Woods, Rosie, and McPherson (2011) report themes from a qualitative study of individuals with stroke participating in a 6 week VR game intervention. A range of perspectives related to the motivating and challenging nature of the interventions are described.

However, does motivation to participate remain high over the course of a prolonged VR intervention period? Li, Lam-Damji, Chau, and Fehlings (2009) investigated how children with CP used a home-based VR system and reported that the number of minutes played per day decreased over time. They suggested that more game variety may be needed to sustain children's interest. Golomb et al. (2011) describe a lengthy tele-rehabilitation intervention using a VR gaming system and custom made sensor glove. They concluded that a variety of tactics were needed to sustain the engagement of their adolescent participants to continue to practice over time.

An additional factor to consider with respect to motivation and motor learning is the optimal level of cognitive effort required to engage in the VR task. Volkening et al. (2011) explored the motivation of 12 subacute stroke patients playing VR games of differing challenge levels. Users achieved the greatest amount of physical practice (in terms of number of repetitions) in the easiest scenario, but rated this scenario as lowest on the motivation scale, finding that it was boring and of insufficient cognitive demand. The most challenging VR scenario, although rated as motivating, was too difficult to result in many repetitions. It was the more moderate VR scenario that was rated as the most motivating because it achieved the appropriate level of cognitive and physical effort. These findings illustrate the importance of matching not only a user's physical abilities but also his or her cognitive abilities to the VR task in terms of sustaining motivation to practice.

3.3 How Might Training in a Virtual Environment Transfer to Improved Performance of Tasks in the Physical Environment?

Transfer is a central concept in motor learning, defined as: "the gain (or loss) in the capability for performance in one task as a result of practice or experience on some other task" (Schmidt & Lee, 2011, p. 465). Achieving transfer of learning is of central importance within rehabilitation (Holden & Todorov, 2002). VR applications used to train complex skills in surgical, flight, or military situations have demonstrated that it is possible to learn skills in VEs and then transfer this learning into skilled performance in the real world (Bossard, Kermarrec, Buche, & Tisseau, 2008; Holden, 2005). The evidence of transfer of training from VEs to PEs in healthy subjects can be found elsewhere (Bossard et al., 2008; Holden, 2005; Rose et al., 2000).

What conditions and attributes within a VE may facilitate transfer? Transfer will be facilitated if the interaction with the VE and the cognitive processing required for task performance is similar to that required in the PE (Rose et al., 1998), or if the VE provides important information for learning and increases practice salience (Rose et al., 2000). Transfer may be facilitated when the VE requires the learner to adapt to changing demands, problem-solve different solutions to tasks, learn from mistakes, simplify and segment tasks, and repeat variable complex situations (Bossard et al., 2008). VEs that can be individualized—for example, by replicating the users' home environment or modifying stimulus presentation according to user needs and capabilities—should enhance transfer and generalization of learning (Schultheis & Rizzo, 2001).

Transfer of learning to performance in the PE may even be enhanced when subjects train in VEs as compared to training in physical environments. Rose et al. (2000) studied healthy participants and found that when interference tasks were added to a new task in the PE, those who had practiced in a VE performed better as compared to those who had trained in the PE. The authors suggest that the characteristics of the VE training may have better prepared participants to deal with interferences in the real world.

What evidence do we have that skills trained in VEs transfer to activities in the physical world for people with disabilities? Few studies rigorously examine transfer, and studies differ in terms of the level of the task involved and also how transfer is measured (Rose et al., 2000). Studies have demonstrated differing levels of evidence of transfer from VE training to the real world by evaluating post-training performance on standardized tests of motor function, functional activities such as overground and community walking and stair climbing, activities of daily living, and gait speed. Results of these studies are described in Chap. 6.

3.4 How Might Training in a Virtual Environment Hinder Motor Learning?

Features of some VR systems may be detrimental to motor learning for a number of reasons, particularly in clients with neurological impairments. Firstly, commercially available game-based VR systems where there are a small number of training options without the possibility of individualizing treatment parameters or manipulate challenge levels may limit accessibility of VE training in individuals with motor or cognitive impairments, rendering the VR tasks too frustrating, difficult, or physically impossible. Secondly, the motor learning literature suggests that feedback is beneficial in the early stages of learning a motor skill but should not be relied upon throughout training (Winstein, Pohl, & Lewthwaite, 1994). Reliance on the abundant, immediate or consistent feedback provided by some VEs may cause dependence on the conditions of VE practice for successful performance. Thirdly, VR gaming systems may provide inaccurate (Deutsch et al., 2011) or discouraging feedback (Lange et al., 2012). For example, the KP feedback provided by the Nintendo Wii games may not accurately reflect the movements made by the user (Deutsch et al., 2011) and games may not elicit the specific movements that are impaired or that should be promoted in neurological populations (Gordon & Okita, 2010). More information about the quality of movement made in different VEs can be found in Chap. xx of this volume. Small improvements in movement patterns may not be identified in terms of eliciting game success. Lastly, the abundance of visual and auditory feedback within certain VEs may be too overwhelming for clients with cognitive, memory, or attention impairments in motor learning processes (Levac et al., 2011).

3.5 How Can Clinicians Emphasize Motor Learning Within VR-Based Therapy?

The interactive nature of most rehabilitation interventions suggests that the therapist will be an important factor in treatment effectiveness (Whyte & Hart, 2003). Although it is clear that VR systems rely on hardware and software, their use in all rehabilitation situations requires clinicians to make decisions about the appropriateness of the intervention for the client, as well as the implementation of treatment parameters and progression through different levels of the game or task (Levac & Galvin, 2013). Clinicians must also consider issues relating to safety, cost, and evidence for effectiveness in comparison to other types of interventions. While Mirelman et al. (2009) argue that VEs that provide motivating and interpretable feedback do not require a clinician to be present at all times, the use of VR can also amplify and enhance the expertise and effectiveness of clinicians (Rizzo & Kim, 2005). The automaticity of task delivery within VEs may allow the clinician to better concentrate on observing movement performance and promoting effective strategies, even if the task is complex (Laufer & Weiss, 2011; Weiss et al., 2006). Lange et al. (2012) suggest that as VR systems become more ubiquitous, the primary role for the therapist will be in promoting transfer of rehabilitation gains to real-world performance.

The following recommendations are provided to illustrate how clinicians can promote motor learning within VR-based therapy (Table 3.2):

1. Take the time to become familiar with practicalities and features of the VR system and its applications to understand the attributes that may take advantage of motor learning variables or that may hinder motor learning. Therapists have identified a need for training as a factor limiting the effective use of VR systems in practice (Glegg et al., 2013; Levac et al., 2011). For certain VR systems, resources exist to assist clinical decision-making. For example, Deutsch et al. (2011)

Table 3.2 Recommendations for clinicians

Recommendations	Details
Become familiar with the VR system	Dedicate time for training Take advantage of existing resources in the literature to inform training
Keep abreast of the scientific literature	Appraise the evidence as to how training in the VE can promote motor learning outcomes of retention, transfer, and generalization
Take a client-centered approach	Consider the intersection between a VR system's affordances and the client's impairments in motor learning processes
Set goals according to ICF levels	In addition to impairment-focused goals, set goals that relate to increased participation in functional activities
Emphasize learning not performance	Focus on transfer and generalization of skills being practiced in the VE to real-life activities and settings
Be aware of and mitigate for potentially challenging features of commercially available VR systems	Make practice task-oriented Ensure optimal movement quality Mitigate negative feedback Use therapeutic adaptations
Add therapeutic adaptations to target transfer and generalization	Change conditions of the physical environment
Modify and progress task challenges as individuals improve	Modify VR system parameters or physical environment factors to progress challenge
Set up home or delegated therapy programs according to motor learning principles and have a plan for monitoring programs and evaluating outcomes	Organize practice schedule according to conditions that promote motor learning Ensure assistants are well trained in the VR tasks Make a plan to monitor performance, progress challenge, and evaluate learning

have described each Nintendo Wii game, analyzed the games for the feedback provided (specifically, knowledge of performance and knowledge of results), and outlined the impairments that each game targets to inform clinicians in making decisions about which games to implement in therapy (Deutsch et al., 2011). Galvin and Levac (2011) also provide a descriptive analysis and initial classification framework of several VR systems used in pediatric rehabilitation with the intent of supporting therapist decision-making about system use.

2. Continually keep abreast of advances in the scientific literature to appraise the level of evidence as to how training in the VE of interest can promote transfer of learning to real-life functional activities.
3. Take a client-centered approach by considering the intersection between a VR system's affordances and the client's capabilities as they relate to potential impairments in motor learning processes (Galvin & Levac, 2011). Because of specific cognitive, memory, or attention impairments, some clients may not be the best candidates for using certain VR systems (Levac et al., 2011).
4. Set client-centered goals for VR-based therapy that target different levels of the International Classification of Functioning, Disability, and Health: impairments in body structures and function, activity limitations, or participation restrictions.

5. Consider the difference between "performance" and "learning" by recognizing that improved performance within a therapy session is considered to be learning only when the improvements are retained over time (Newell, Yeuo-The, & Gottfried, 2001). Rather than focusing on a client's performance during the therapy session, focus on how the skills being practiced in the VE can transfer to use in real-life activities and settings. This may involve considering what the client needs to learn in the VE in order to function in the real world, highlighting similarities between movements in the VE and those required in the real world, or asking the client to brainstorm and problem-solve about similarities between the VR task and functional skills required in daily life.
6. Additional considerations apply when using commercially available gaming systems that were not designed for rehabilitation, as there is much less opportunity to grade the level of task difficulty. If games are fantasy-based, the clinician needs to "help bridge the link between the gaming world and the real world" (Gordon & Okita, 2010, p. 183). Observing the client's movement is paramount, as these systems offer much potential for compensation in the form of "cheating" and avoidance of therapeutically beneficial movement (Lange et al., 2012; Lewis & Rosie, 2012). Patients may be able to use smaller range of joint movements to achieve success at the VR task, particularly when they are playing in a "competition" as opposed to a "simulation" mode (Deutsch et al., 2011). This is particularly the case for the Nintendo Wii in which the remote control captures movement acceleration as opposed to spatial position changes (Deutsch et al., 2011). As such, it may be relevant to limit unsupervised practice and to use hands-on techniques to prevent inappropriate movements.
7. Add therapeutic adaptations that may help to target transfer and generalization to real world. For example, therapists can change the support surface on which clients play VR games by having them stand on a BOSU ball or balance board.
8. As the client's skills improve, continually modify tasks through progression and manipulation of available system options to individualize and target different challenge levels.
9. The above considerations also apply to tele-rehabilitation. When setting up therapy programs to be delivered at home, consider motor learning principles relevant to structure of the practice schedule, be aware of the potential for compensatory movement strategies, and monitor progression of difficulty or challenge over time (Table 3.2).

3.6 Model of VR-Based Rehabilitation

Weiss et al. (2006) present a model (Fig. 3.1) using concepts from the International Classification of Functioning, Disability, and Health to guide the use of VR in rehabilitation. The model illustrates that the goal of using VR in rehabilitation is to assist the client in regaining independent function in the real world. Characteristics or factors of the VE (including the attributes discussed in this chapter) interact with clients'

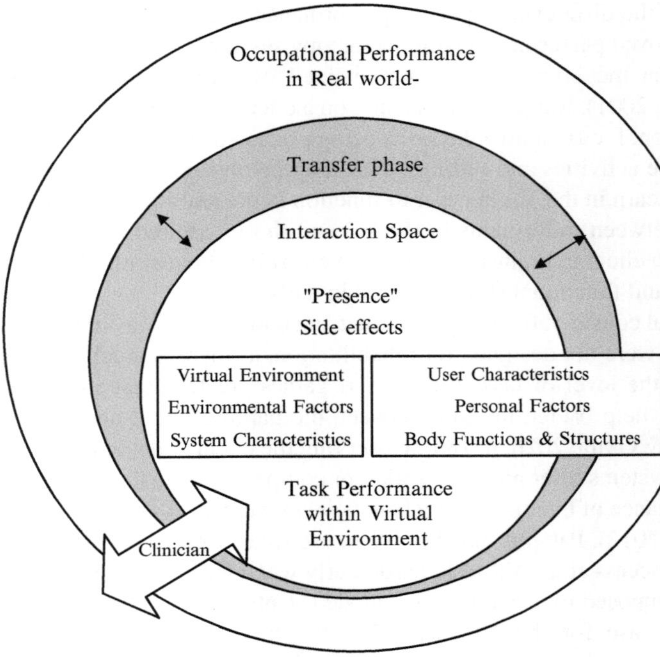

Fig. 3.1 A model of VR-based rehabilitation within the context of terminology from the International Classification of Functioning, Disability, and Health concepts. Reproduced with permission from: Weiss, P.L., Kizony, R., Feintuch, U., & Katz, N. (2010). Virtual Reality Applications in Neurorehabilitation. In Selzer, M., Clarke, S., Cohen, L., Duncan, P., & Sage, F. (Eds). *Textbook of Neural Repair and Rehabilitation*, *Volume 2*: *Medical Neurorehabilitation* (pp. 182–197). Cambridge: Cambridge University Press. DOI: http://dx.doi.org/10.1017/CBO9780511545078.015

personal characteristics to determine task performance within the VE. The model indicates that the clinician plays a key role in facilitating the transfer phase from task performance within the VE into occupational performance in the real world.

3.7 Future Research Directions

Much remains to be discovered about how training in a VE can promote motor learning in rehabilitation clients. Researchers need to clearly identify the skills being trained in the VE that will be transferred to the PE and how this will be measured (Rose et al., 2000). VR intervention studies should include longer-term motor learning outcomes such as retention of learning and transfer and generalization of skills learned in VR therapy to real-life activities, including outcomes measured at the ICF activity and participation levels (Sandlund, McDonough, & Hager-Ross, 2009; Weiss et al., 2006). A motor learning theoretical framework may assist researchers in linking the impact of the motor learning variables evident within VR interventions to improved outcomes (Levac et al., 2012). Little is known about which training conditions best facilitate transfer (Sveistrup, 2004). Ultimately, it is important to understand whether training in a VE is more effective with respect to achieving motor learning than training in the real world (Holden, 2005).

It will be important to develop and evaluate methods for training clinicians to implement VR-based therapy (Levac & Galvin, 2013). This includes educational opportunities related to how a clinician structures VR interventions, provides additional instructions and feedback, or progresses and modifies the intervention. Research is needed to develop guidelines that will support clinicians in (1) identifying optimal dosing requirements and treatment parameters for different outcomes; (2) evaluating how much practice or feedback is most beneficial; and (3) determining which particular motor learning variables, demonstrated to varying degrees in different VEs, are most important for improving rehabilitation outcomes.

Finally, the role of user motivation to participate in VE training from the user's perspective requires exploration. Studies should explore the link between user motivation and training outcomes, how motivation may differ between ecologically valid versus game-based VEs, and how motivation might change over a course of therapy.

3.8 Conclusions

Rehabilitation interventions that maximize functional neuroplastic change after CNS injury provide abundant, intensive, motivating, and meaningful task practice (Kleim & Jones, 2008). VR-based rehabilitation interventions can exploit the capacity of the CNS for functional reorganization and mediate recovery through neuroplasticity. Motor learning concepts form the basis of the scientific rationale for the integration of VE training into rehabilitation practice. This chapter has described and summarized the evidence for the attributes of VR technologies that align with the motor learning variables of practice, feedback, observational learning, and motivation. The conditions under which training in a VE might lead to improvements in real-life skills are discussed, as are features of VR systems that may be detrimental for motor learning.

VR-based therapy can be provided in a variety of rehabilitation settings, including research laboratories, clinics, the community, and homes. Clinicians play a crucial role in structuring, delivering, progressing, and monitoring interventions in ways that maximize transfer of improvements to real-life functional skills. Suggestions for how therapists can use VR to promote motor learning have been provided. Given that VR systems vary substantially in terms of the extent to which attributes of motor learning can be manipulated, the practitioner must be familiar with the system he/she is using and keep up to date with new developments. This may be challenging in such a rapidly changing field.

Effective rehabilitation approaches should provide task-oriented training, individual feedback, goal-tailored exercise schedules, frequent movement repetition, engaging and fun gaming scenarios, individualized interventions, and feedback directed towards motor learning (Timmermans, Seelen, Willmann, & Kingma, 2009). VR-based therapy can include all of these elements. Research to evaluate which attributes and practice conditions most promote skill transfer will enhance the promise of VR-based therapy as a rehabilitation intervention that can improve performance of functional real-life skills in a wide variety of rehabilitation clients.

References

Adamovich, S. V., August, K., Merians, A. S., & Tunik, E. (2009). A virtual reality-based system integrated with fmri to study neural mechanisms of action observation-execution: A proof of concept study. *Restorative Neurology and Neuroscience, 27*(3), 209–223.

Adamovich, S. V., Fluet, G. G., Tunik, E., & Merians, A. S. (2009). Sensorimotor training in virtual reality: A review. *Neurorehabilitation, 25*(1), 29–44.

Ballester, B. R., Bermudez, I., Badia, S., & Verschure, P. (2011). *The effect of social gaming in virtual reality based rehabilitation of stroke patients. International Conference on Virtual Rehabilitation, Zurich, Switzerland.* Washington, DC: IEEE.

Barnett, M. L., Ross, D., Schmidt, R. A., & Todd, B. (1973). Motor skills learning and the specificity of training principle. *Research Quarterly, 44*(4), 440–447.

Bermudez, I., Badia, S., Samaha, H., Garcia Morgade, A., & Verschure, P. F. (2011). *Exploring the synergies of a hybrid BCI-VR neurorehabilitation system: Monitoring and promoting cortical reorganization through mental and motor training. International Conference on Virtual Rehabilitation, Zurich, Switzerland.* Washington, DC: IEEE.

Bernhardt, J., Dewey, H., Thrift, A., & Donnan, G. (2004). Inactive and alone: Physical activity within the first 14 days of acute stroke unit care. *Stroke, 35*(4), 1005–1009.

Bossard, C., Kermarrec, G., Buche, C., & Tisseau, J. (2008). Transfer of learning in virtual environments: A new challenge? *Virtual Reality, 12*, 151–161.

Brutsch, K., Koenig, A., Zimmerli, L., Mrillat-Koeneke, S., Riener, R., Jncke, L., et al. (2011). Virtual reality for enhancement of robot-assisted gait training in children with central gait disorders. *Journal of Rehabilitation Medicine, 43*(6), 493–499.

Bryanton, C., Bosse, J., Brien, M., McLean, J., McCormick, A., & Sveistrup, H. (2006). Feasibility, motivation, and selective motor control: Virtual reality compared to conventional home exercise in children with cerebral palsy. *Cyberpsychology & Behavior, 9*(2), 123–128.

Buccino, G., Solodkin, A., & Small, S. L. (2006). Functions of the mirror neuron system: Implications for neurorehabilitation. *Cognitive and Behavioral Neurology, 19*, 55–63.

Cameirao, M. S., Badia, S. B., Oller, E. D., & Verschure, P. F. (2010). Neurorehabilitation using the virtual reality based rehabilitation gaming system: Methodology, design, psychometrics, usability and validation. *Journal of Neuroengineering & Rehabilitation, 7*, 48.

Cirstea, M. C., Ptito, A., & Levin, M. F. (2003). Arm reaching improvements with short-term practice depend on the severity of the motor deficit in stroke. *Experimental Brain Research, 152*(4), 476–488.

Deutsch, J. E. (2009). Virtual reality and gaming systems to improve walking and mobility for people with musculoskeletal and neuromuscular conditions. *Studies in Health Technology & Informatics, 145*, 84–93.

Deutsch, J. E., Borbely, M., Filler, J., Huhn, K., & Guarrera-Bowlby, P. (2008). Use of a low-cost, commercially available gaming console (Wii) for rehabilitation of an adolescent with cerebral palsy. *Physical Therapy, 88*(10), 1–12.

Deutsch, J. E., Brettler, A., Smith, C., Welsh, J., John, R., Guarrera-Bowlby, P., et al. (2011). Nintendo Wii sports and Wii fit game analysis, validation, and application to stroke rehabilitation. *Topics in Stroke Rehabilitation, 18*(6), 701–719.

Eng, K., Siekierka, E., Pyk, P., Chevrier, E., Hauser, Y., Cameirao, M., et al. (2007). Interactive visuo-motor therapy system for stroke rehabilitation. *Medical & Biological Engineering & Computing, 45*(9), 901–907.

Feintuch, U., Raz, L., Hwang, J., Josman, N., Katz, N., Kizony, R., et al. (2006). Integrating haptic-tactile feedback into a video-capture-based virtual environment for rehabilitation. *Cyberpsycology & Behavior, 9*(2), 129–132.

Flynn, S., Palma, P., & Bender, A. (2007). Feasibility of using the Sony PlayStation 2 gaming platform for an individual poststroke: A case report. *Journal of Neurologic Physical Therapy, 31*(4), 180–189.

Gaggioli, A., Meneghini, A., Morganti, F., Alcaniz, M., & Riva, G. (2006). A strategy for computer-assisted mental practice in stroke rehabilitation. *Neurorehabilitation & Neural Repair, 20*(4), 503–507.

Galvin, J., & Levac, D. (2011). Facilitating clinical decision-making about the use of virtual reality within paediatric motor rehabilitation: Describing and classifying virtual reality systems. *Developmental Neurorehabilitation, 14*(2), 112–122.

Glegg, S., Holsti, L., Velikonja, D., Ansley, B., Brum, C., & Sartor, D. (2013). Factors influencing therapists' adoption of virtual reality for brain injury rehabilitation. *Journal of Cybertherapy and Rehabilitation, 16*(5), 385–401.

Golomb, M. R., McDonald, B. C., Warden, S. J., Yonkman, J., Saykin, A. J., Shirley, B., et al. (2010). In-home virtual reality videogame telerehabilitation in adolescents with hemilplegic cerebral palsy. *Archives of Physical Medicine and Rehabilitation, 91*, 1–8.

Golomb, M. R., Warden, S. J., Fess, E., Rabin, B., Yonkman, J., Shirley, B., et al. (2011). Maintained hand function and forearm bone health 14 months after an in-home virtual-reality videogame hand telerehabilitation intervention in an adolescent with hemiplegic cerebral palsy. *Journal of Child Neurology, 26*(3), 389–393.

Gordon, A. M., & Magill, R. A. (2011). Motor learning: Application of principles to pediatric rehabilitation. In S. K. Campbell (Ed.), *Physical therapy for children* (3rd ed., p. 157). Philadelphia, PA: Saunders.

Gordon, A. M., & Okita, S. Y. (2010). Augmenting pediatric constraint-induced movement therapy and bimanual training with video gaming technology. *Technology and Disability, 22*, 179–191.

Harris, K., & Reid, D. (2005). The influence of virtual reality play on children's motivation. *Canadian Journal of Occupational Therapy, 72*, 21–29.

Hibbard, P. B., & Bradshaw, M. F. (2003). Reaching for virtual objects: Binocular disparity and the control of prehension. *Experimental Brain Research, 148*, 196–201.

Holden, M. K. (2005). Virtual environments for motor rehabilitation: Review. *Cyberpsychology and Behavior, 8*(3), 187–211.

Holden, M. K., & Todorov, E. (2002). Use of virtual environments in motor learning and rehabilitation. In K. M. Stanney (Ed.), *Handbook of virtual environments: Design, implementation, and applications* (pp. 999–1026). London: Lawrence Elbraum.

Holden, M., Todorov, E., Callahan, J., & Bizzi, E. (1999). Virtual environment training improves motor performance in two patients with stroke: Case report. *Neurology Report, 23*(2), 57–67.

Huber, M., Rabin, B., Docan, C., Burdea, G., Nwosu, M., Abdelbaky, M., et al. (2008). *PlayStation 3-based tele-rehabilitation for children with hemiplegia. International Conference on Virtual Rehabilitation, 2008, Vancouver, BC.* Washington, DC: IEEE.

Jack, D., Boian, R., Merians, A. S., Tremaine, M., Burdea, G. C., Adamovich, S. V., et al. (2001). Virtual reality-enhanced stroke rehabilitation. *IEEE Transactions on Neural Systems & Rehabilitation Engineering, 9*(3), 308–318.

Jang, S. H., You, S. H., & Hallett, M. (2005). Cortical reorganization and associated functional motor recovery after virtual reality in patients with chronic stroke: An experimenter-blind preliminary study. *Archives of Physical Medicine and Rehabilitation, 86*, 2218–2223.

Kizony, R., Levin, M. F., Hughey, L., Perez, C., & Fung, J. (2010). Cognitive load and dual-task performance during locomotion poststroke: A feasibility study using a functional virtual environment. *Physical Therapy, 90*(2), 252–260.

Kleim, J., & Jones, T. (2008). Principles of experience-dependent neural plasticity: Implications for rehabilitation after brain damage. *Journal of Speech, Language & Hearing Research, 51*(1), S225–S239.

Koenig, A., Wellner, M., Koneke, S., Meyer-Heim, A., Lunenburger, L., & Riener, R. (2008). Virtual gait training for children with cerebral palsy using the lokomat gait orthosis. *Studies in Health Technology & Informatics, 132*, 204–209.

Krakauer, J. W. (2006). Motor learning: Its relevance to stroke recovery and neurorehabilitation. *Current Opinion in Neurology, 19*(1), 84–90.

Krakauer, J. W., Carmichael, S. T., Corbett, D., & Wittenberg, G. F. (2012). Getting neurorehabilitation right: What can be learned from animal models? *Neurorehabilitation and Neural Repair, 26*(8), 923–931.

Lange, B., Koenig, S., Chang, C., McConnell, E., Suma, E., Bolas, M., et al. (2012). Designing informed game-based rehabilitation tasks leveraging advances in virtual reality. *Disability and Rehabilitation, 34*(22), 1863–1870.

Laufer, Y., & Weiss, P. L. (2011). Virtual reality in the assessment and treatment of children with motor impairment: A systematic review. *Journal of Physical Therapy Education, 25*(1), 59–71.

Lee, T. D., Swinnen, S. P., & Serrien, D. J. (1994). Cognitive effort and motor learning. *QUEST, 46*, 328–344.

Lehto, N. K., Marley, T. L., Ezekiel, H. J., Wishart, L. R., Lee, T. D., & Jarus, T. (2001). Application of motor learning principles: The physiotherapy client as a problem-solver. IV. Future directions. *Physiotherapy Canada, 53*(2), 109–114.

Levac, D., & Galvin, J. (2013). When is virtual reality 'therapy'? *Archives of Physical Medicine & Rehabilitation, 94*(4), 795–798. doi:10.1016/j.apmr.2012.10.021. pii: S0003-9993(12)01078-7.

Levac, D., Miller, P., & Missiuna, C. (2011). Usual and virtual reality video game-based physiotherapy interventions for children and youth with acquired brain injuries. *Physical and Occupational Therapy in Pediatrics, 32*(2), 180–195.

Levac D, Missiuna C, Wishart L, DeMatteo C, Wright V. (2011). Documenting the content of physical therapy for children with acquired brain injury: Development and validation of the Motor Learning Strategy Rating Instrument. *Physical Therapy, 91*(5):689–99.

Levin, M. F. (2011). Can virtual reality offer enriched environments for rehabilitation? *Expert Review of Neurotherapeutics, 11*(2), 153–155.

Lewis, G. N., & Rosie, J. A. (2012). Virtual reality games for movement rehabilitation in neurological conditions: How do we meet the needs and expectations of users? *Disability & Rehabilitation, 34*(22), 1880–1886.

Lewis, G. N., Woods, C., Rosie, J. A., & McPherson, K. M. (2011). Virtual reality games for rehabilitation of people with stroke: Perspectives from the users. *Disability & Rehabilitation Assistive Technology, 6*(5), 453–463.

Li, W., Lam-Damji, S., Chau, T., & Fehlings, D. (2009). The development of a home-based virtual reality therapy system to promote upper extremity movement for children with hemiplegic cerebral palsy. *Technology and Disability, 21*, 107–113.

Magdalon, E. C., Michaelson, S. M., Quevedo, A. A., & Levin, M. F. (2011). Comparison of grasping movements made by healthy subjects in a 3-dimensional immersive virtual versus physical environment. *Acta Psychologica, 138*(1), 126–134.

Miller, S., & Reid, D. (2003). Doing play: Competency, control, and expression. *Cyberpsychology & Behavior, 6*(6), 623–632.

Mirelman, A., Bonato, P., & Deutsch, J. E. (2009). Effects of training with a robot-virtual reality system compared with a robot alone on the gait of individuals after stroke. *Stroke, 40*(1), 169–174.

Mirelman, A., Patritti, B. L., Bonato, P., & Deutsch, J. E. (2010). Effects of virtual reality training on gait biomechanics of individuals post-stroke. *Gait & Posture, 31*(4), 433–437.

Molier, B. I., Van Asseldonk, E. H., Hermens, H. J., & Jannink, M. J. (2010). Nature, timing, frequency and type of augmented feedback; does it influence motor relearning of the hemiparetic arm after stroke? A systematic review. *Disability and Rehabilitation, 32*, 1799–1809.

Mouawad, M. R., Doust, C. G., Max, M. D., & McNulty, P. A. (2011). Wii-based movement therapy to promote improved upper extremity function post-stroke: A pilot study. *Journal of Rehabilitation Medicine, 43*(6), 527–533.

Mumford, N., & Wilson, P. H. (2009). Virtual reality in acquired brain injury upper limb rehabilitation: Evidence-based evaluation of clinical research. *Brain Injury, 23*(3), 179–191.

Newell, K. M., Yeuo-The, L., & Gottfried, M. K. (2001). Time scales in motor learning and development. *Psychological Review, 108*(1), 57–82.

Nithianantharajah, J., & Hannan, A. J. (2006). Enriched environments, experience-dependent plasticity and disorders of the nervous system. *Nature Reviews. Neuroscience, 7*(9), 697–709.

Parsons, T. D., Rizzo, A. A., Rogers, S., & York, P. (2009). Virtual reality in paediatric rehabilitation: A review. *Developmental Neurorehabilitation, 12*(4), 224–238.

Perani, D., Fazio, F., Borghese, N. A., Tettamanti, M., Ferrari, S., Decety, J., et al. (2001). Different brain correlates for watching real and virtual hand actions. *NeuroImage, 14*(3), 749–758.

Petrosini, L., Graziano, A., Mandolesi, L., Neri, P., Molinari, M., & Leggio, M. G. (2003). Watch how to do it! new advances in learning by observation. *Brain Research - Brain Research Reviews, 42*(3), 252–264.

Ploughman, M. (2002). A review of brain neuroplasticity and implications for the physiotherapeutic management of stroke. *Physiotherapy Canada, 54*(3), 164–176.

Rizzo, A., & Kim, G. J. (2005). A SWOT analysis of the field of virtual reality rehabilitation and therapy. *Presence, 14*(2), 119–146.

Robertson, J. V. G., & Roby-Brami, A. (2010). Augmented feedback, virtual reality and robotics for designing new rehabilitation interventions. In J. P. Didier & E. Bigand (Eds.), *Rethinking physical and rehabilitation medicine: New technologies induce new learning strategies* (pp. 223–245). Paris: Springer.

Rose, F. D., Attree, E. A., Brooks, B. M., & Johnson, D. A. (1998). Virtual environments in brain damage rehabilitation: A rationale from basic neuroscience. In G. Riva, B. K. Wiederhold, & M. Molinari (Eds.), *Virtual environments in clinical psychology and neuroscience*. Amsterdam, The Netherlands: Ios Press.

Rose, F. D., Attree, E. A., Brooks, B. M., Parslow, D. M., Penn, P. R., & Ambihaipahan, N. (2000). Training in virtual environments: Transfer to real world tasks and equivalence to real task training. *Ergonomics, 43*(4), 494–511.

Sandlund, M., McDonough, S., & Hager-Ross, C. (2009). Interactive computer play in rehabilitation of children with sensorimotor disorders: A systematic review. *Developmental Medicine & Child Neurology, 51*(3), 173–179.

Schmidt, R. A. (1991). *Motor learning principles for physical therapy. Contemporary Management of Motor Problems: Proceedings of the II Step Conference* (p. 49). Alexandria, Va: Foundation for Physical Therapy.

Schmidt, R. A., & Lee, T. D. (2011). *Motor control and learning: A behavioral emphasis* (5th ed.). Champaign, IL: Human Kinetics.

Schuler, T., Brutsch, K., Muller, R., van Hedel, U. J., & Meyer-Heim, A. (2011). Virtual realities as motivational tools for robotic assisted gait training in children: A surface electromyography study. *Neurorehabilitation, 28*(4), 401–411.

Schultheis, M. T., & Rizzo, A. A. (2001). The application of virtual reality technology in rehabilitation. *Rehabilitation Psychology, 46*, 296–311.

Snider, L., Majnemer, A., & Darsaklis, V. (2010). Virtual reality as a therapeutic modality for children with cerebral palsy. *Developmental Neurorehabilitation, 13*(2), 120–128.

Subramanian, S. K. (2010). Does provision of extrinsic feedback result in improved motor learning in the upper limb poststroke? A systematic review of the evidence. *Neurorehabilitation Neural Repair, 24*(2), 113–124.

Subramanian, S. K., Lourenço, C. B., Chilingaryan, G., Sveistrup, H., & Levin, M. F. (2013). Adaptive arm-motor recovery using a virtual reality intervention in chronic stroke: Randomized control trial. *Neurorehabilitation Neural Repair, 27*(1), 13–23.

Sveistrup, H. (2004). Motor rehabilitation using virtual reality. *Journal of NeuroEngineering and Rehabilitation, 1*(1), 10. doi:10.1186/1743-0003-1-10.

Timmermans, A. A., Seelen, H. A., Willmann, R. D., & Kingma, H. (2009). Technology-assisted training of arm-hand skills in stroke: Concepts on reacquisition of motor control and therapist guidelines for rehabilitation technology design. *Journal of Neuroengineering & Rehabilitation, 6*, 1. doi:10.1186/1743-0003-6-1.

Tunik, E., Saleh, S., Bagce, H., Merians, A., & Adamovich, S. V. (2011). *Mirror feedback in virtual reality elicits ipsilesional motor cortex activation in chronic stroke patients. International Conference on Virtual Rehabilitation, Zurich, Switzerland.* Washington, DC: IEEE.

Volkening, K., Bergmann, J., Muller, F., Ziherl, J., Novak, D., Mihelj, M., et al. (2011). *Cognitive demand in a VR-enriched arm training and its relation to performance, motivation and cognitive abilities. International Conference on Virtual Rehabilitation, Zurich, Switzerland.* Washington, DC: IEEE.

Walker, M. L., Ringleb, S. I., Maihafer, G. C., Walker, R., Crouch, J. R., Van Lunen, B., et al. (2010). Virtual reality-enhanced partial body weight-supported treadmill training poststroke: Feasibility and effectiveness in 6 subjects. *Archives of Physical Medicine & Rehabilitation, 91*(1), 115–122.

Wang, M., & Reid, D. (2011). Virtual reality in pediatric neurorehabilitation: Attention deficit hyperactivity disorder, autism and cerebral palsy. *Neuroepidemiology, 36*(1), 2–18.

Weiss, P. L., & Katz, N. (2004). The potential of virtual reality for rehabilitation. *Journal of Rehabilitation Research and Development, 41*(5), vii–x.

Weiss, P. L., Kizony, R., Feintuch, U., Rand, D., & Katz, N. (2006). Virtual reality applications in neurorehabilitation. In M. E. Selzer, L. Cohen, F. H. Gage, & S. Clarke (Eds.), *Textbook of neural repair and rehabilitation* (pp. 182–197). Cambridge, England: University Press.

Weiss, P. L., Rand, D., Katz, R., & Kizony, R. (2004). Video capture virtual reality as a flexible and effective rehabilitation tool. *Journal of Neuroengineering Rehabilitation, 1*(1), 12.

Whyte, J., & Hart, H. (2003). It's more than a black box; It's a Russian doll: Defining rehabilitation treatments. *American Journal of Physical Medicine and Rehabilitation, 82*(8), 639–652.

Winstein, C. J., Pohl, P. S., & Lewthwaite, R. (1994). Effects of physical guidance and knowledge of results on motor learning: Support for the guidance hypothesis. *Research Quarterly for Exercise & Sport, 65*(4), 316–323.

Wishart, L., Lee, T., Ezekiel, H. J., Marley, T., & Lehto, N. K. (2000). Application of motor learning principles: The physiotherapy client as a problem solver. 1. Concepts. *Physiotherapy Canada, Summer, 52*, 229–232.

You, S. H., Jang, S. H., Kim, Y. H., Kwon, Y. H., Barrow, I., & Hallett, M. (2005). Cortical reorganization induced by virtual reality therapy in a child with hemiparetic cerebral palsy. *Developmental Medicine & Child Neurology, 47*(9), 628–635.

Zwicker, J. G., & Harris, S. R. (2009). Reflection on motor learning theory in pediatric occupational therapy practice. *Canadian Journal of Occupational Therapy, 76*(1), 29–37.

Chapter 4
Vision, Perception, and Object Manipulation in Virtual Environments

Robert V. Kenyon and Stephen R. Ellis

Objective To present aspects of human vision and human perception that affect the user interface to a virtual environment. To examine those aspects that need to transfer the visual information in the physical world to the virtual world.

4.1 Introduction

In many stroke and traumatic brain injury cases, patients relearn lost motor skills by repeatedly performing the same task again and again. The tasks that are performed can be limited by the physics of the environment and the equipment available to the therapist. Thus, training exercises using tasks related to activities of daily living may be missing or inadequate even though such training has been shown to be an important part of the rehabilitation regimen (Dean & Shepherd, 1997; Nudo & Friel, 1998; Nudo, 1999). In addition, the repetition of the task can prove to be a burden on the patient, for example, due to the monotony of the situation. Providing a variety of challenges to the patient using different environments can prove to be an

R.V. Kenyon, P.T., Ph.D. (✉)
Department of Computer Science, University of Illinois at Chicago,
851 S. Morgan St., SEO bldg. Rm 1133, Chicago, IL 60607, USA
e-mail: kenyon@uic.edu

S.R. Ellis
Human Systems Integrations Division, Advanced Controls and Displays Laboratory,
NASA Ames Research Center, Moffett Field, CA 94035-1000, USA
e-mail: stephen.r.ellis@nasa.gov

P.L. (Tamar) Weiss et al. (eds.), *Virtual Reality for Physical and Motor Rehabilitation*, Virtual Reality Technologies for Health and Clinical Applications,
DOI 10.1007/978-1-4939-0968-1_4,

important component in the adherence of patients to their rehabilitation regimen and improvement in their condition (Hanlon, 1996; Jarus & Gutman, 2001). This is important since recovery has been shown to be positively related to the number of times a patient repeats the training tasks (Taub, Uswatte, & Pidikiti, 1999).

Virtual environments (VEs) are not constrained by the physics of the real world and can adapt very rapidly to almost any situation. This inherent versatility of VE is an influential factor in its acceptance and use in rehabilitation. The ability to display any one of a number of different environmental scenarios, as well as tasks, in a matter of minutes or even seconds provides the therapist with maximum flexibility in retraining the patient's perceptual and motor system (Patton, Dawe, Scharver, Muss-Ivaldi, & Kenyon, 2004). However, VEs fall short of the real world because they do not contain all the visual, tactile, auditory, and other sensory cues found in the physical world. For example, for persons to interact effectively with objects in the environment, it is necessary for them to first know where the object is relative to themselves, e.g., right, left, up, down, what size it is, and what distance it is from them. These are attributes that we determine from the physical environment without really paying much attention to the process. In a VE the ease at which we process and use visual and other information sources may not be as natural due to the limitations of rendering this kind of environment. These VE limitations are associated with spatial and temporal display tolerances of VEs that must be understood for specific rehabilitation applications.

The overall purpose of this chapter is to provide readers with information that will help them utilize a VE. While VEs have been developed to convey a variety of sensory information, e.g., haptic, auditory, or kinesthetic, VEs are predominantly a source of visual information. Therefore, understanding limitations of the VE and how these limitations impact perceptions generated by the user's visual system is important for deciding how and when to apply this technology. For example, some VE applications are too ambitious and do not achieve their desired effect due to current limitations of technology and the characteristics of the sensory systems that are activated by the VE. In order to understand how VEs might be useful for rehabilitation it is important to be clear about what they are and how they are different from related technologies such as interactive computer graphics. What we discuss here are some aspects of human vision that have an important bearing on how users perceive the synthetic environment.

4.1.1 What Is a Virtual Environment?

Virtual environment displays [a.k.a, virtual reality (VR)] are interactive, computer graphics-based, head-referenced displays that create the illusion that their users are in a place other than where they physically are. This illusion is created through the operation of three types of equipment: (1) sensors, such as head-mounted position trackers that measure head position and orientation; (2) effectors, such as a stereoscopic display that presents visually realistic depth information; and

(3) special-purpose hardware to link the output of the sensors to inputs for the effectors so that they may produce sensory effects resembling those experienced by inhabitants of a physical environment (Ellis, 1994).

In a VE this linkage is accomplished by a simulation computer. In a head-mounted teleoperator display, a display closely related to a VE display, the linkage is accomplished by the robot manipulators, vehicles, control systems, sensors, and cameras at a remote work site. Both VE and telerobot-type displays may provide useful human machine interfaces for rehabilitation. The common important element that distinguishes them from normal computer graphics is that they are inherently multimodal. These displays do not just present visual information but also coordinate it with haptic, kinesthetic, auditory, or vestibular stimuli. This coordination is what provides the VE with its potentially great rehabilitative power, but it also makes the design of such interfaces more challenging since the sensory information being displayed must be not only of high fidelity but also correctly intercorrelated among the sensory modalities.

The definition of a virtual environment requires three distinct operations. First, the shape and kinematics of the actors and object need to be specified via a modeling program. Second, the modes and rules of interactions of all actors and objects need to be established for all possible interactions among them and with the environment itself. Third, the extent and character of the enveloping environment need to be specified. A number of different names have been used to describe virtual environment research. Some like the oxymoronic "virtual reality" originally suggested much higher performance than the then current technology could generally provide at the time. But progress in sensor and display technologies during the past 49 years since Sutherland's (Sutherland, 1965) introduction of the idea has now made many of the suggested applications of the technology practical, including especially some in rehabilitation medicine. Nevertheless, successful application still depends upon the detailed performance of the VE system with respect to the human user's physical, physiological, perceptual, and motor capabilities. This display technology works by developing a real-time, interactive, personal simulation (Foley, 1987) of the content, geometry, and dynamics of a work environment directly analogous to that used for traditional vehicle simulation (Cardullo, 1993; Rolfe & Staples, 1986) (Fig. 4.1). But unlike vehicle simulation, typical virtual environment simulation is unmediated. The users themselves are placed in an environment, not in a vehicle that is in an environment, and the hardware producing the simulation is usually worn rather than entered.

Since VEs are inherently multimodal with at least one nonvisual sense being paired with vision, curiosity naturally arises regarding the necessary performance requirements for the various sensory displays. Figure 4.1 gives a sense of the dimensions' ranges of fidelity that may need to be considered in the design and implementation. The denoted values in this figure are neither optimal nor minimal, but correspond to estimates for each value chosen by developers because they were adequate to support some practical work at the time the table was published (Ellis, 1994). This table provides a rough description of the characteristics underlying communication channels that connect user actions with either environmental response in teleoperation systems or simulated environmental response in virtual environment systems.

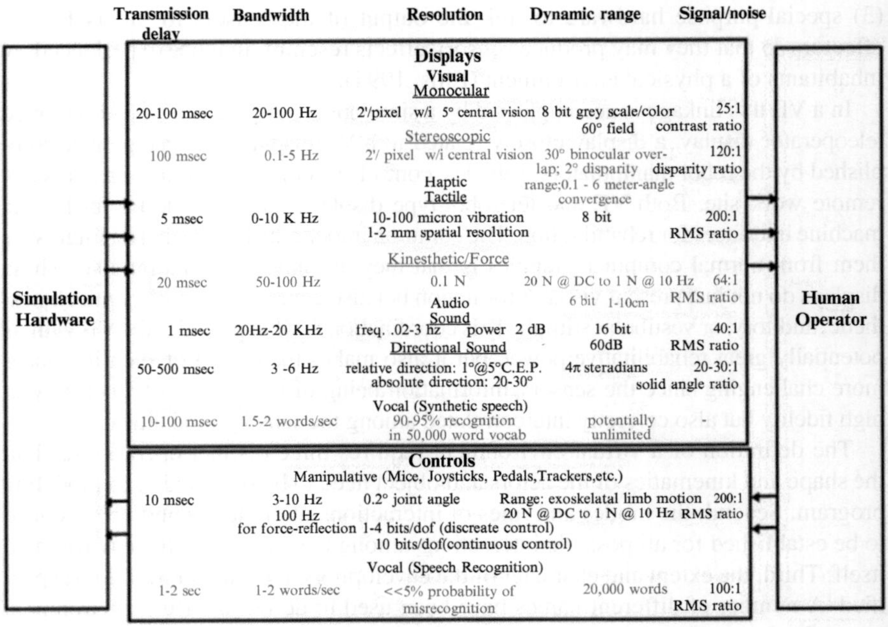

Fig. 4.1 Information flows within a virtual environment (VE)

VEs enjoy such a wide range of applications that providing a single description of perceptions and actions that occur in the VE as well as in the physical world is impossible. One must first understand how the actor will use the VE before specifying the visual requirements for a VE application or predicting what perceptions would be applicable to such a condition. Unfortunately, there is no universal solution to such a problem: "the devil is in the details." Therefore, to know if a VE is suitable for a rehabilitation situation you should first know what information you expect to convey to the actor through the interface. Then you can address the relevant perceptions that would be needed in the VE to be faithful to their counterpart in the physical world. Addressing the relevant perceptions and interactions would essentially provide an approach to populating a table like that included in Fig. 4.1 with values that would support a specific application. The nature and requirements of some of the sensory communication channels identified in this figure are considered in more detail below.

4.1.2 *Visual Acuity vs. Display Resolution*

One of the constraints to faithfully rendering real-world objects in a VE is the resolution of the display system. Ideally, to provide the human observer with the same environmental fidelity that he or she receives in physical world, VE displays should match the resolution of the human visual system (Febretti et al., 2013). The standard dot separation visual acuity of the human is 1 min of arc (30 cycles/deg) and is commonly referred to as 20/20 vision [Snellen Chart] (Colenbrander, 2013). Consequently, the visual angle of a pixel would need to match this 1 min of arc resolution. This can be a difficult challenge for many VE systems.

Display resolution can be calculated by dividing the number of pixels [horizontal or vertical] into the visual field of view [FOV] that those pixels span, i.e., deg/pixel of the display [see Cruz-Neira, Sandin, Defanti, Kenyon, and Hart (1992) for complete discussion]. Consequently, if the display resolution is fixed, then the deg/pixel can be manipulated by changing the viewer's distance from the display. Given a fixed number of pixels, the resolution of deg/pixel can be increased by reducing the FOV or decreased by increasing the FOV. In many applications the user strives to maximize both of these parameters in an effort to match both the resolution and FOV of the human visual system. This trade-off is one of the important limitations that VE users must face when designing their application in VE and is driven by the application at hand.

Display resolution in a VE is sometimes compared to that of the standard human visual acuity. However, we must be careful when linking display resolution to human visual resolution since contemporary pixels on displays are produced in sharp focus and a person with a normal visual acuity would see the pixels on the display in focus, not blurred. Acuity loss is due to the addition of Gaussian noise as a consequence of the undersampling of the image, thus interfering with some of the frequency content of the image (Crow, 1977; Shannon, 1949).

4.2 Stereovision Requirement and Implications

User interaction with proximal virtual objects is a chief attribute provided by most VE applications that can impact system performance. Most users require that the VE provide stereovision to work effectively with objects at close range. This one characteristic alone creates a series of constraints affecting the virtual environment (Kenyon, DeFanti, & Sandin, 1995). Stereovision requires that the user's current head position and orientation in the space be known to the image-generating software so that the correct perspective views for each eye can be presented (Cruz-Neira et al., 1992). Without such information the stereo presentation of the world appears distorted and moves incompatibly with what we consider real. Such unexpected distortions of the environment can interfere with the user's sense of "presence" or "suspension of disbelief" (Slater, Khanna, Mortensen, & Yu, 2009; Slater, Usoh, & Steed, 1994). This is a strong component that can change a user's performance in VE. In the past, rendering time and tracking latency were a powerful combination that could have adverse effects on performance. However, with the current state of high-end computers, the rendering time has diminished significantly to the point that usually the position tracker communication delay is the main constraint on presentation. But with the increase in computer power the complexity and sophistication of the generated images have also increased. The net result is that rendering times [update rate] have remained about the same but the image quality has gone up dramatically. It is also important to distinguish between rendering time [update rate] and system latency. System latency manifests itself as (1) a *transport* delay due to intrinsic delays in sensor and displays and (2) *communication* delays between the user and image generation and environmental simulation. Total system delay has been identified by Professor Frederick Brooks, Turing Award winner and pioneer in the field of VE, as one of the most important factors influencing performance and acceptance of virtual environment interfaces (Brooks, 1999). Fortunately, this problem can be managed to some extent through signal processing and interfacing techniques (Jung, Adelstein, & Ellis, 2000).

4.2.1 Stereovision and Its Limitations in the VE

The introduction of stereovision in a VE provides many advantages and some drawbacks. Clearly, adding stereo allows a more natural perception of near-object cues from the visual environment. Size, distance, location, and navigation to the objects become more familiar and less ambiguous to the user. However, there are system performance penalties to be paid. Two independent viewpoints must be presented to the user [right eye; left eye] for stereovision to be enabled. In most head-mounted displays (HMDs), each eye views a separate visual channel where the resolution and frame rate are fixed. Such systems show display characteristics that differ little from monoscopic to stereoscopic presentations. However, projection-based systems that need to show two independent viewpoints on the same screen can exhibit significant changes in display performance. To produce independent views, some projection-based systems use shutter glasses in conjunction with synchronized field sequential video to present the right and then the left eye information in the scene. Other systems use polarized stereo to present the stereo pair (Febretti et al., 2013). This has the effect of reducing vertical resolution by 50 %, e.g., from 1,024 horizontal lines to 512 lines. In addition, to prevent 30 Hz flickering of the stereo image that usually accompanies a single frame refresh rate of 60 Hz, the refresh rate must be increased to 120 Hz for a virtually flicker-free stereo rate of 60 Hz for the highest vertical resolution.

The quantizing of depth resulting from sampling the scene can adversely affect an observer's perceptions and can lead to an error in a viewer's depth perception of virtual objects (Hodges & Davis, 1993; Pfautz, 1996). For example, if a VE stereo display system has a resolution of 1280×1024 pixels, the effects of this limitation can be shown in a simplistic case where a point object is being displayed in a projection-based system such as a CAVE® (Fig. 4.2). If we make the size of the point object to be rendered less than a pixel, then to display this object in the VE projection-based system we have to light up two pixels (one for the left and one for the right eye) in order for a viewer to see the object in stereo. This condition, as shown in Fig. 4.2, can produce large depth intervals. This effect can be modulated in projection-based systems when viewers move away from a screen, thus reducing the size of the pixel's visual angle and thereby reducing the quantizing error. However, this is not an option for HMDs since the visual angle of the pixel is fixed. An additional type

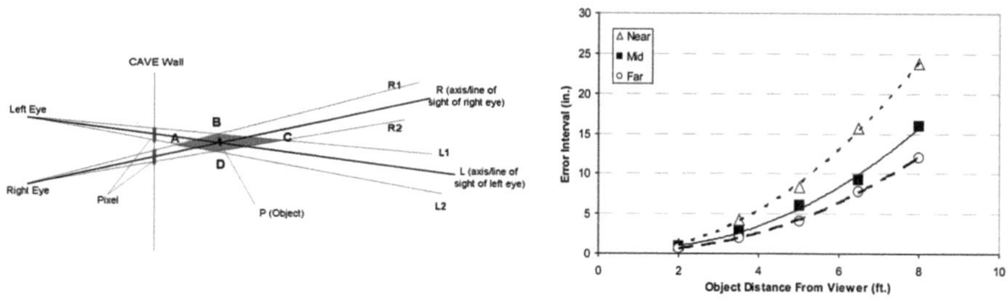

Fig. 4.2 Object P can be perceived at any depth between A and C before a pixel boundary is reached (*left*). The graph (*right*) shows the error interval for various viewer distances from the projection screen and object distances from the user. In a worst-case scenario (*right*) the depth error interval [A–C] can be as large as 23.79 in. (near = 4 ft; mid = 6 ft; far = 8 ft eye relief from a 1280 × 1024 projection screen) (Kenyon et al., 2007)

of depth error can be introduced during object motion in stereo display systems that use time multiplexing in which the displays of the left and right eye's view are relatively delayed with respect to each other (Hoffman, Karasev, & Banks, 2011).

4.2.2 *Viewer-Centered Perspective*

In most vehicle simulation environments, the operator's perspective view is fixed to the *heading of the vehicle* and not to the operator's direction of gaze. For example, in most flight simulators, the eye point used for the visual perspective, while located close to the expected location of the pilot's head, is fixed to the axis of the vehicle and not to the pilot's head direction. This situation results in only one correct viewing point for the rendering of the visual scene. Movements of the head and eyes to locations away from the direction of projection can result in a somewhat distorted stereo-perspective view for the actor. However, if the viewer located at the correct geometric eye point simply rotates about the eye point, there ideally should be no rendering distortions, i.e., the issue is translation. Also, with translation the motion parallax of the image, especially with respect to near physical objects such as frame of the window formed by the display, is not correct. There are also optical effects if there is a lens in front of the monitor to make virtual object appear at infinity [infinity optical system] (LaRussa & Gill, 1978). The problem is not essentially a heading problem, but a position problem. Stereovision exacerbates this perspective problem because of the apparent size changes when head movement is not tracked.

In the CAVE and other head-tracked virtual environments, the perspective view is generated using the direction of projection determined by the measured position and orientation of the *actor's head* (Hughes et al., 2013). As mention previously, without this feature the farther the user is from the true center of projection for each eye the more geometric distortion appears in the image of objects. The need to track the user's head and therefore the eyes, can add a great disadvantage to the performance of the system. This is because the generation of the images [update rate] in the past has been at the mercy of the head-tracking instrument's performance. When inefficiently interfaced to the graphics systems, head-tracking systems can add long, and in some cases unacceptable, delays between user motion and the resultant motion on the screen. Fortunately, efficient tracker interface techniques that can substantially reduce the full system display lags have been demonstrated (Ellis, Mania, Adelstein, & Hill, 2004; Jacoby, Adelstein, & Ellis, 1996). In addition to these delays, these systems are nonlinear near the edges of the tracker range. Nonlinear errors can distort the image so that objects appear to fly away from the observer as they are approached. To counteract these effects and make this environment useful for training physical world tasks, calibration of the tracker within the working space is needed (Ghazisaedy, Adamczyk, Sandin, Kenyon, & Defanti, 1995). This can add more complexity to these systems and more computations per image, though the costs of such correction can now be assigned to very fast graphics cards largely removing the problem. Though the perceived visual stability that low latency rendering can provide may not always be required for sensory–motor rehabilitation, it is worth noting that even very small rendering lags on the order of 10 ms can be detected by human users (Ellis et al., 2004) and that sensory–motor adaptation is impaired by visual–haptic delays (Held, Efstathiou, & Greene, 1966).

4.3 Oculomotor Interactions

The extrinsic eye muscles control the direction of gaze and therefore the area of the world that is seen by the visual system. However, this is only part of the story. The quality of the visual perception as we gaze from one object to the next is also a function of the synergy among three centers of the oculomotor system: pupil, accommodation, and vergence systems (see Semmlow (1981) for review). These three systems are collectively referred to as the near triad, and they are lumped together because they interact in such a way as to aid each in performing their function when we gaze at objects in the physical world (Donders & Moore, 1864; Hering, 1977; Maddox, 1886). However, when one moves into the virtual world, these synergistic systems can corrupt our vision of the objects and instead of aiding one another they can be pitted against each other.

4.3.1 Accommodation and Vergence

In the physical world we shift our gaze toward objects at different locations and distances from us without much notice of what occurs within the motor control portion of the visual system. As we move our gaze from object to object, our oculomotor system changes focus (accommodation) and direction of gaze for each eye (vergence and/or version) so that the object of interest remains clear and single.[1]

[1] There is also a link to the pupil system, but in most cases that effect is very small and is overshadowed by vergence and accommodation.

The coordinated or the synkinetic relationship between the human pupil system, accommodative system, and vergence eye movement system was reported by Johannes Muller (1826). He observed that if one eye were covered, and the viewing eye changed fixation from a far to a near target along its line of sight, the covered eye rotated inward. To be more specific, covering one eye removes the binocular stimulus to vergence [binocular disparity] so that any resulting vergence would be due to accommodation. A concomitant link from vergence to accommodation has also been found whereby changes in vergence will affect the level of accommodation (Fincham & Walton, 1957). In the physical world, these two linkages aid each system to keep objects clear and single; however, this is not always true in a VE.

In current VE systems, all virtual objects produce the same accommodative stimulus or demand to the eye regardless of their perceived distance from the user since the image is projected onto a screen that is either optically fixed, as in an HMD, or at a fixed location from the observer, in projection-based systems. This disconnect between accommodative demand and vergence demand can disrupt our perception due to the link between the elements of the near triad (Semmlow & Hung, 1983). When a subject looks at the VE scene projected onto the screen in front of them, the blur signal that drives accommodation is determined by the optics of the eye and the distance the subject's eye is from the projected object. For example, a virtual object is rendered to appear 2 ft from the eye but the wall upon which it is generated is 6 ft from the eye. In this example, the object's depth as measured by the disparity between the two eyes does not equal the accommodative demand (blur on the retina); therefore, the vergence and accommodative signals are not consistent. To further complicate this situation, for large discrepancies between these two systems, vergence would drive accommodation away from its demand point [the wall] or vice versa. This can result in the virtual object appearing either double and clear or single and blurred (Kenyon et al., 1995). However, in cases where all the objects are far from the eye (>2 m) there may be little concern for such discrepancies since the accommodative demand is about 0.5 diopters and that is close to the "resting" accommodation for humans (Hoffman, Girshick, Akeley, & Banks, 2008).

4.3.2 *Coexisting Physical and Virtual Objects*

One of the advantages that projection-based and augmented reality systems afford users is the ability to see both physical and virtual objects simultaneously. This permits the user to directly view his/her own body, limbs, and hands or those of another person in the environment. Consequently, we do not need to spend energy on modeling or rendering poor replicas of the real thing. This approach improves graphics performance and manual task performance (Kenyon & Afenya, 1995). The size and location of physical and virtual objects introduce the ability to interact with objects from both worlds making the environment a more powerful tool for prototyping and for realistic interactions with objects in the environment. But the synkinetic relationship can produce anomalies in the visual world when virtual and physical objects coexist (Banks, Akeley, Hoffman, & Girshick, 2008; Kenyon et al., 1995). For example, in projection-based systems, physical objects can occlude virtual objects but the reverse is not true.

HMD-based augmented reality (AR) display systems do not suffer from this problem since the image is projected a few millimeters in front of the viewer's eye. HMD AR systems have a different rendering distortion in that it is difficult to place a virtual object *behind* a physical object if they have common sight lines. The occlusion distance cue tends to make the virtual object appear in front of the physical one. But the specific interaction depends upon the particular viewing conditions and users' ability to focus which degrades with age (Ellis & Menges, 1998). In fact, in many systems of all types, conflict between accommodative and convergence stimuli furnished by adjacent physical and virtual objects within the work space can lead to eye strain and visibility problems within the environment (Wann, Rushton, & Mon-Williams, 1995). In some HMD systems, accommodative demand can be estimated and compensated for by changes in accommodative demand required by the HMD optics (Hoffman et al., 2008; Rolland, Krueger, & Goon, 2000).

In 3-D projection-based systems like the CAVE and for AR VE systems (Johnson et al., 2000), interactions with concurrent physical and virtual objects are a natural consequence of their design. However, the optical characteristics of the physical and virtual objects can be very different. A physical object a foot away from you produces convergence, accommodative, and stereo stimuli that are all in accord. Virtual objects can produce congruent convergence and stereo stimuli for an object a foot away, but the accommodative stimulus is determined by the optical system of the VE. Consequently, it is possible for vergence and accommodation to be in conflict with each other when physical and virtual objects exist simultaneously within a VE's working space. When you introduce a physical object near the location of a virtual object, and if there is a large difference in the stimulus to accommodation for each object, the visual result can be that one of the two objects becomes blurred and appear doubled. For example, while sitting in a real chair at a virtual table you pick up a virtual soda can on the table with your real hand, the virtual can's optical distance is at the screen while your hand is at arm's length. If you attended to the can, your hand could be out of focus and perhaps doubled while the can would be clear and single. If you now attended to your hand, the can would be blurred and doubled and the virtual can would be clear and single. This dual, forced-choice condition placed on the user when interacting with both physical and virtual objects may limit how we apply this technology and can also be associated with distance judgment errors (Ellis & Menges, 1998). Interestingly, with high contrast and high luminance displays this may be slightly compensated for by the increase in depth of focus due to contraction of the pupil of the eye.

Prospects for training users to differentially accommodate so that both objects can be seen clearly are not promising. However, many people can learn to see both near and far objects simultaneously in focus when one eye wears a distance correction and the other eye wears a near correction (monovision). Schor, Landsman, and Erickson (1987) have found that presbyopic contact lens patients with monocular corrections could see clearly at all distances by suppressing blur that occurs regionally between corresponding retinal areas. This intraocular suppression of blur over corresponding areas of the retina is believed to be the main mechanism for the successful use of monovision. Thus, a monocular corrective lens worn by the user might prove to be a solution to the anomaly produced by coexisting physical and virtual objects. Monovision has the unfortunate side effect, however, of a loss of stereopsis in most users.

4.4 Peripheral and Central Vision Influences on Perception

The interaction of visual and vestibular sensory information can profoundly affect our sense of motion within a VE. When the FOV is larger than 20°–40°, the peripheral visual field is activated and motion of objects in the ambient field produces vection, the illusion of self-motion, in the subject (Dichgans & Brandt, 1972; Dichgans, Held, Young, & Brandt, 1972; Hulk & Rempt, 1983). This effect has been utilized for a variety of situations from parlor entertainment to flight simulation. A human operator's performance with only a central FOV display can be dramatically improved if veridical motion cues are added or if the FOV is expanded to cover the peripheral retina (Kenyon & Kneller, 1993). The addition of physical motion stimulates the vestibular sensors that produce velocity or lead information that aids the operator during tracking (Shirley & Young, 1968). However, neurophysiological studies have found that visual motion on the peripheral retina can effect changes in the activity of cells that also carry vestibular motion information from the semicircular canals (Waespe & Henn, 1977). This observation suggests that presentation of images that extend into the far periphery provides the opportunity for the peripheral retina to utilize this velocity information in a manner similar to vestibularly sensed motion and, in turn, provide the human operator with information that can aid a user's acceptance of the virtual display as real (McGreevy, 1992) much as does a low system response latency (Brooks, 1999). A virtual environment with a restricted FOV may have reduced perceptual effects, but visual motion without concomitant physical motion can induce motion or simulator sickness (Kennedy, Hettinger, & Lilienthal, 1990).

4.4.1 Importance of Size Constancy for the Perception of Objects

When we use a VE system we presume that many of the important attributes afforded by the physical world will be available. However, that is not always the case unless the proper visual cues are generated in the VE. Environments lacking such information can lead to distorted perceptions of the virtual world. One of these important attributes is size constancy. Descartes (1637) first described the phenomenon known as "size constancy" where an object is perceived as being the same size regardless of its distance from the observer even though the retinal size of the object shrinks with increasing distance from the observer. The absence of size constancy can result in virtual objects being perceived as too large, too small, too close, too far away, or dynamically changing size as the viewing distance changes. These misperceptions greatly affect the utility of the virtual world in providing an environment in which to learn and to manipulate objects. Therefore, it is important for us to know what cues are needed for size constancy so that people's perceptions in the virtual world mimic those in the physical world. For example, in many reaching/grasping tasks used for upper body rehabilitation, knowing the size and distance to the virtual object is an important component for training so that they may open their hand enough to surround the object and attach it to their hand so that it can be manipulated (Connelly et al., 2010; Luo, Kenyon, Kline, Waldinger, & Kamper, 2005).

Many studies of the perceived size of objects in the physical world have been performed (see Sedgwick (1986) for review). Holway and Boring (1941) showed that removal of various visual cues would cause a reliance on the physical optics of the situation. They showed that as the number of cues to depth is reduced, performance suffers and subjects adopt a size judgment that is based on the visual size of the object on the retina also known as visual angle (VA) size judgments. Gilinsky (1951) quantified this phenomena for both optical and perceptual cases showing that size constancy can be affected by the conditions of the experiment and the instructions. Furthermore, Leibowitz and Dato (1966) showed that removing stereovision had little to no effect on performance; performance was only affected by the removal of monocular depth cues. Consequently, if there are very few contours and visible points, stereovision alone is remarkably ineffective at producing size constancy in the physical world.

Initially, size constancy was not demonstrated in the VE. A study by Eggleston, Janson, and Aldrich (1996) using a HMD found that their subjects relied on a visual angle approach in sizing objects. That is, instead of the perceived size of the object remaining the same regardless of its distance, the object size perceived by the subject shrank with increasing distance of the object from the subject. Baitch and Smith (2000) showed similar results for a single object that was approximately 15 in. from the subject using a CAVE (Cruz-Neira et al., 1992) system that provided stereovision but no head tracking or surrounding items in the environment to support the object's position in space. This may have been due to the characteristics and limitations of this synthetic environment. These results lead to a concern that some perceptions that appear readily in the physical world may not materialize in the virtual world. For example, a VE needs to have a very good dynamic response for motion parallax information to be useful for accurate hand localization of virtual targets (McCandless, Ellis, & Adelstein, 2000).

Using a CAVE system, Kenyon, Sandin, Smith, Pawlicki, and Defanti (2007) compared the effect of two different scenes on the perception of size constancy. One scene was a virtual environment (ENV) with a number of surrounding items accompanying a virtual textured coke bottle whose size could be manipulated (Fig. 4.3, left). The second scene (No-ENV) was of an environment where no surrounding items were provided and only the coke bottle was visible (Fig. 4.3, right). In both scenes they incorporated stereovision, perspective rendering, head-tracked projection centers, texture mapping, diffuse and specular lighting effects using a Gouraud shading algorithm (Gouraud, 1971), and hidden surface removal to visualize the objects in the scene.

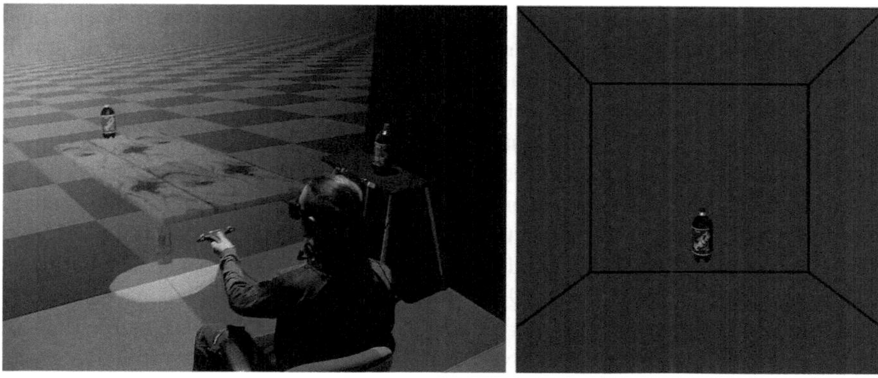

Fig. 4.3 Visual scenes for sizing bottles in the VE. The position and initial size of the bottle are randomly presented to the subject. (*Left*) Experimental setup for the ENV condition with the physical coke bottle to the right of the subject and the virtual scene. (*Right*) Visual scene for sizing bottles in the No-ENV task. Both the table and the floor are removed leaving only the grey background and the bottle for the subjects to perform this task. The *dark lines* in the figure represent the edges of the CAVE walls (Kenyon et al., 2007)

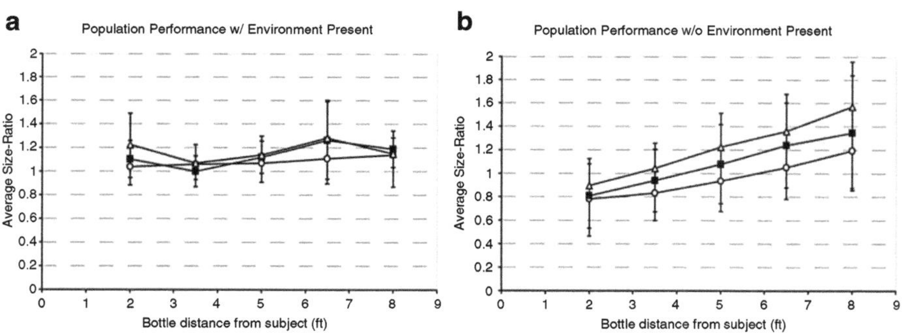

Fig. 4.4 (*Left*) Size ratio is plotted as a function of the position of the bottle from the subject. The size ratio values maintain a value that hovers about 1 for the different bottle positions from the subject indicating the approximate size constancy performance. (*Right*) The rise in the size ratio with increasing bottle distance indicates that subjects are relying more on visual angle than size constancy. Size ratio defined as perceived/true bottle size. Size constancy size ratio = 1 (Kenyon et al., 2007)

The ability of subjects to set the virtual bottle to the correct size (a size ratio of 1) was best in the condition where a number of objects accompanied and supported the position of the bottle (Fig. 4.4, left). Not only was performance consistent with that for size constancy, but also the task was easier to perform according to subject reports. In contrast, the mean size ratio for the No-ENV condition (Fig. 4.4, right) increased as the bottle position receded from the subject. The size ratio settings for this condition ranged between 0.4 and 1.6 for the bottle distance of 2–8 ft from the subject.

In 2 of the 12 subjects no size constancy was seen in the two environments, and 2 subjects showed size constancy in both environments. Therefore, while most will respond well to more cues to depth, not all subjects will be amenable to these cues. It is possible that the surrounding objects could have sizes that were knowable to the subject and they used these internal image size ratios to help estimate size changes of bottle. Further research is needed to substantiate this hypothesis.

In this study, stereovision was provided in each environment but did not seem to be sufficient for most of the subjects when surrounding objects were removed from the scene as in the No-ENV condition. This result in VE is consistent with that shown by Leibowitz and Dato (1966) (Fig. 4.5) where in the physical world stereovision alone is not a strong cue for size constancy. In addition, Combe, Posselt, and Kemeny (2008) using projection-based, HMD, and AR systems found, at most, a 5.5 % underestimation in size for their systems. As has been shown in both the VE and physical world, cues such as perspective, obstruction, relative size, and texture are all important for this percept (Gilinsky, 1951; Harvey & Leibowitz, 1967; Holaday, 1933; Koh & Charman, 1999). This has important implications for VE since the addition of stereovision is an expensive complication to the use of the system. Therefore, if people are within proximity of the rendered center of projection for the scene, the need for stereo cues to produce size constancy can be much reduced if not eliminated. In fact, stereovision may serve primarily as an image segregation function where overlapping objects are more easily identified due to their differing distances from the observer. This image segregation function is particularly evident in the Julesz random dot stereograms (Julesz, 1971). In fact, disparity may be explicitly used for declutter purposes in information displays (Julesz, 1971; Peterson, Axholt, & Ellis, 2009).

4.4.2 Effectiveness of Motion Parallax and Stereovision for Size Constancy

Given the apparently lesser role of stereovision in size constancy one might speculate whether another monocular cue to depth might have a more important influence in producing size constancy when viewing a non-stereo image. If such a cue existed, then perhaps the complexity of the image needed to generate size constancy could be reduced. One possible candidate is motion parallax. Motion parallax is the optical change of the visual field of an observer which results from a change in viewing position during head movements or locomotion (Gibson, 1950). Motion parallax, like stereovision, is primarily useful for image segregation and relative depth. Motion parallax is a monocular cue to depth that is often seen used in the animation of wire-frame objects to convey three-dimensional structures when displayed on a two-dimensional display. In addition, when a user feels unsure about an object's distance, he/she usually tries to look at the object from different perspectives by moving his/her own position. This introduces observer-generated motion parallax. Meanwhile,

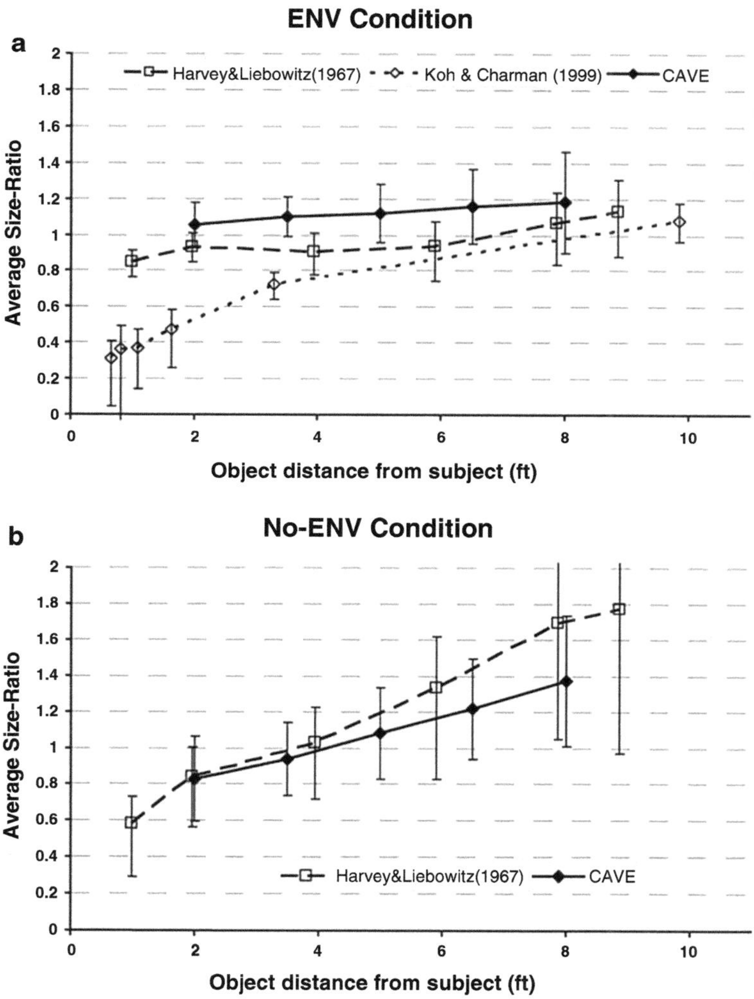

Fig. 4.5 (*Left*) Transformed data from Harvey and Leibowitz (1967) [*dashed line*] to our size-ratio format [*solid line*]. A close relationship is seen in their data and ours from the CAVE. Comparison of these data to Koh and Charman (1999) [*dotted line*] shows some agreement, but at close positions there is a large deviation from our data. (*Right*) Comparison of Harvey and Liebowitz [*dashed line*] to our No-ENV [*solid line*] data show good agreement in data (Kenyon et al., 2007)

it is not uncommon that the user will also manipulate the object itself to get a better observation, and VE-generated motion parallax is consequently produced. Given the propensity of 2D displays for VE systems it is important to understand whether motion parallax is a stronger cue than stereovision to support size constancy.

Huber, Stringer, Davies, and Field (2004) performed experiments under the applied contexts of minimal access surgery (MAS) tasks and studied the effects of stereoscopy and observer-produced motion parallax for distance judgment. Results indicated that stereoscopy confers a considerable performance advantage, while providing motion parallax information was not beneficial. Experiments by Beall, Loomis, Philbeck, and Fikes (1995), where subjects judged the size of objects whose visual dimension varied fourfold, concluded that absolute motion parallax only weakly determined the visual scale of nearby objects. Rondot, Lessard, and Robert (1995) studied distance perception during a teleoperation task. Their results suggested that stereoscopy and motion parallax were of equal significance in distance judgment, and users' performance varied largely between HMD and projected screen settings. Additional studies where motion parallax was a component showed inconsistent effects of motion parallax. Ikehara, Cole, and Merritt (1992) compared the results of different experimental methodologies for size–distance perception tests. They argued that for size and distance perception studies, point light sources and rods could produce different results, but the difference was not significant enough to change their conclusions.

Xun Luo, Kenyon, Kamper, Sandin, and DeFanti (2007), using similar visual conditions as Kenyon et al. (2007), studied size constancy when three different motion parallax conditions were applied: no motion parallax with head and scene still (No-MP), motion parallax generated by the VE with head still and the virtual scene moved 1 ft with a 4 ft/s peak velocity at 0.25 Hz (Passive-MP), and motion parallax generated by the lateral movement of the viewer with the same virtual scene movement (Active-MP). Size ratio settings for all three motion parallax settings overlapped in mean value and standard deviations. When scene texture was rich and stereovision was turned off, subjects' performance fell between the size constancy and visual angle conditions. Consequently, this research showed that motion parallax, produced by moving the virtual environment or by observer motion alone, is not a significant factor in determining size constancy performance.

These observations tended to suggest that observer-generated and VE-generated motion parallax, when grouped together, do have some effect on a subject's performance for size constancy, but these effects were reduced when the richness of the scene decreased. When the scene was poor, all three kinds of motion parallax would have no observable effect on the subjects' size constancy performance. Thus, both stereoscopic viewing and motion parallax help with the performance of manipulative interaction within a virtual environment but as cited earlier, for the effects of motion parallax to be fully manifest it must be presented with sufficiently low full system latency (McCandless et al., 1999, 2000).

These size constancy behaviors in a VE are similar to those in the physical world that have shown that a subject's performance lies on continuum between size constancy and visual angle and that this performance is a function of the cues that are present in the scene. In Fig. 4.6 we show where one might expect a subject's performance to lie given the cues presented. This figure shows that the dominant condition for size constancy is a feature-rich scene with stereovision. That is followed by a rich scene and monocular condition. Notice that under sparse visual conditions stereovision modestly improves performance compared to monocular viewing.

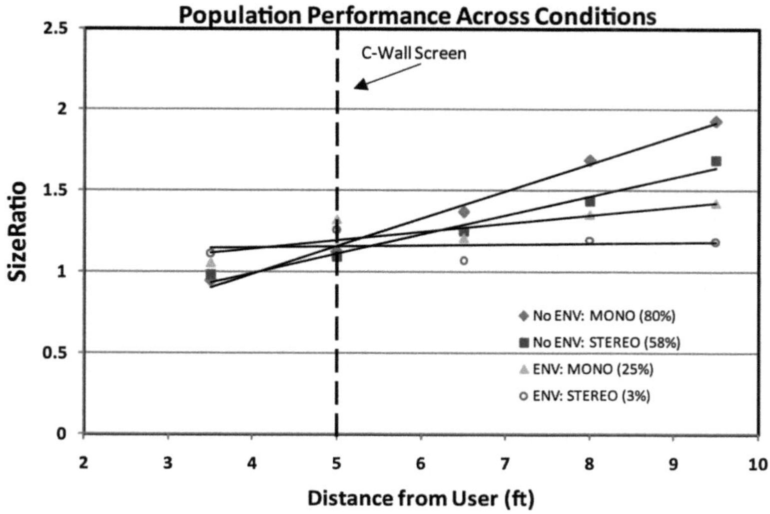

Fig. 4.6 Averaged fitted slopes for four combinations of scene complexity and stereovision conditions with their associated size ratios vs. user distance from the virtual object for each condition. C-wall refers to VE projection screen (Luo et al., 2007)

4.4.3 Role of Accommodation in Size Constancy

Other forces may be at work that inhibit size constancy in VE. Since there is a conflict between accommodation and vergence in most VE conditions, some have pointed to the fixed stimulus to accommodation as the factor that could adversely affect size constancy. In fact, accommodation has been suspected as a contributor to size illusions in virtual environments due to the lack of appropriate accommodative stimuli for the objects displayed. As we explained previously, the amount of accommodative demand for an object at the same distance in the virtual and physical worlds is not necessarily the same (Kenyon et al., 1995; Neveu, Blackmon, & Stark, 1998; Robinett & Rolland, 1992). Consequently, the CAVE and other forms of virtual environments can cause the user to endure conflicts between accommodation and vergence for objects in the scene or experience perceptual errors due to the lack of an appropriate relationship between accommodation and distances of the virtual objects (Peli, 1995; Rolland, Gibson, & Ariely, 1995; Wann et al., 1995). Because of this lack of synergy between the accommodation and other visual information, and accommodation's role in a person's estimate of distance to an object (Leibowitz & Moore, 1966), this mismatch could be an important factor in the lack of size constancy when many monocular cues are absent from the virtual scene but stereovision remains. However, initial experiments indicate that accommodation mismatch plays little or no role in the perception of size constancy. Kenyon, Phenany, Sandin, and Defanti (2008) opened the loop on accommodation using an artificial pinhole pupil resulting in a depth of focus that encompassed the projection screen and the virtual objects. Accordingly, accommodation would not be driven by the image on the wall nor the object close to the user since they are both in focus on the retina. Also, any changes in vergence that would affect accommodation through its synkinetic connection would not affect target blur. Their results showed that opening the loop on accommodation did not restore size constancy in the sparse image condition, as it would be expected to do if accommodation was influential in reducing size constancy.

Finally, in consideration of the impact of stereoscopic display and motion parallax on a user's interaction with a virtual environment, it is also important to distinguish perceptual impact from sensory–motor interaction. This contrast goes back to the old "two visual systems" discussion in which researchers contrasted the system that identified "what" was in the visual field from the one that identified "where" something might be (e.g., Bridgeman, Kirch, and Sperling (1981)). In this connection it is noteworthy that though stereoscopic vision or motion parallax might not have a major impact on perceptual aspects of VE, they can, when presented with sufficient dynamic fidelity, provide information for precise manipulative interaction with virtual objects through the mechanisms of disparity or motion parallax nulling, respectively, during a reaching movement (Ellis & Menges, 1998; McCandless, Ellis, & Adelstein, 1999).

4.5 Designing a VE for Rehabilitation Purposes

The design and implementation of VE imagery may seem straightforward, but like any visual design there is much art involved and this fact should not be underestimated. Many times researchers must team up with artists to satisfy the requirements of the rehabilitation goals. Production of useful computer-generated imagery usually requires the competence of someone who is comfortable in the use of sophisticated rendering software. However, some of the programing demands can be reduced through the use of script-based rendering systems or of a language with high-level functionality ("The Alice Project", 2013; "Unity Technologies Inc.", 2013). This trend to simplify environment design and avatar actions continues due to the demand for VE systems in rehabilitation and many other areas of application. Thus, future rendering systems will probably further unburden the developer's reliance on specialized computer graphics programing to produce the environments that they require.

The technology in this area is moving so rapidly that in-depth discussion of current use of VE for rehabilitation would be outdated in a short time. However, the principles we have addressed here can prove instructive. A good example of an abundant use of monocular cues to depth and stereopsis is seen in Fig. 4.7 (Tsoupikova, Stoykov, Kamper, & Vick, 2012; Tsoupikova et al., 2013). For this rehabilitation visual scene the researchers have placed many redundant cues to depth that aid the user in judging the location, distance, and size of the objects

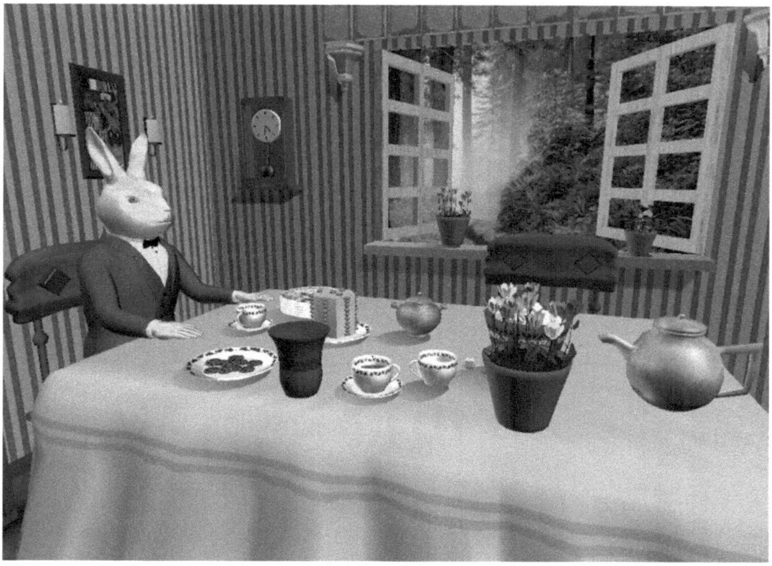

Fig. 4.7 The March Hare from "Alice in Wonderland" rendered as an avatar therapist guides the patient through the moves and acquisition of objects to fulfil the training prescription for this rehabilitation. The user is able to interact with a number of objects shown in the table (Tsoupikova et al., 2013)

presented to the actor. The choice of environment is also important since cartoonlike environments are more acceptable to the user than are poorly designed realistic scenes; see for example, "The Uncanny Valley" (Mori, 1970). Inadequate real scenes lack realistic behaviors of physical properties of the scene such as reflections, object movements, and interactions to name only a few (Seyama & Nagayama, 2007; Wages, Grünvogel, & Grützmacher, 2004). However, obviously fictitious scenes can more effectively draw the user into the scene or the story (Manning, 1998; McCloud, 1994). In the scene shown in Fig. 4.7 we have a cartoon environment for the actors to perform their tasks. In addition, the scene is drawn with shadows and lighting, all of which confirm the physics of the situation. Both the strong monocular cues and stereo cues work together to provide the user with information that will aid them in performing their rehabilitation task.

The need for various cues in the environment is driven by the rehabilitation task to be performed. Some patients undergoing rehabilitation may also have perceptual difficulties as a result of their injury. The distortions that appear in VEs may be exaggerated in these users and make them more susceptible to anomalies that otherwise would not be significant to others. In one sense, making the environment a close rendition of the physical world may be needed for some cases of using VE in rehabilitation. Alternatively, cues that cause such anomalies may need to be reduced or removed from the environment to make it more useful for training.

Acknowledgements The Electronic Visualization Laboratory (EVL) at the University of Illinois at Chicago specializes in the design and development of high-resolution visualization and virtual reality display systems, collaboration software for use on multi-gigabit networks, and advanced networking infrastructure. These projects are made possible by major funding from the National Science Foundation (NSF) awards CNS-0115809, CNS-0224306, CNS-0420477, SCI-9980480, SCI-0229642, SCI-9730202, SCI-0123399, ANI-0129527, and EAR-0218918 as well as the NSF Information Technology Research (ITR) cooperative agreement (SCI-0225642) to the University of California San Diego (UCSD) for "The OptIPuter" and the NSF Partnerships for Advanced Computational Infrastructure (PACI) cooperative agreement (SCI-9619019) to the National Computational Science Alliance. EVL also receives funding from the State of Illinois, General Motors Research, the Office of Naval Research on behalf of the Technology Research, Education, and Commercialization Center (TRECC), and Pacific Interface Inc. on behalf of NTT Optical Network Systems Laboratory in Japan.

References

Baitch, L., & Smith, R. C. (2000). *Physiological correlates of spatial perceptual discordance in a virtual environment.* Paper presented at the Proceedings Fourth International Projection Technology Workshop, Ames, Iowa.

Banks, M. S., Akeley, K., Hoffman, D. M., & Girshick, A. R. (2008). Consequences of incorrect focus cues in stereo displays. *Journal of the Society for Information Display, 24*(7), 7.

Beall, A. C., Loomis, J. M., Philbeck, J. W., & Fikes, T. G. (1995). *Absolute motion parallax weakly determines visual scale in real and virtual environments.* Paper presented at the Proc. SPIE.

Bridgeman, B., Kirch, M., & Sperling, A. (1981). Segregation of cognitive and motor aspects of visual function using induced motion. *Perception & Psychophysics, 29*(4), 336–342.

Brooks, F. P. (1999). What's real about virtual reality? *IEEE Computer Graphics and Applications, 19*(6), 16–27.

Cardullo, F. (1993). *Flight simulation update 1993*. Binghamton, NY: Watson School of Continuing Education.

Colenbrander, A. (2013). Measuring vision and vision loss. In W. Tasman & E. A. Jaeger (Eds.), *Duane's ophthalmology* (Vol. 5). Philadelphia, PA: Lippincott Williams & Wilkins.

Combe, E., Posselt, J., & Kemeny, A. (2008). *1: 1 Scale perception in virtual and augmented reality.* Paper presented at the 18th International Conference on Artificial Reality and Telexistence.

Connelly, L., Jia, Y., Toro, M. L., Stoykov, M. E., Kenyon, R. V., & Kamper, D. G. (2010). A pneumatic glove and immersive virtual reality environment for hand rehabilitative training after stroke. *IEEE Transactions on Neural Systems and Rehabilitation Engineering, 18*(5), 551–559.

Crow, F. C. (1977). The aliasing problem in computer-generated shaded images. *Communications of the ACM, 20*(11), 799–805.

Cruz-Neira, C., Sandin, D., Defanti, T., Kenyon, R., & Hart, J. (1992). The CAVE audio-visual environment. *ACM Transactions on Graphics, 35*, 65–72.

Dean, C. M., & Shepherd, R. B. (1997). Task-related training improves performance of seated reaching tasks after stroke a randomized controlled trial. *Stroke, 28*(4), 722–728.

Descartes, R. (1637). *La Dioptrique, discours VI: De la vision* (Vol. 1). Cambridge, England: Cambridge University Press. 1985.

Dichgans, J., & Brandt, T. (1972). Visual-vestibular interaction and motion perception. *Bibliotheca Ophthalmologica, 82*, 327–338.

Dichgans, J., Held, R., Young, L. R., & Brandt, T. (1972). Moving visual scenes influence the apparent direction of gravity. *Science, 178*(4066), 1217–1219.

Donders, F. C., & Moore, W. D. (1864). *On the anomalies of accommodation and refraction of the eye: With a preliminary essay on physiological dioptrics* (Vol. 22). London: The New Sydenham Society.

Eggleston, R. G., Janson, W. P., & Aldrich, K. A. (1996). *Virtual reality system effects on size-distance judgements in a virtual environment.* Paper presented at the Virtual Reality Annual International Symposium, 1996, Proceedings of the IEEE 1996.

Ellis, S. R. (1994). What are virtual environments? *IEEE Computer Graphics and Applications, 14*(1), 17–22.

Ellis S. R., Mania, K, Adelstein, B. D., & Hill, M. (2004). Generalizeability of latency detection in a variety of virtual environments. *Proceedings of the Human Factors and Ergonomics Society* pp. 1836–1841.

Ellis, S. R., & Menges, B. M. (1998). Localization of virtual objects in the near visual field. *Human Factors, 40*(3), 415–431.

Febretti, A., Nishimoto, A., Thigpen, T., Talandis, J., Long, L., Pirtle, J., et al. (2013). *CAVE2: A hybrid reality environment for immersive simulation and information analysis.* Paper presented at the Proceedings of IS&T/SPIE Electronic Imaging, San Francisco, CA.

Fincham, E. F., & Walton, J. (1957). The reciprocal actions of accommodation and convergence. *The Journal of Physiology, 137*(3), 488–508.

Foley, J. D. (1987). Interfaces for advanced computing. *Scientific American, 257*(4), 126–135.

Ghazisaedy, M., Adamczyk, D., Sandin, D., Kenyon, R., & Defanti, T. (1995, March 11–15). *Ultrasonic calibration of a magnetic tracker in a virtual reality space.* Paper presented at the Proceedings of the IEEE Annual Virtual Reality International Symposium (VRAIS), Raleigh, NC.

Gibson, J. J. (1950). *The perception of the visual world.* Boston, MA: Houghton Mifflin.

Gilinsky, A. S. (1951). Perceived size and distance in visual space. *Psychological Review, 58*(6), 460–482.

Gouraud, H. (1971). Continuous shading of curved surfaces. *IEEE Transactions on Computers, 100*(6), 623–629.

Hanlon, R. E. (1996). Motor learning following unilateral stroke. *Archives of Physical Medicine and Rehabilitation, 77*(8), 811–815.

Harvey, L. O., Jr., & Leibowitz, H. W. (1967). Effects of exposure duration, cue reduction, and temporary monocularity on size matching at short distances. *Journal of the Optical Society of America, 57*(2), 249–253.

Held, R., Efstathiou, A., & Greene, M. (1966). Adaptation to displaced and delayed visual feedback from the hand. *Journal of Experimental Psychology, 72*(6), 887.

Hering, E. (1977). *The theory of binocular vision* (B. Bridgeman & L. Stark, Eds.). New York, NY: Springer.

Hodges, L. H., & Davis, E. T. (1993). Geometric considerations for stereoscopic virtual environments. *Presence, 2*, 34–43.

Hoffman, D. M., Girshick, A. R., Akeley, K., & Banks, M. S. (2008). Vergence-accommodation conflicts hinder visual performance and cause visual fatigue. *Journal of Vision, 8*(3), 33. doi:10.1167/8.3.33.

Hoffman, D. M., Karasev, V. I., & Banks, M. S. (2011). Temporal presentation protocols in stereoscopic displays: Flicker visibility, perceived motion, and perceived depth. *Journal of the Society for Information Display, 19*(3), 271–297. doi:10.1889/JSID19.3.271.

Holaday, B. E. (1933). Die Grössenkonstanz der Sehdinge bei Variation der inneren und äusseren Wahrnehmungsbedingungen. *Archive für die gesamte Psychologie, 88*, 419–486.

Holway, A. H., & Boring, E. G. (1941). Determinants of apparent visual size with distance variant. *The American Journal of Psychology, 54*(1), 21–37.

Huber, J. W., Stringer, N. S., Davies, I. R., & Field, D. (2004). *Only stereo information improves performance in surgical tasks.* Paper presented at the Medical Imaging 2004.

Hughes, J., Van Dam, A., McGuire, M., Sklar, D., Foley, J., Feiner, S., et al. (2013). *Computer graphics: Principal and practice* (3rd ed.). Reading, MA: Addison Wesley.

Hulk, J., & Rempt, F. (1983). Vertical optokinetic sensations by limited stimulation of the peripheral field of vision. *Ophthalmologica, 186*(2), 97–103.

Ikehara, C. S., Cole, R. E., & Merritt, J. O. (1992). Effects of test structure on depth perception measurement tasks. *Proc. SPIE Stereoscopic Displays and Applications III, 1669*

Jacoby, R. H., Adelstein, B. D., & Ellis, S. R. (1996). *Improved temporal response in virtual environments through system hardware and software reorganization.* Paper presented at the Electronic Imaging: Science & Technology.
Jarus, T., & Gutman, T. (2001). Effects of cognitive processes and task complexity on acquisition, retention, and transfer of motor skills. *Canadian Journal of Occupational Therapy, 68*(5), 280–289.
Johnson, A., Sandin, D., Dawe, G., DeFanti, T., Pape, D., Qiu, Z., et al. (2000). *Developing the Paris: Using the cave to prototype a new VR display.* Paper presented at the Proceedings of IPT 2000: Immersive Projection Technology Workshop.
Julesz, B. (1971). *Foundations of cyclopean perception.* Chicago, IL: University of Chicago Press.
Jung, J. Y., Adelstein, B. D., & Ellis, S. R. (2000). *Discriminability of prediction artifacts in a time-delayed virtual environment.* Paper presented at the Proceedings of the Human Factors and Ergonomics Society Annual Meeting.
Kennedy, R. S., Hettinger, L. J., & Lilienthal, M. G. (1990). Simulator sickness. In G. H. Crampton (Ed.), *Motion and space sickness* (pp. 317–341). Boca Raton, FL: CRC Press.
Kenyon, R. V., & Afenya, M. B. (1995). Training in virtual and real environments. *Annals of Biomedical Engineering, 23*(4), 445–455.
Kenyon, R. V., DeFanti, T. A., & Sandin, D. J. (1995). Visual requirements for virtual environment generation. *Journal of the Society for Information Display, 3*, 211–214.
Kenyon, R., & Kneller, E. (1993). The Effects of Field-of-View Size on the Control of Roll Motion. *IEEE Trans. Systems, Man and Cybern, 23*, 183–193.
Kenyon, R. V., Phenany, M., Sandin, D., & Defanti, T. (2008). Accommodation and size-constancy of virtual objects. *Annals of Biomedical Engineering, 36*(2), 342–348. doi:10.1007/s10439-007-9414-7.
Kenyon, R. V., Sandin, D., Smith, R., Pawlicki, R., & Defanti, T. (2007). Size-constancy in the CAVE. *Presence, 16*(2), 172–187.
Koh, L. H., & Charman, W. N. (1999). Size constancy and angular size matching in size perception of near objects. *Optometry and Vision Science, 76*(4), 241–246.
LaRussa, J. A., & Gill, A. T. (1978). The holographic Pancake Window™. In L. Beiser (Ed.), *Proceedings of the Society of Photo-Optical Instrumentation Engineers.* Volume 162. Visual Simulation & Image Realism (pp. 120–129). Bellingham, WA: Society of Photo-Optical Instrumentation Engineers.
Leibowitz, H. W., & Dato, R. A. (1966). Visual size-constancy as a function of distance for temporarily and permanently monocular observers. *The American Journal of Psychology, 79*(2), 279–284.
Leibowitz, H., & Moore, D. (1966). The role of changes in accommodation and convergence in the perception of size. *Journal of the Optical Society of America, 56*, 1120–1123.
Luo, X., Kenyon, R., Kamper, D., Sandin, D., & DeFanti, T. (2007). *The effects of scene complexity, stereovision, and motion parallax on size constancy in a virtual environment.* Paper presented at the Virtual Reality Conference, 2007, VR'07, IEEE.
Luo, X., Kenyon, R. V., Kline, T., Waldinger, H. C., & Kamper, D. G. (2005, June 28–July 1). *An augmented reality training environment for post-stroke finger extension rehabilitation.* Paper presented at the IEEE 9th International Conference on Rehabilitation Robotics (ICORR), Chicago, IL, USA.
Maddox, E. E. (1886). Investigations in the relation between convergence and accommodation of the eyes. *Journal of Anatomy and Physiology, 20*(Pt 3), 475.
Manning, A. D. (1998). Understanding comics: The invisible art. *IEEE Transactions on Professional Communication, 41*(1), 66–69. doi:10.1109/TPC.1998.661632.
McCandless, J. W., Ellis, S. R., & Adelstein, B. D. (1999). *The effect of accommodative demand, motion parallax and age on virtual object localizations.* Paper presented at the Proceedings of the Human Factors and Ergonomics Society Annual Meeting.
McCandless, J. W., Ellis, S. R., & Adelstein, B. D. (2000). Localization of a time-delayed, monocular virtual object superimposed on a real environment. *Presence (Camb), 9*(1), 15–24.

McCloud, S. (1994). *Understanding comics*. New York, NY: HarperCollins.
McGreevy, M. W. (1992). The presence of field geologists in Mars-like terrain. *Presence, 1*(4), 375–403.
Mori, M. (1970). The uncanny valley (K. F. MacDorman & T. Minato, Tans). *Energy, 7*(4), 33–35.
Muller, J. (1826). *Elements of physiology* (W. Baly, Trans. Vol. 2). London: Taylor & Walton.
Neveu, C., Blackmon, T., & Stark, L. (1998). Evaluation of the effects of a head-mounted display on ocular accommodation. *Presence, 7*(3), 278–289.
Nudo, R. J. (1999). Recovery after damage to motor cortical areas. *Current Opinion in Neurobiology, 9*(6), 740–747.
Nudo, R., & Friel, K. (1998). Cortical plasticity after stroke: Implications for rehabilitation. *Revue Neurologique, 155*(9), 713–717.
Patton, J. L., Dawe, G., Scharver, C., Muss-Ivaldi, F. A., & Kenyon, R. (2004, September). *Robotics and virtual reality: A perfect marriage for motor control research and rehabilitation.* Paper presented at the IEEE Engineering in Medicine and Biology Society Conference (EMBC), San Francisco, CA, USA.
Peli, E. (1995). Real vision and virtual reality. *Optics & Photonics News, 6*, 28–34.
Peterson, S. D., Axholt, M., & Ellis, S. R. (2009). Objective and subjective assessment of stereoscopically separated labels in augmented reality. *Computers & Graphics, 33*(1), 23–33. doi:10.1016/j.cag.2008.11.006.
Pfautz, J. D. (1996). *Distortion of depth perception in a virtual environment application.* (Ph.D.), Massachusetts Institute of Technology, Cambridge.
Robinett, W., & Rolland, J. P. (1992). A computational model for the stereoscopic optics of a head-mounted display. *Presence, 1*(1), 45–62.
Rolfe, J. M., & Staples, K. J. (1986). *Flight simulation*. London: Cambridge University Press.
Rolland, J. P., Gibson, W., & Ariely, D. (1995). Towards quantifying depth and size perception in virtual environments. *Presence, 4*(1), 24–29.
Rolland, J. P., Krueger, M. W., & Goon, A. (2000). Multifocal planes head-mounted displays. *Applied Optics, 39*(19), 3209–3215.
Rondot, P., Lessard, J., & Robert, J.-M. (1995). *Study of motion parallax in depth perception with a helmet-mounted display system used in teleoperation.* Paper presented at the Photonics East'95.
Schor, C., Landsman, L., & Erickson, P. (1987). Ocular dominance and the interocular suppression of blur in monovision. *American Journal of Optometry and Physiological Optics, 64*(10), 723–730.
Sedgwick, H. (1986). Space perception. In K. R. Boff, L. Kaufman, & J. P. Thomas (Eds.), *Handbook of perception and human performance* (Vol. 1, pp. 21–1 – 21–57). New York, NY: Wiley.
Semmlow, J. L. (1981). Oculomotor response to near stimuli: The near triad. In B. Zuber (Ed.), *Models of oculomotor behavior and control* (1st ed., pp. 162–191). Boca Raton, FL: CRC Press.
Semmlow, J., & Hung, G. (1983). The near response: Theories of control. In C. Schor & K. Ciuffreda (Eds.), *Vergence eye movements: Basic and clinical aspects* (pp. 175–195). Boston, MA: Butterworths.
Seyama, J. I., & Nagayama, R. S. (2007). The uncanny valley: Effect of realism on the impression of artificial human faces. *Presence, 16*(4), 337–351. doi:10.1162/pres.16.4.337.
Shannon, C. E. (1949). Communication in the presence of noise. *Proceedings of the IRE, 37*(1), 10–21.
Shirley, R. S., & Young, L. R. (1968). Motion cues in man-vehicle control effects of roll-motion cues on human operator's behavior in compensatory systems with disturbance inputs. *Man-Machine Systems, IEEE Transactions, 9*(4), 121–128.
Slater, M., Khanna, P., Mortensen, J., & Yu, I. (2009). Visual realism enhances realistic response in an immersive virtual environment. *IEEE Computer Graphics and Applications, 29*(3), 76–84. doi:10.1109/mcg.2009.55.

Slater, M., Usoh, M., & Steed, A. (1994). Depth of presence in virtual environments. *Presence, 3*(2), 130–144.
Sutherland, I. E. (1965). The ultimate computer display. *International Federation of Information Processing, 2*, 506.
Taub, E., Uswatte, G., & Pidikiti, R. (1999). Constraint-induced movement therapy: A new family of techniques with broad application to physical rehabilitation—A clinical review. *Journal of Rehabilitation Research and Development, 36*(3), 237–251.
The Alice Project. (2013). From http://www.alice.org/
Tsoupikova, D., Stoykov, N., Kamper, D., & Vick, R. (2012). Virtual reality environment assisting post stroke hand rehabilitation: Case report. *Studies in Health Technology and Informatics, 184*, 458–464.
Tsoupikova, D., Stoykov, N., Vick, R., Li, Y., Kamper, D., & Listenberger, M. (2013). *Use of virtual reality to promote hand therapy post-stroke.* Paper presented at the IS&T/SPIE Electronic Imaging.
Unity Technologies Inc. (2013). From http://unity3d.com/unity/
Waespe, W., & Henn, V. (1977). Neuronal activity in the vestibular nuclei of the alert monkey during vestibular and optokinetic stimulation. *Experimental Brain Research, 27*(5), 523–538.
Wages, R., Grünvogel, S. M., & Grützmacher, B. (2004). How realistic is realism? Considerations on the aesthetics of computer games. In M. Rauterberg (Ed.), *Entertainment computing–ICEC 2004* (pp. 216–225). Heidelberg: Springer.
Wann, J. P., Rushton, S., & Mon-Williams, M. (1995). Natural problems for stereoscopic depth perception in virtual environments. *Vision Research, 35*(19), 2731–2736.

Chapter 5
Sensorimotor Recalibration in Virtual Environments

W. Geoffrey Wright, Sarah H. Creem-Regehr, William H. Warren, Eric R. Anson, John Jeka, and Emily A. Keshner

Objective To present a range of expert annotated overviews on topics related to using VR technology to reveal the sensorimotor integration process and to help in the understanding of how sensorimotor integration occurs to support motor planning and performance.

W.G. Wright
Departments of Physical Therapy and Biomedical Engineering,
Temple University, Philadelphia, PA 19130, USA
e-mail: wrightw@temple.edu

S.H. Creem-Regehr
Department of Psychology, University of Utah,
380 S. 1530 E., Room 502, Salt Lake City, UT 84112, USA
e-mail: sarah.creem@psych.utah.edu

W.H. Warren
Department of Cognitive, Linguistic, and Psychological Sciences, Brown University,
Box 1821, Providence, RI 02912, USA
e-mail: bill_warren@brown.edu

E.R. Anson
Department of Kinesiology, University of Maryland, College Park,
MD 20742, USA
e-mail: eanson1@umd.edu

J. Jeka
Department of Kinesiology, Temple University, 1800 N Broad St,
Philadelphia, PA 19122, USA
e-mail: jjeka@temple.edu

E.A. Keshner (✉)
Department of Physical Therapy and Department of Electrical and Computer Engineering,
Temple University, 3307 N. Broad ST, Philadelphia, PA 19140, USA
e-mail: ekeshner@temple.edu

P.L. (Tamar) Weiss et al. (eds.), *Virtual Reality for Physical and Motor Rehabilitation*, Virtual Reality Technologies for Health and Clinical Applications,
DOI 10.1007/978-1-4939-0968-1_5, © Springer Science+Business Media New York 2014

5.1 Sensory Feedback Can Fool You

If we don't see and touch an object, is it real? In the allegory of the cave (on which the acronym CAVE was based), Plato describes prisoners chained in a cave, unable to turn their heads. All they can see is the wall of the cave. Behind them burns a fire. Such prisoners would mistake appearance for reality. They would think the objects they see on the wall (the shadows) were real; they would know nothing of the real causes of the shadows. Such it is with back projection virtual reality. What we see are projected images, not real objects, yet we still respond with physical actions that are appropriate to the images we perceive. The unique characteristic of the virtual environment that propels us to respond is the overwhelming influence of vision. The coupling of the visual and motor system plays a critical role in the vast repertoire of healthy, adaptive motor behavior. In fact, visual perception and plans for action are so intimately connected that they could reflect a single cerebral function (Trevarthan, 1968).

It is not clear how the CNS processes multiple sensory signals to organize response behaviors. Studies of self-motion perception go back at least as far as Ernst Mach's (1875) investigations into these phenomena, and reports of vection and inversion illusions date to at least the nineteenth century (Wood, 1895). Although the contemporary technology for testing the interaction of visual and vestibular senses was much more limited than today, they were able to discern that there must be a sense organ specifically capable of detecting inertial forces and that visual input alone was capable of inducing a sense of self-motion. When there is some unexpected visual situation, such as a tilting room, a mismatch between signals produces a sensory conflict where we cannot distinguish between visual field motion and motion of the body (Dichgans, Held, Young, & Brandt, 1972; Lackner & DiZio, 1988). For instance, if you have even been sitting in a train and sensed your train pulling out of the station, only to realize that it's the train next to you that is pulling away, while yours remained stationary, then you experienced illusory self-motion. Whether it's a conscious recognition or an unconscious resolution of the sensory conflict, the absence of the acceleration or vibration that would normally coincide with actual movement may be what causes this illusion of self-motion to dissipate so quickly.

Resolving ambiguity between motion of objects in the world and motion of oneself is not a simple switch between inputs but reflects the interdependence between multisensory delays and thresholds (Lambrey & Berthoz, 2003). A growing body of evidence suggests that even nonvisual and non-vestibular aspects of VE immersion, such as audition and cognition, play an important role in self-motion perception (Riecke, 2009; Wright, DiZio, & Lackner, 2006). In this chapter, five experts from the fields of postural and locomotor control present the work they have engaged in to understand how the brain uses multiple pathways of sensory feedback to organize movement behavior. Each will discuss how virtual reality may help us understand or engage the mechanisms underlying sensorimotor integration.

5.2 Perception of Self-Motion and Motor Responses During Visual–Vestibular Discordance (W. Geoffrey Wright)

The focus of our research over the last few years has been the investigation into how visual and inertial motion detection interacts to induce a sense of self-motion, and how this subsequently affects perceptual and motor processing. One term that deserves elaboration here because of its complementary role relative to visual input is "inertial motion detection." This refers to sensory processing involved in the detection of self-movement that is sensitive to acceleration (e.g., vestibular, mechanoreceptors, visceral fluid shift). When we use the more common term "vestibular," such as when referring to "visual–vestibular conflict," we acknowledge that this only refers to a part of the process of inertial motion detection. Disentangling vestibular and somatosensory contributions to self-motion detection is an area of great interest, especially for clinical applications. However, it is important to recognize that the vestibular representation starts off as head-centered, while the rest of the inertial detectors require a whole-body representation. Additionally, both the head-centered vestibular and the head-centered visual representations must eventually be represented in body coordinates in order to effectively interact with the environment. One way to avoid a visual–vestibular conflict is to simply design VEs that only move at constant velocity and never turn. However, this makes for an uninteresting virtual experience, and more importantly limits ecological validity. Therefore, in order to investigate how the brain resolves sensory and/or motor discordance, we must put the sensory inputs in conflict. Using sinusoidal stimulation is how we have typically approached this in our research.

The visual–vestibular discordance has been systematically adjusted by passively moving the subjects in a pattern that either matches the visual input or does not (Wright, DiZio, & Lackner, 2005; Wright et al., 2006; Wright, Schneider, & Glasauer, 2009). The frequency of oscillation in many of our studies was 0.1–0.5 Hz, which was selected in order to keep the visual, vestibular, and somatosensory stimuli within the dynamic range of all three systems, with none dominating (Angelaki, 1998; Xerri, Borel, Barthelemy, & Lacour, 1988). This too is important when employing dynamic VE, because high-frequency visual motion is by itself unlikely to induce high-frequency self-motion; however, when added to low-frequency visual motion, it can enhance low-frequency or steady-state self-motion perception (Palmisano, Gillam, & Blackburn, 2000).

In one study we combined visual and vestibular stimulation, and seated individuals wearing a head-mounted display (HMD) were exposed to various combinations of 0.2 Hz vertical linear oscillation and visual scene motion (Wright et al., 2005). In conditions in which subjects were only exposed to visually depicted motion while actually sitting stationary (Fig. 5.1a, b), we found that even low amplitude vertical visual oscillation induced the perception of vertical self-oscillation. The reported self-motion was closely entrained with the spatial and temporal properties of the

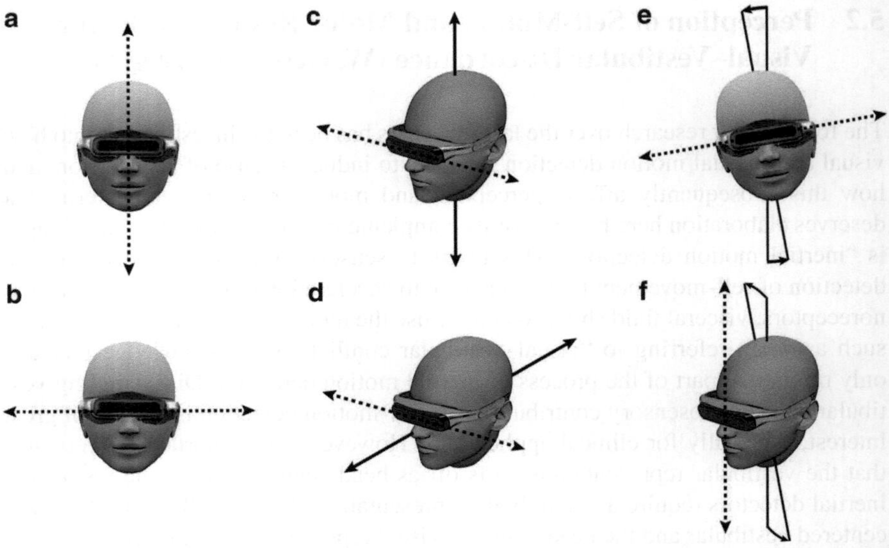

Fig. 5.1 Linear sinusoidal VE motion viewed in HMD (*dotted lines*) while subject sat stationary or was exposed to passive physical motion (*solid lines*). (**a**) VE scene depicting low-frequency (~0.2 Hz) vertical linear motion while subject sat stationary. (**b**) Horizontal visual oscillation viewed by stationary subject. (**c**) Low-frequency horizontal visual oscillation combined with vertical oscillation of subject. (**d**) Low-frequency horizontal visual oscillation combined with horizontal linear oscillation of subject along naso-occipital axis. (**e**) Low-frequency horizontal visual oscillation combined with actual roll-tilt of subject about the naso-occipital axis. (**f**) Low-frequency vertical visual oscillation combined with actual roll-tilt of subject about the naso-occipital axis

visual stimulus despite the visual–vestibular conflict occurring because of the sinusoidal visual acceleration. In conditions, when the visual input stimulation was also combined with some phase-locked sinusoidal vestibular stimulation, self-motion perception increased significantly. This occurred regardless of whether the amplitude of physical oscillation matched the visual amplitude or not. If the visual and vestibular were phase-shifted relative to what is experienced in the real world (i.e., 180° phase shift), then the sensory input that dominated the self-motion perception depended on the relative amplitudes of the visual and vestibular stimulation. However, it is notable that the highest amplitudes of visual scene motion were almost completely dominant even if the actual motion platform oscillation was equal in magnitude but 180° out-of-phase from normal (Wright et al., 2005). If the subject was asked to view a horizontally oscillating VE scene while being exposed to phase-matched vertical linear oscillation (Fig. 5.1c), then the largest component of self-motion was horizontal. Perhaps even more interesting was that as the amplitude of real vertical acceleration increased (i.e., the motion platform amplitude was increased), the conviction that the direction of perceived self-motion was *horizontal* increased significantly as well (Wright, 2009). These findings together show that when viewing a VE that depicts an accurate representation of the physical test environment, the visual input tends to dominate over vestibular input in determining one's perceived spatial position relative to external space. However, even in the presence of increasing sensory conflict, spatial mapping of inertial inputs may be completely labile, while amplitude coding of the input intensifies the perceived self-motion, independent of direction.

In other studies designed to assess how perceived self-orientation and self-motion combine to affect one's manual motor behavior, seated individuals wearing an HMD viewed either horizontal or vertical sinusoidal linear translation (±1 m at 0.25 Hz) while sitting in a motion apparatus capable of roll-tilting (Wright & Glasauer, 2003; Wright & Glasauer, 2006; Wright et al., 2009; Wright & Schneider, 2009). In one study (Wright & Schneider, 2009), unbeknownst to the subject, the motion apparatus remained stationary at all times (Fig. 5.1b). The subjects' task was to align a handheld object to perceived vertical using their unconstrained arm. The kinematics of the hand and handheld object showed automatic, unconscious translation of the arm in the direction and phase of the visually depicted motion. For subjects that perceived compelling self-motion, the motor responses were significantly greater. In a series of other studies that combined actual roll-tilt about the subject's naso-occipital axis with visually depicted linear translation (Wright & Glasauer, 2003, 2006; Wright et al., 2009), we were able to induce a much more compelling sense of self-motion that followed the visual motion, despite the fact that the subject only tilted and did not actually translate (Fig. 5.1e, f). In these conditions, the magnitude of the arm's motor response was commensurately larger and entrained with the direction of perceived self-motion and orientation. The effect of constant velocity virtual visual rotation on reaching trajectory had been previously shown (Cohn, DiZio, & Lackner, 2000), but our studies revealed that even during visual–vestibular conflict, an integrated representation of self-motion and associated gravitoinertial forces could be formed and used to guide motor behavior. Together these studies show that automatic upper extremity manual responses which are controlled by descending cortical, reticulo-, and vestibulospinal tracts can be affected by immersion in a dynamically moving VE, much like automatic postural behavior can be (Keshner & Kenyon, 2000).

The distinction between motor responses of upper extremity distal appendages and axial musculature is important. Axial (and proximal) musculature, which is integral to postural control and head stabilization, has bilateral descending innervation, whereas arms and legs have a much greater proportion of descending tracts involved in unilateral, independent volitional control. Therefore, we hypothesized that head control may differ from upper extremity control in how it is affected by visual–vestibular conflict. To investigate this further, we use dynamic VR visual stimulation in combination with passive sinusoidal linear motion to test head stabilization under these conditions (Wright, Agah, Darvish, & Keshner, 2013). Healthy subjects were seated in a linear sled capable of horizontally accelerating the subject along the naso-occipital axis (anterior–posterior—A/P). The subjects wore a very lightweight HMD (<0.5 kg) while being exposed to a range of sinusoidal frequencies (0.1–1.1 Hz) and amplitudes (0.02–1.5 m) both visually and inertially (i.e., physically). The direction of linear visual motion within the VE either matched the direction of the sled motion or did not, while the moments of peak speed of the visual and physical inputs were synchronized. The results of this stimulation were that head kinematics showed a complex interaction dependent on weighting of visual and physical inputs that changed with the sled driving frequency. The most striking findings relevant to visual–vestibular conflict occurred when subjects viewed a horizontally oscillating visual scene, while exposed to physical A/P oscillation (i.e., sled motion—Fig. 5.1d). The head response showed a yaw response that was absent when viewing A/P visual motion. Moreover, if the visual scene was close-up (i.e., near depth of field and spatially dense) then the effect was greater. From these findings we surmised that visual flow could organize lateral cervical responses despite being discordant with inertial input. Thus, at least some similarity with upper extremity motor control during visual–vestibular conflict exists, in that unintended, involuntary or reflexive motor responses can occur in a VE, which may not be present in traditional training environments.

5.2.1 Using Visual–Vestibular Discordance to Adapt Postural Behavior

Our latest research focuses on how to use visual–vestibular discordance to induce a motor effect that does not disappear as soon as the conflicting sensory stimulation is removed. Our interest is driven largely by the current thrust to show how motor rehabilitation in a VE can be retained once an individual returns to the real world. The first step in this process is determining whether the phasic effects can adapt over time in a VE. We approached this problem by measuring aftereffects following an extended period of exposure to discordant visual–vestibular stimulation. The type of stimulation we used, called cross-axis adaptation (Trillenberg, Shelhamer, Roberts, & Zee, 2003; Wei & Angelaki, 2001), involved linear visual stimulation along one axis (e.g., sinusoidal A/P visual translation), while also being exposed to sinusoidal linear translation of the support surface along an orthogonal axis (e.g., mediolateral—M/L).

Pilot data was collected to test whether cross-axis adaptation of discordant sensorimotor conditions could be induced in whole-body postural tasks. Subjects ($n=7$) were asked to stand on a moveable platform with force plates (Neurocom, Clackamas, OR) placed within a three-walled virtual CAVE (VEPO laboratory). Center-of-pressure (COP) measurements were collected and compared across conditions. The VE was a graphically rendered, realistic visual scene that included three-dimensional depth information (e.g., texture gradient, occlusion, and foreshortening), orientation cues, and dynamic parallax during motion.

The experiments followed a standard adaptation protocol: baseline, adaptation, and post-adaptation (which is a repeat of the baseline condition to measure aftereffects). During baseline measurements standing subjects viewed the VE scene as it was linearly oscillated sinusoidally at 0.2 Hz at an amplitude equivalent to 3 m in the A/P direction. This type of visual stimulus has been shown to induce postural

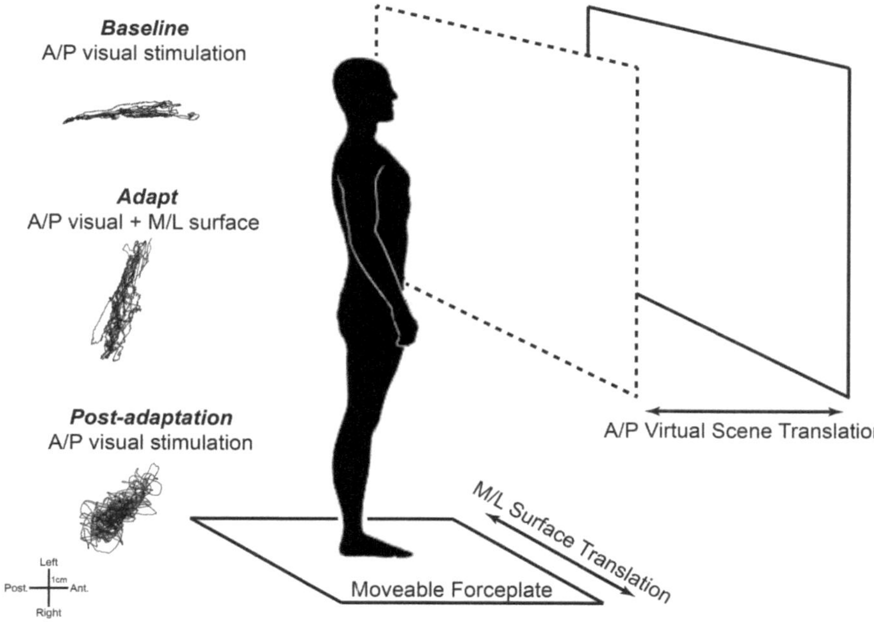

Fig. 5.2 Cross-axis stimulation during whole-body postural task. Subject views A/P sinusoidal visual translation during baseline (*upper COP trace*), combined A/P visual motion with M/L sinusoidal surface translation (*middle trace*), and again only A/P sinusoidal visual translation during post-adaptation (*bottom trace*). The aftereffect of postural adaptation to the cross-axis stimulation during adaptation persists in the post-adaptation phase

entrainment (Lishman & Lee, 1973). To reduce postural stability in the A/P direction and induce automatic postural compensations, the surface was also COP sway-referenced in the A/P tilt direction. This manipulation was intended to increase weighting of the visual and vestibular channels and reduce reliance on somatosensory input (Peterka, 2002). During 5 min of adaptation, subjects concurrently viewed the same A/P oscillating VE scene while the support surface sinusoidally translated 20 cm along the M/L axis at a frequency and phase matched to that of the VE scene. The post-adaptation phase was a repeat of the baseline condition, which allowed for a comparison of pre- and post-adaptation to determine if adaptation to the combined cross-axis stimuli had occurred.

The results revealed that the amplitude of M/L COP motion in baseline compared to the post-adaption condition showed a significant increase in M/L COP movement in the post-adaptation phase ($p<0.05$). A power spectral density analysis showed there to be a significant increase ($p<0.01$) at the 0.2 Hz frequency of M/L COP. In many cases, the axis of COP sway was ~45° between the A/P and M/L axes, even though subjects were viewing only A/P optic flow during the post-adaptation phase (Fig. 5.2). This aftereffect decayed quickly, but in some cases was still present for many minutes after the cross-axis stimulation had been removed.

These results suggest that prolonged cross-axis stimulation induces a sensorimotor recalibration causing motor responses that the postural system assumes will help maintain stability. In other words, much like the adaptations using prism glasses (Hardt, Held, & Steinbach, 1971; Held & Freedman, 1963; Morton & Bastian, 2004; Stratton, 1896), immersion in a VE can cause sensorimotor adaptations that are retained even after discordant sensory stimuli are removed.

5.3 Perceptual-Motor Recalibration: What Have We Learned from Virtual Reality? (Sarah H. Creem-Regehr)

Almost 20 years ago, Rieser, Pick, Ashmead, and Garing (1995) demonstrated that locomotion is calibrated to our perceptual experiences, and furthermore, that locomotion recalibrates to changing environmental circumstances. Using a clever "real world" paradigm involving a treadmill placed on a trailer pulled by a tractor, they decoupled the normal relationship between visual and biomechanical information for self-motion. A participant could walk on the treadmill and be pulled at a rate slower or faster than they were walking, allowing for visual flow to be mismatched to their speed of walking. These studies showed us that given a brief experience with a new relationship between perceptual and motor information for self-motion, actors will then change the way they dynamically update space—they recalibrate their walking as informed by the newly learned perceptual-motor relationship. A pre/posttest paradigm was used. Actors first performed a visually directed walking task, in which they viewed a target on the ground, closed their eyes, and walked to the location of the target. This task, known as *blind walking*, is proposed to recruit dynamic spatial updating, keeping track of one's own changing spatial position with respect to the environment. Numerous studies have shown that people are very good at this task, relying on a continuously updated representation of space, tied to their own action through the space even without visual feedback (Loomis, Da Silva, Fujita, & Fukusima, 1992; Rieser, Ashmead, Taylor, & Youngquist, 1990). After the pretest, individuals participated in an adaptation phase, in which they experienced faster or slower visual flow relative to their walking speed on the treadmill-trailer apparatus. A posttest followed, similar to the pretest. The results showed that posttest walking changed as a function of the adaptation condition. After experiencing a visually faster condition, participants would then stop short of the target in the posttest. Likewise, after a visually slower condition, participants would overshoot the target.

Our laboratory and others have further pursued perceptual-motor calibration of locomotion in numerous virtual environment settings and designs (see Chap. 8). It is important to ask, what more can virtual environments tell us about the integration of perceptual and motor systems beyond Rieser and colleagues' elegant study? I consider there to be two types of contributions of virtual reality to the study of perceptual-motor relationships. The first is the use of VEs as a *methodology* to address theoretical questions that cannot be easily addressed in the real world.

The second is the use of VEs for their *applied outcome* that can inform future use of technology for important applications such as architectural design, education, and rehabilitation.

Several projects in our laboratory replicated and expanded on the early recalibration results with virtual environments (VEs) with both theoretical and applied goals in mind. We found that perceptual-motor recalibration occurs using VE adaptation methods for walking, turning, and wheelchair locomotion (Kuhl, Creem-Regehr, & Thompson, 2008; Kunz, Creem-Regehr, & Thompson, 2013; Mohler, Creem-Regehr, & Thompson, 2006; Mohler et al., 2007). We have used two different virtual environment technologies. The first is the Sarcos Treadport (Hollerbach, Xu, Christensen, & Jacobsen, 2000), a custom built treadmill-based virtual environment (VE) comprised of a $6' \times 10'$ walking surface, coupled to computer graphics presented on three $8' \times 8'$ projection screens, oriented to provide an approximately 180° field of view. The bottom of the screens is even with the walking surface. The display used did not support stereo. Translational position of viewpoint is based on sensed body position. In Mohler et al. (2007) we used the Treadport initially for both applied and basic research questions. First, we asked whether a learned perception-action coupling presented on the treadmill-VE would be similar to effects seen in the real world, investigating whether walking in the real world could be altered by a mismatch between visual flow and biomechanical walking speed. Participants walked without vision to previously viewed targets on the floor of a real world hallway in pre- and posttest. During the adaptation period, they walked on the Treadport for 10 min while viewing a graphical "endless hallway," a high-quality graphics model of a real world hallway. In a *visually slower* condition, the visual speed was 0.5× the walking speed; in a *visually same* condition the visual speed was matched to the walking speed; and in a *visually faster* condition, the visual speed was 2× the walking speed. The results replicated Rieser et al. (1995), showing an overshoot in blind walking to targets in the visually slower condition, a slight overshoot in the visually same condition, and an underestimation in distance walked in the visually faster condition (see Fig. 5.3 for a schematic of the results). These findings support the claim that adaptation in a virtual environment can transfer to real world locomotion. The results are consistent with the explanation that actors will spatially update their representation of the environment as a function of the learned relationship between sensory and motor information for self-motion.

Second, we addressed an open question of whether recalibration effects are caused by a change in the magnitude of optic flow alone, or also by a change in perceived self-motion. Unlike our previous studies using a realistic hallway model, a more stylized hallway display was used in order for viewers to see a rendering of a smaller hallway moving at a slower visual speed and a larger hallway moving at a faster visual speed, but with the same average magnitude of optic flow. This is a good example of using VEs as a methodology to create an experience that could not be accomplished with real world manipulations. Using the same paradigm, participants showed similar recalibration of locomotion as in the previous study, providing evidence that perception of self-motion (informed by visual cues outside of the magnitude and distribution of optic flow) can change perceptual-motor calibration.

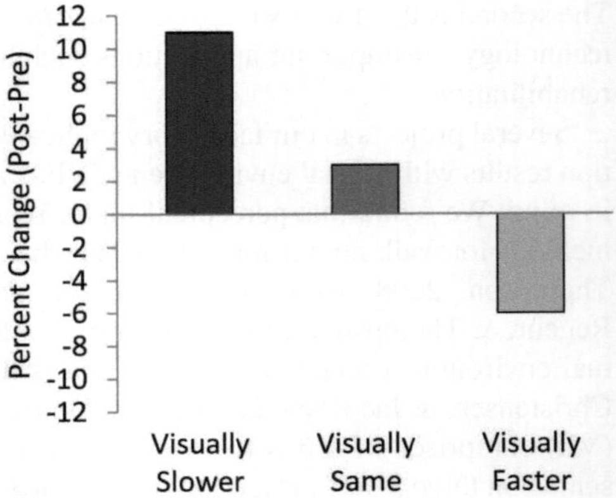

Fig. 5.3 Results adapted from Mohler et al. (2007), Experiment 1, showing recalibration effects as percent change in walking distance in the real world after treadmill-VE adaptation

More recently, we used the Treadport to examine another theoretical question about the use of motor simulation in imagined locomotion (Kunz, Creem-Regehr, & Thompson, 2009). While there has been a body of evidence from behavioral and functional neuroimaging methods suggesting that imagined and executed actions share similar underlying mechanisms, these claims have typically focused on arm and hand movements (e.g., reaching, grasping). Locomotion is a particularly interesting example of imagined movement because it involves both simulated full-body movement and the concurrent updating of environmental spatial information. We reasoned that if imagined locomotion relies on the same perceptual-motor mechanisms as real locomotion, we should find similar recalibration effects for an imagined walking task. This would provide further support that imagined walking is supported by motor simulation processes. Using a similar pre/posttest paradigm, we asked participants to view targets on the ground in the real world, but instead of actual walking, they were asked to imagine walking to the target and to indicate when they had reached it by starting and stopping a handheld timer. We used a design including visually faster (2×) and visually slower (0.5×) adaptation phases while participants walked on the treadmill at 1.3 m/s, with pre- and posttest imagined walking. The results showed that imagined walking was recalibrated similarly to real locomotion, supporting shared motor mechanisms for real and imagined walking. Posttest imagined walking time increased in the visually slower condition and decreased in the visually faster condition, compared to pretest (see Fig. 5.4).

In more recent and current work, our laboratory uses head-mounted display virtual environments (HMD-VE) to examine space perception and related perceptual-motor recalibration questions (Fig. 5.5). Participants view the VE using an NVIS nVisor SX HMD with an approximately 42°×32° field of view. There is 100 % stereo overlap between the two eyes. HMD optical pincushion distortion is corrected using a GPU shader program without introducing additional latency (Kuhl, Thompson, & Creem-Regehr, 2009). Three degree-of-freedom positional tracking is done optically using a Worldviz PPT-H camera-based tracking system (presently

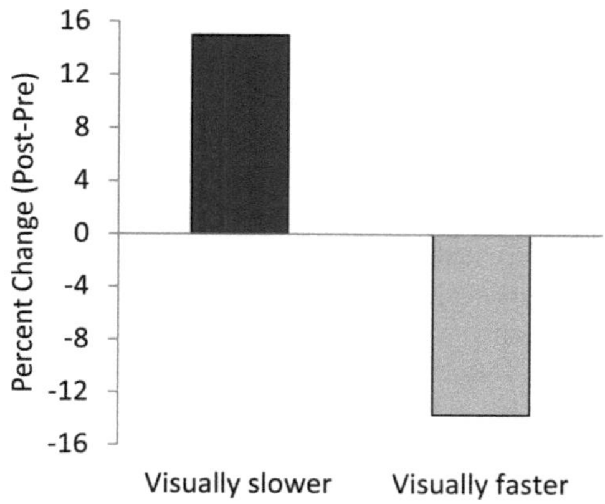

Fig. 5.4 Results adapted from Kunz, Creem-Regehr, & Thompson, (2009) showing the percent change for imagined walking time as a function of the visually slower and visually faster conditions

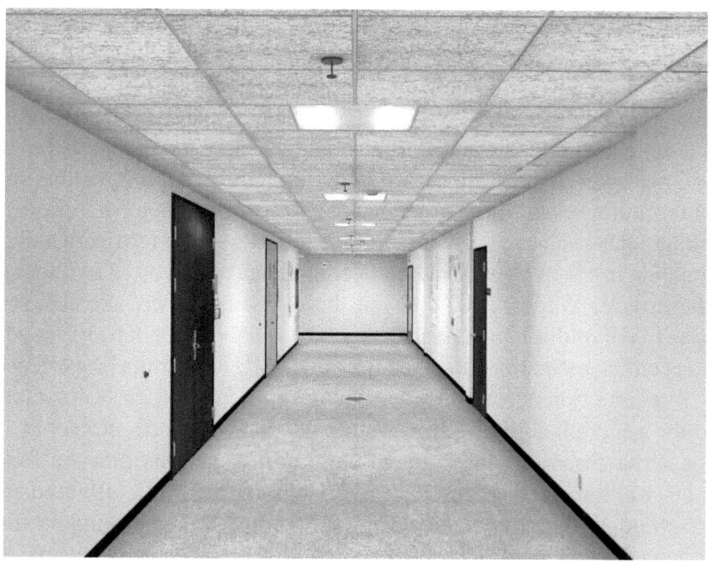

Fig. 5.5 Virtual hallway viewed through the HMD (from Kunz et al., 2013)

eight cameras), and three degree-of-freedom orientation is done with a combination of optical tracking for yaw using the PPT-H system and accelerometers for pitch and roll using an Intersense IC3 orientation sensor.

One of the consistent findings in our laboratory over past decade is an underestimation of distance found in the HMD-VE compared to the real world. Using multiple response measures, we have found that viewers perceive and act as if distances are shorter than they are intended to be. A body of work has aimed to try to understand this systematic distance compression effect by examining factors inherent to the technology (Chap. 6)—such as stereo viewing, reduced field of view, and the mechanics of the head-mounted display (Creem-Regehr, Willemsen, Gooch, & Thompson, 2005; Willemsen, Colton, Creem-Regehr, & Thompson, 2009), the influence of pictorial cues—such as those corresponding with the quality of graphics (Kunz, Wouters, Smith, Thompson, & Creem-Regehr, 2009; Thompson et al., 2004), and the response measures used to indicate perception—such as walking, throwing, and verbal reports (Geuss, Stefanucci, Creem-Regehr, & Thompson, 2012; Kunz, Wouters et al., 2009, Sahm, Creem-Regehr, Thompson, & Willemsen, 2005). Several years ago, we explored whether different types of feedback within the HMD-VE would influence distance estimations. In Mohler et al. (2006), we found more evidence for perceptual-motor recalibration, this time with only a "matched" VE condition. Using a pre/posttest paradigm all within the HMD, we found that an adaptation period that involved eyes open walking through a virtual hallway influenced later blind walking accuracy within the HMD. In other words, several minutes of walking within the immersive VE led to an increase in distance walked in a blind walking task, eliminating most of the compression effect seen in other studies.

In addition to perceptual-motor recalibration, Mohler et al. (2006) suggest that there are other mechanisms influencing VE distance judgments given feedback from eyes open walking. In this work, we found that the feedback also made verbal reports of distance more accurate, a somewhat surprising finding given that verbal reports of distance do not involve dynamic spatial updating. One possibility is that in addition to perceptual-motor recalibration, feedback leads to a cognitive correction applied to distance judgments such as a corrective rule (e.g., "targets are farther than they appear so I must adjust my walk/report"). This account is also supported by other laboratories (Richardson & Waller, 2007). Given these findings, there are still some open questions as to the multiple mechanisms by which people adapt to VE experience.

In one recent investigation, we used the HMD-VE to examine the effects of recalibration of locomotion across different locomotion modalities. Kunz et al. (2013) examined the generalizability of locomotion adaptation effects. Rieser et al. (1995) argued for a functional organization of calibration—actions that are functionally equivalent to walking to targets (such as side-stepping) were recalibrated after adaptation to forward walking on the treadmill. Blind throwing and blind rotations were not influenced by the recalibration of locomotion. However, others have demonstrated that recalibration may be limb-specific or that the transfer of adaptation effects from walking to side-stepping or crawling is weak.

We explored this question of generalizability in two ways. First, we established that the effects seen in walking extended to wheelchair locomotion. Participants who were normal walkers (and who had little experience with using wheelchairs) performed pre- and posttest blind wheelchair locomotion to previously viewed targets on the ground in the real world. The adaptation in the HMD-VE involved wheelchair locomotion within a virtual hallway with visual flow presented at 0.5× (visually slower) or 2× (visually faster) actual speed of wheeling. As in previous studies, we found a strong recalibration effect, showing overestimation in distance wheeled after the visually slower condition and an underestimation in distance wheeled after the visually faster condition (see Fig. 5.6). Second, we asked whether

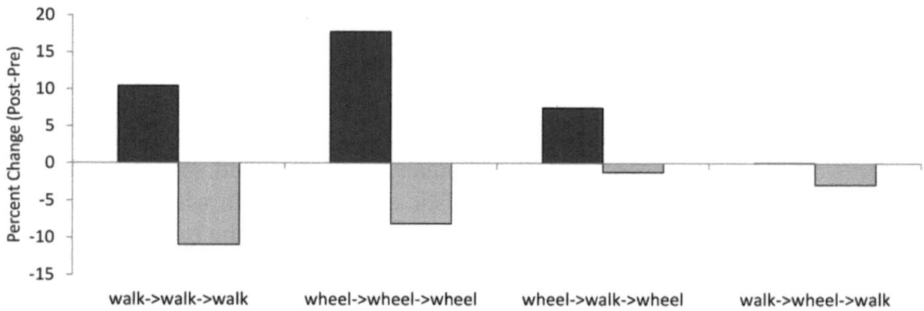

Fig. 5.6 Results adapted from Kunz et al. (2013) showing recalibration effects for four locomotion conditions: from *left* to *right*, walking pre/posttest with walking adaptation, wheelchair pre/posttest with wheelchair adaptation, wheelchair pre/posttest with walking adaptation, and walking locomotion pre/posttest with wheelchair adaptation

adaptation in one locomotion modality (walking or wheeling) would transfer to the other modality. This design addressed the question of whether perceptual-motor calibration is functionally or biomechanically defined. Participants performed wheeling in the pre/posttest, but walking in the adaptation period, or the reverse. As Fig. 5.6 shows, the effects for recalibration from walking to wheeling were smaller than in the matched modalities. However, there was no evidence for a recalibration effect from wheeling to walking. Taken together, this study and our earlier work show that dynamic spatial orientation is influenced by the learned relationship between perceptual and motor information for self-motion. This generalizes to locomotion modalities that are less experienced, as seen in wheelchair locomotion, but only strongly when the adaptation and response modalities match.

In summary, our work on perceptual-motor recalibration in virtual environments suggests that people adapt their actions to changing environment circumstances, similar to the real world. From an applications viewpoint, there are clear advantages to this. Viewers within virtual environments will quickly learn to adjust their actions to feedback so that they may act more accurately. Given evidence that spatial layout and scale in VEs is not always perceived as intended, the ability to calibrate one's actions over short time frames is likely important for use of VEs in applications where absolute scale matters. Perceptual-motor calibration mechanisms may also work to facilitate or rehabilitate actions that may be impaired because of injury or other causes. At the same time, the evidence that perceptual-motor calibration transfers from the VE into the real world could have some negative implications as well. Consider an application where a VE is used for training of a real world space. If individuals calibrate their actions to the VE, there is the possibility of error or biases in performance when back in the real world. Understanding the mechanisms underlying the change in behavior seen after feedback in VEs may help to identify circumstances when VE training might be most helpful. Furthermore, from a theoretical viewpoint, the recalibration paradigm that we have used has helped to answer several related questions about the processes underlying dynamic spatial orientation and action representations.

5.4 Studying the Control of Locomotion in Ambulatory Virtual Reality (William H. Warren)

Research in the Virtual Environment Navigation Lab (VENLab) at Brown University focuses on the multisensory control of human locomotion and spatial navigation. The purpose of the lab is to create naturalistic environments in which visual information can be manipulated during ongoing locomotion, and the resulting behavior measured. Ambulatory VR allows us not only to manipulate environmental objects with ease, but also to test theories of perceptual-motor control by breaking the laws of physics and optics. To that end, participants in the VENLab walk freely in an open 12×15 m area while wearing a head-mounted display (HMD). Head position is recorded with a hybrid ultrasonic/inertial tracking system (60 Hz) and used to update the stereoscopic HMD (63° H × 55° V, 1280×1024 pixels, 60 Hz) with a latency of 50 ms. Interactive virtual worlds are generated on a graphics PC and transmitted to the display using HD-TV technology, so the HMD is completely wireless. In addition, a 16-camera motion capture system is available to record gait kinematics or drive virtual avatars.

A primary project in the lab is the development of a *pedestrian model*, a dynamical model that characterizes human locomotor behavior. Based on experiments in the VENLab, each elementary behavior—such as steering to a goal—is modeled as a dynamical system, with attractors and repellers that determine the path of locomotion (Fajen & Warren, 2003). For example, to steer to a goal at a distance d_g, we treat the agent's current direction of travel (the heading direction ϕ) as if it were attached to the goal direction (ψ_g) by a damped spring (with stiffness k_g and damping b; see Fig. 5.7):

$$\ddot{\phi} = -b\dot{\phi} - k_g\left(\phi - \psi_g\right)\left(e^{-c_1 d_g} + c_2\right) \tag{5.1}$$

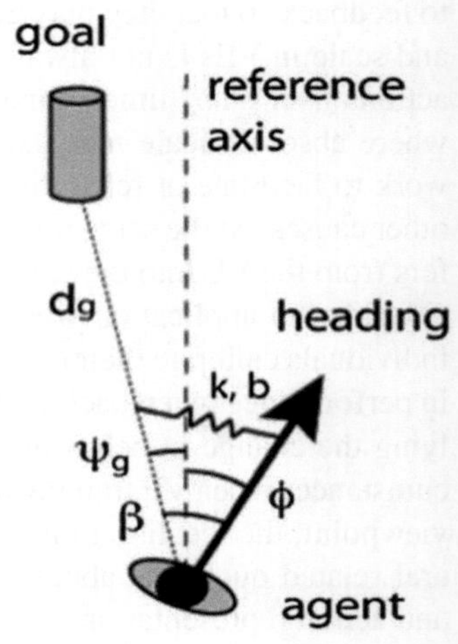

Fig. 5.7 Steering to a goal

This model brings the heading into alignment with the goal as the agent travels forward. The locomotor path thus emerges from the interaction between agent and environment on-line, rather than being explicitly planned.

To guide walking, the locomotion model requires sensory information about the current direction of heading and the visual direction of the goal, that is, the heading error ($\phi - \psi_g$). Potential information for the current walking direction includes vestibular information from the otoliths and proprioceptive information from the lower limbs, collectively known as *idiothetic information*. There is also visual heading information in the form of *optic flow*, the pattern of motion available at the eye of a moving observer (Gibson, 1950, 1958; Warren, 1998, 2008). Such information would act to modulate the dynamics of locomotor behavior and yield adaptive paths of locomotion.

To test whether humans use visual or idiothetic information about heading to control walking, we created a virtual environment in which the optic flow pattern was displaced by 10° from the actual walking direction. Thus, if a participant aligned the idiothetic heading with the goal, the optic flow would indicate a 10° heading error. This result has indeed been reported in several studies (Harris & Bonas, 2002; Rushton, Harris, Lloyd, & Wann, 1998), implying that optic flow plays no role in the control of walking; however, only environments with relatively sparse optic flow were tested in these experiments. In contrast, if the participant aligned the optic flow with the goal, the visual heading error would be 0°. In a key study (Warren, Kay, Zosh, Duchon, & Sahuc, 2001), we observed both effects: as the structure of the scene increased, the visual heading error decreased from nearly 10° with an isolated target, to about 2° with a rich forest-like environment. These findings indicate that both idiothetic information and optic flow are used to control walking, with the flow becoming more dominant as the visual structure increases (see also Bruggeman, Zosh, & Warren, 2007; Butler, Smith, Campos, & Bülthoff, 2010; Harris & Carre, 2001; Turano, Yu, Hao, & Hicks, 2005; Saunders & Durgin, 2011).

Combining visual and idiothetic information for heading is a robust control strategy that ensures successful steering under varying conditions. Warren et al. (2001) proposed that these two sources of information for heading error are linearly combined:

$$\phi - \psi_g = w_{\text{idio}}\left(\phi_{\text{idio}} - \psi_g\right) + w_{\text{flow}}\left(\phi_{\text{flow}} - \psi_g\right) \tag{5.2}$$

where optic flow is weighted by the visual structure s and the flow rate v, with normalized weights: $w_{\text{idio}} = 1/(1+s+v)$, $w_{\text{flow}} = (s+v)/(1+s+v)$. To derive a control law for locomotion, this information can simply be substituted into the locomotion model (Fajen & Warren, 2003):

$$\ddot{\phi} = -b\dot{\phi} - k_g\left[w_{\text{idio}}\left(\phi_{\text{idio}} - \psi_g\right) + w_{\text{flow}}\left(\phi_{\text{flow}} - \psi_g\right)\right]\left(e^{-c_1 d_g} + c_2\right) \tag{5.3}$$

We recently tested this model in two experiments (Unpublished communication). First, we varied the conflict between the optic flow and the actual walking direction over a wide range, from 5° to 25°, as participants walked to a visible goal (Fig. 5.8).

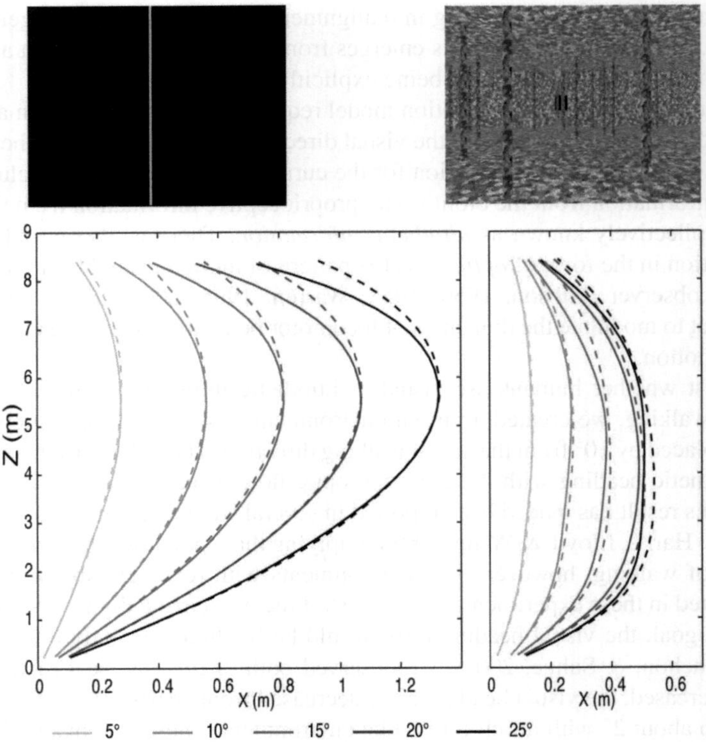

Fig. 5.8 Mean paths of locomotion for humans (*solid*) and simulations (*dotted*) when steering to an isolated target (*left*) or in a rich visual environment (*right*). Paths are more curved with a larger displacement of the optic flow (5–25°)

As expected, the observed heading error was a constant proportion of the optic flow displacement, but the weights depended on the visual structure of the environment. In the rich forest environment, optic flow dominated: least-squares fits of the walking trajectories yielded a flow weight of 0.8 and an idiothetic weight of 0.2 over the whole range of displacements (mean RMS heading error = 0.7°, mean $R^2 = 0.95$). In contrast, with a target alone, idiothetic information dominated with a weight of 0.7, and a flow weight of 0.3 (RMSE = 0.55°, $R^2 = 0.45$). Thus, optic flow and idiothetic information appear to be linearly combined over a large range of displacements, while the flow weight depends on the richness of optic flow.

In a second experiment, we tested whether the flow weight also depends on the rate of optic flow. It has been shown that perceptual judgments of heading are more reliable as the flow rate increases from walking to running speeds (Warren, Morris, & Kalish, 1988), so one might expect that the contribution of flow to locomotor control would likewise increase. To vary the flow rate while holding the physical walking speed (and hence idiothetic information) constant, we manipulated the visual gain in the HMD (gain = 0.5, 1.0, 2.0, 4.0). That is, if the observer walked at a normal speed, the optic flow rate could be half, equal to, twice, or four times the physical speed, corresponding to a slow walk to a fast run. As expected, as the flow rate increased, the heading error decreased. Fits of the walking trajectories yielded flow weights that rose from 0.8 to nearly 1.0 with a gain of 4 (mean $R^2=0.97$).

In sum, both optic flow and idiothetic information for heading are used to guide walking, but their relative contribution depends on the richness and rate of the flow. It is an open question as to whether this information is integrated at the level of heading perception or at the level of locomotor control (see also Chap. 8). Our perceptually based pedestrian model has been expanded to include behaviors such as target interception, avoidance of stationary and moving obstacles, and pedestrian interactions (Fajen & Warren, 2007; Warren & Fajen, 2008) (see also Moussaïd, Helbing, & Theraulaz, 2011; Ondrej, Pettré, Olivier, & Donikian, 2010). These components can be linearly combined to generate locomotor paths through complex environments. We are currently studying interactions such as matching the speed and heading of neighbors, with the ultimate aim of understanding the collective behavior of human crowds (Bonneaud, Rio, Chevaillier, & Warren, 2012; Bonneaud & Warren, 2012; Rio, Bonneaud, & Warren, 2012). We are also beginning to use VR methods to study the assessment of functional mobility and visual-locomotor impairment (Gérin-Lajoie, Ciombor, Warren, & Aaron, 2010; Kiefer, Bruggeman, Woods, & Warren, 2012; Kiefer, Rhea, & Warren, 2013).

5.5 Virtual Reality Balance Training in Rehabilitation (Eric R. Anson and John Jeka)

Augmented reality feedback (ARF) or virtual reality (VR) systems have recently become more prominent as a rehabilitative mechanism (Chap. 3, Man, 2010), and the application of ARF/VR for improved balance control has become more widespread (Bohil, Alicea, & Biocca, 2011). VR applications for balance training that were once too expensive to be incorporated into rehabilitation have begun to make their way into daily rehabilitation practice. Moreover, new VR tools are developing that foster balance rehabilitation during walking, where most falls occur, that may be more effective in reducing fall risk.

Computer-controlled VR treatments have an advantage over the traditional rehabilitation treatments: the ability to manipulate sensory information in a specific, controlled manner (Chap. 3). Accuracy of sensory information can be intentionally manipulated to facilitate sensory reweighting. Recently, video gaming systems have increased the availability of low tech VR (i.e., Wii Fit, Nintendo, Kyoto, Japan) to the general public and several reports have demonstrated improved balance control following training using interactive gaming systems (Bateni, 2012; Deutsch, Borbely, Filler, Huhn, & Guarrera-Bowlby, 2008; Young, Ferguson, Brault, & Craig, 2010).

It has long been known that postural control is influenced by the availability and accuracy of sensory input (Nashner, 1981). Investigations over the last decade have illustrated how the fusion of multisensory inputs is a critical component of upright balance when sensory information is absent (Oie, Kiemel, & Jeka, 2002; Peterka, 2002). Visual feedback has been used to improve postural control during standing; however, the carryover effects of visual ARF during standing have not been consistently reported. Some authors reported reduced sway or improved movement control (Cheng, Wang, Chung, & Chen, 2004; Davlin-Pater, 2010; Sihvonen, Sipilä, & Era, 2004), while others reported no additional effect or limited carryover to walking (Barclay-Goddard, Stevenson, Poluha, Moffatt, & Taback, 2005; Van Peppen, Kortsmit, Lindeman, & Kwakkel, 2006; Walker, Brouwer, & Culham, 2000). Since the majority of falls occur during walking, and standing balance training with VR inconsistently results in carryover it is only natural that this technology be applied to walking (Chaps. 8 and 9).

It has been suggested that the use of VR gaming as part of rehabilitation will improve motivation and compliance for exercise attendance, but not all older adults prefer this therapeutic modality (Laver, Ratcliff, George, Burgess, & Crotty, 2011). While these systems are low cost and have promising results, particularly when VR is used to augment traditional therapies (Bateni, 2012), a limitation to these types of VR is that they are not designed to engage the ARF while walking. An additional limitation of the gaming systems is that they provide nonspecific interaction with an onscreen avatar, and multiple body positions allow the user to be successful in the game.

Until recently it has been challenging to provide VR or ARF during walking, but advances in head-mounted displays and more realistic computer-generated images now allow for the provision of augmented visual information about body movement *during walking*. Inconsistent carryover from training with VR or ARF during standing to walking and other daily activities suggests that incorporating VR or ARF during walking may be more appropriate. Individuals who survived a stroke were able to demonstrate improved community ambulation on an obstacle course following VR training on a treadmill that included ARF related to obstacle clearance while walking (Yang, Tsai, Chuang, Sung, & Wang, 2008). Improved control of trunk and leg motion during over-ground walking following ARF in a VR environment has been demonstrated in an individual with transfemoral amputation (Darter & Wilken, 2011). Other applications of ARF provided during walking have demonstrated improved control of trunk motion and improved balance using torso vibration vests or a head-mounted visual, vibration, and sound feedback device (Verhoeff, Horlings, Janssen, Bridenbaugh, & Allum, 2009; Wall, Wrisley, & Statler, 2009).

Mobility improvements measured via time to complete an obstacle course and number of penalties (striking an obstacle) were reported for an experimental group that walked on a treadmill while viewing a VR scene with rotational motion that was not consistent with the direction of treadmill walking (Buccello-Stout et al., 2008). The improvement in obstacle course navigation was interpreted as a sensorimotor adaptation from training with the incongruent VR environment. Individuals with mild traumatic brain injuries (mTBI) have been able to demonstrate improved walking balance after VR training (Gottshall, Sessoms, & Bartlett, 2012). Ongoing clinical trials are being conducted to investigate the comparative effectiveness of training with the Wii Fit vs. traditional vestibular rehabilitation (Meldrum et al., 2012).

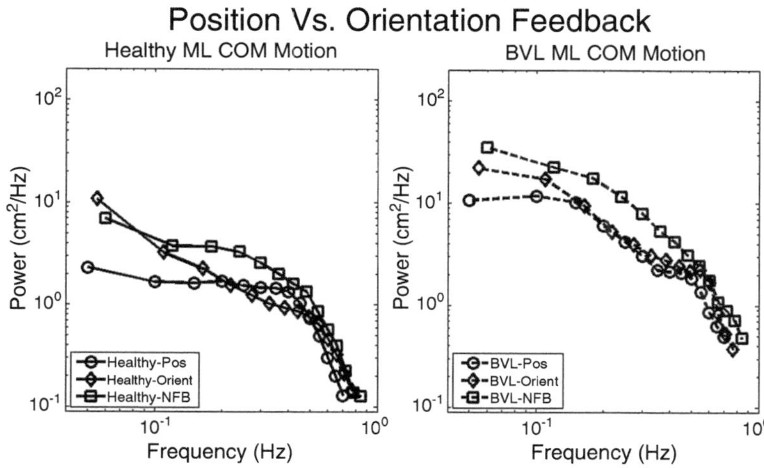

Fig. 5.9 Mediolateral COM movement variability is shown to decrease for the frequency range below 0.4 Hz during treadmill walking with feedback. The no feedback (NFB) condition is represented by the squares in both plots. COM translation feedback (represented by the *circles*) resulted in the greatest reduction in mediolateral COM movement variability, but trunk orientation feedback (represented by the *diamonds*) also resulted in reduced mediolateral COM movement variability. With feedback, individuals with BVL (*dashed lines* in the *right hand plot*)

We have investigated the beneficial effects of providing ARF during walking that is specific to trunk motion. We have demonstrated that there is a reduction in variability of center of mass (COM) translation when visual feedback is present compared to when it is absent for healthy young and older adults (Anson, Agada, Fleming, Kiemel, & Jeka, 2010; Green et al., 2010. In these experiments, we presented a cursor representing COM translation overlaid on a bulls-eye. Providing the ARF error signal (displacement of the cursor from the center of the bulls-eye) led to a reduction in movement variability. Movement variability during trials when the individuals saw just the bulls-eye without the cursor was no different than in no feedback conditions with the TV screen covered (Green et al., 2010).

We have also demonstrated that individuals with bilateral vestibular loss (BVL) demonstrate improved control of COM translation during treadmill walking (see Fig. 5.9) regardless of the type of feedback. In this experiment, we presented either COM translation (red lines) or trunk angle orientation (black lines) with respect to vertical displayed as two-dimensional cursor motion on a bulls-eye with the center representing the middle of the treadmill for translation or perfectly upright for orientation. The feedback conditions are contrasted with a no feedback condition with the monitor turned off (blue lines). The individuals with BVL were able to demonstrate improved control of COM translation, demonstrated by reduction in low-frequency variability. Interestingly mediolateral COM translation improved regardless of the type of feedback presented, but the magnitude of improvement was greater when the feedback provided was specific to COM translation.

5.6 Conclusions

Of great importance to the continued use of virtual reality in rehabilitation is identification of the similarity of responses within a virtual environment to those in a physical environment. The studies discussed in this chapter are all supportive of transference for both perceptual-motor adaptation and motor relearning. Wright illustrated how sensorimotor adaptations are retained after acting within the virtual environment, although unintended motor responses could appear in a VE that may not be present in more traditional training environments. Creem-Regehr identified perceptual-motor recalibration in the VE based on the learned relationships between the virtual world motion and their own motion, and Anson and Jeka tell us that these relationships can be learned even in individuals with sensory loss. According to Warren, the relative contribution of specific sensory signals depends on the richness and rate of the optic flow. Thus, in the VE our processes of adaptation to changing environment circumstances are similar to those in the physical world; however, we still need to fine-tune the sensory array before we can expect motor responses to be equivalent.

References

Angelaki, D. E. (1998). Three-dimensional organization of otolith-ocular reflexes in rhesus monkeys. III. Responses to translation. *Journal of Neurophysiology, 80*(2), 680–695.

Anson, E., Agada, P., Fleming, H., Kiemel, T., & Jeka, J. (2010). Visual feedback to improve postural control during locomotion in the healthy elderly. *Parkinsonism & Related Disorders, 16*(Suppl 1), S79–S80.

Barclay-Goddard, R., Stevenson, T., Poluha, W., Moffatt, M., & Taback, S. (2005). Force platform feedback for standing balance training after stroke. *Stroke, 36*(2), 412–413.

Bateni, H. (2012). Changes in balance in older adults based on use of physical therapy vs the Wii Fit gaming system: A preliminary study. *Physiotherapy, 98*, 211–216.

Bohil, C., Alicea, B., & Biocca, F. (2011). Virtual reality in neuroscience research and therapy. *Nature Reviews. Neuroscience, 12*, 752–762.

Bonneaud, S., Rio, K., Chevaillier, P., Warren, W. H., et al. (2012). Accounting for patterns of collective behavior in crowd locomotor dynamics for realistic simulations. In Z. Pan (Ed.), *Lecture notes in computer science: Transactions on edutainment VII* (Vol. 7145, pp. 1–11). Heidelberg: Springer.

Bonneaud, S., & Warren, W. H. (2012). A behavioral dynamics approach to modeling realistic pedestrian behavior. *Proceedings of the 6th International Conference on Pedestrian and Evacuation Dynamics, Zurich, Switzerland* (pp. 1–14).

Bruggeman, H., Zosh, W., & Warren, W. H. (2007). Optic flow drives human visuo-locomotor adaptation. *Current Biology, 17*, 2035–2040.

Buccello-Stout, R., Bloomberg, J., Cohen, H., Whorton, E., Weaver, G., & Cromwell, R. (2008). Effects of sensorimotor adaptation training on functional mobility in older adults. *Journal of Gerontology: Psychological Sciences, 63B*(5), P295–P300.

Butler, J. S., Smith, S. T., Campos, J. L., & Bülthoff, H. H. (2010). Bayesian integration of visual and vestibular signals for heading. *Journal of Vision, 10*, 1–13.

Cheng, P., Wang, C., Chung, C., & Chen, C. (2004). Effects of visual feedback rhythmic weight-shift training on hemiplegic stroke patients. *Clinical Rehabilitation, 18*(7), 747–753.

Cohn, J. V., DiZio, P., & Lackner, J. R. (2000). Reaching during virtual rotation: context specific compensations for expected coriolis forces. *Journal of Neurophysiology, 83*(6), 3230–3240.

Creem-Regehr, S. H., Willemsen, P., Gooch, A. A., & Thompson, W. B. (2005). The influence of restricted viewing conditions on egocentric distance perception: Implications for real and virtual indoor environments. *Perception, 34*, 191–204.

Darter, B., & Wilken, J. (2011). Gait training with virtual reality-based real time feedback: Improving gait performance following transfemoral amputation. *Physical Therapy, 91*(9), 1385–1394.

Davlin-Pater, C. (2010). The effects of visual information and perceptual style on static and dynamic balance. *Motor Control, 14*, 362–370.

Deutsch, J., Borbely, M., Filler, J., Huhn, K., & Guarrera-Bowlby, P. (2008). Use of a low-cost, commercially available gaming console (Wii) for rehabilitation of an adolescent with cerebral palsy. *Physical Therapy, 88*, 1196–1207.

Dichgans, J., Held, R., Young, L. R., & Brandt, T. (1972). Moving visual scenes influence the apparent direction of gravity. *Science, 178*, 1217–1219.

Fajen, B. R., & Warren, W. H. (2003). Behavioral dynamics of steering, obstacle avoidance, and route selection. *Journal of Experimental Psychology: Human Perception and Performance, 29*, 343–362.

Fajen, B. R., & Warren, W. H. (2007). Behavioral dynamics of intercepting a moving target. *Experimental Brain Research, 180*, 303–319.

Gérin-Lajoie, M., Ciombor, D. M., Warren, W. H., & Aaron, R. K. (2010). Using ambulatory virtual environments for the assessment of functional gait impairment: A proof-of-concept study. *Gait & Posture, 31*, 533–536.

Geuss, M. N., Stefanucci, J. K., Creem-Regehr, S. H., & Thompson, W. B. (2012). Effect of viewing plane on perceived distances in real and virtual environments. *Journal of Experimental Psychology: Human Perception and Performance, 38*, 1242.

Gibson, J. J. (1950). *Perception of the visual world*. Boston, MA: Houghton Mifflin.

Gibson, J. J. (1958). Visually controlled locomotion and visual orientation in animals. *British Journal of Psychology, 49*, 182–194.

Gottshall, K., Sessoms, P., & Bartlett, J. (2012, August). Vestibular physical therapy intervention: Utilizing a computer assisted rehabilitation environment in lieu of traditional physical therapy. *Proceedings of the Annual International Conference of the IEEE Engineering in Medicine and Biology Society, 2012*, 6141–6144.

Green, J., Anson, E., Agada, P., Rosenberg, R., Fleming, H., & Jeka, J. (2010). Visual feedback improves postural control during locomotion. *Parkinsonism & Related Disorders, 16*(Suppl 1), S81–S82.

Hardt, M. E., Held, R., & Steinbach, M. J. (1971). Adaptation to displaced vision: A change in the central control of sensorimotor coordination. *Journal of Experimental Psychology, 89*, 229–239.

Harris, J. M., & Bonas, W. (2002). Optic flow and scene structure do not always contribute to the control of human walking. *Vision Research, 42*, 1619–1626.

Harris, M. G., & Carre, G. (2001). Is optic flow used to guide walking while wearing a displacing prism? *Perception, 30*, 811–818.

Held, R., & Freedman, S. J. (1963). Plasticity in human sensorimotor control. *Science, 142*, 455–462.

Hollerbach, J. M., Xu, Y., Christensen, R. R., & Jacobsen, S. C. (2000) Design specifications for the second generation Sarcos Treadport locomotion interface. *Haptics Symposium, Proceedings of the ASME Dynamic Systems and Control Division* (DSC-Vol 69-2, pp. 1293–1298). Orlando.

Keshner, E. A., & Kenyon, R. V. (2000). The influence of an immersive virtual environment on the segmental organization of postural stabilizing responses. *Journal of Vestibular Research, 10*, 207–219.

Kiefer, A. W., Bruggeman, H., Woods, R., & Warren, W. H. (2012). Obstacle detection during walking by patients with tunnel vision. *Journal of Vision, 12*, 183.

Kiefer, A. W., Rhea, C. K., & Warren, W. H. (2009). VR-based assessment and rehabilitation of functional mobility. In F. Steinicke et al. (Eds.), *Human walking in virtual environments: Perception, technology and applications*. Heidelberg: Springer.

Kuhl, S. A., Creem-Regehr, S. H., & Thompson, W. B. (2008). Recalibration of rotational locomotion in immersive virtual environments. *ACM Transactions on Applied Perception, 5*, 2–11.

Kuhl, S. A., Thompson, W. B., & Creem-Regehr, S. H. (2009). HMD calibration and its effects on distance judgments. *ACM Transactions on Applied Perception, 6*, 19.

Kunz, B. R., Creem-Regehr, S. H., & Thompson, W. B. (2009). Evidence for motor simulation in imagined locomotion. *Journal of Experimental Psychology: Human Perception and Performance, 35*, 1458–1471.

Kunz, B. R., Creem-Regehr, S. H., & Thompson, W. B. (2013). Does perceptual-motor calibration generalize across two different forms of locomotion? Investigations of walking and wheelchairs. *PLoS One, 8*, e54446.

Kunz, B. R., Wouters, L., Smith, D., Thompson, W. B., & Creem-Regehr, S. H. (2009). Revisiting the effect of quality of graphics on distance judgments in virtual environments: A comparison of verbal reports and blind walking. *Attention, Perception, & Psychophysics, 71*, 1284–1293.

Lackner, J. R., & DiZio, P. (1988). Visual stimulation affects the perception of voluntary leg movements during walking. *Perception, 17*, 71–80.

Lambrey, S., & Berthoz, A. (2003). Combination of conflicting visual and non-visual information for estimating actively performed body turns in virtual reality. *International Journal of Psychophysiology, 50*, 101–115.

Laver, K., Ratcliff, J., George, S., Burgess, L., & Crotty, M. (2011). Is the Nintendo Wii Fit really acceptable to older people?: A discrete choice experiment. *BMC Geriatrics, 11*, 64.

Lishman, J. R., & Lee, D. N. (1973). The autonomy of visual kineasthesis. *Perception, 2*, 287–294.

Loomis, J. M., Da Silva, J. A., Fujita, N., & Fukusima, S. S. (1992). Visual space perception and visually directed action. *Journal of Experimental Psychology, 18*, 906–921.

Mach, E. (1875). *Grundlinien der Lehre von den Bewegungsempfindungen*. Leipzig: Engelmann.

Man, D. (2010). Common issues of virtual reality in neuro-rehabilitation. In Prof. Jae-Jin Kim (Ed.), *Virtual reality*. InTech. ISBN: 978-953-307-518-1, doi: 10.5772/13547. Available from http://www.intechopen.com/books/virtual-reality/common-issues-of-virtual-reality-in-neuro-rehabilitation

Meldrum, D., Herdman, S., Moloney, R., Murray, D., Duffy, D., Malone, K., French, H., Hone, S., Conroy, R., & McConn-Walsh, R. (2012). Effectiveness of conventional versus virtual reality based vestibular rehabilitation in the treatment of dizziness, gait and balance impairment in adults with unilateral peripheral vestibular loss: a randomised controlled trial. *BMC Ear Nose Throat Disord, 12*, 3. doi: 10.1186/1472-6815-12-3.

Mohler, B. J., Creem-Regehr, S. H., & Thompson, W. B. (2006). The influence of feedback on egocentric distance judgments in real and virtual environmnets. In: *Proceedings of the Third SIGGRAPH Symposium on Applied Perception in Graphics and Visualization.*

Mohler, B. J., Thompson, W. B., Creem-Regehr, S. H., Willemsen, P., Pick, Jr. H. L., & Rieser, J. J. (2007) Calibration of locomotion resulting from visual motion in a treadmill-based virtual environment. *ACM Transactions on Applied Perception, 4*, 1–15.

Morton, S. M., & Bastian, A. J. (2004, October). Prism adaptation during walking generalizes to reaching and requires the cerebellum. *Journal of Neurophysiology*, *92*(4), 2497–24509.

Moussaïd, M., Helbing, D., & Theraulaz, G. (2011). How simple rules determine pedestrian behavior and crowd disasters. *Proceedings of the National Academy of Sciences, 108*, 6884–6888.

Nashner, L. M. (1981). Analysis of stance posture in humans. In A. Towe & E. Luschei (Eds.), *Handbook of behavioral neurobiology (vol 5) motor coordination*. New York, NY: Plenum Press.

Oie, K., Kiemel, T., & Jeka, J. (2002). Multisensory fusion: Simultaneous re-weighting of vision and touch for the control of human posture. *Cognitive Brain Research, 14*, 164–176.

Ondrej, J., Pettré, J., Olivier, A.-H., & Donikian, S. (2010). A synthetic-vision based steering approach for crowd simulation. *ACM Transactions on Graphics, 29*(123), 121–129.

Palmisano, S., Gillam, B. J., & Blackburn, S. G. (2000). Global-perspective jitter improves vection in central vision. *Perception, 29*(1), 57–67.

Peterka, R. J. (2002). Sensorimotor integration in human postural control. *Journal of Neurophysiology, 88*(3), 1097–1118.

Richardson, A. R., & Waller, D. (2007). Interaction with an immersive virtual environment corrects users' distance estimates. *Human Factors, 49*, 507–517.

Riecke, B. E. (2009). Cognitive and higher-level contributions to illusory self-motion perception ("vection"): Does the possibility of actual motion affect vection? *Japanese Journal of Psychonomic Science, 28*(1), 135–139.

Rieser, J. J., Ashmead, D. H., Taylor, C. R., & Youngquist, G. A. (1990). Visual perception and the guidance of locomotion without vision to previously seen targets. *Perception, 19*, 675–689.

Rieser, J. J., Pick, H. L., Ashmead, D. H., & Garing, A. E. (1995). Calibration of human locomotion and models of perceptual-motor organization. *Journal of Experimental Psychology: Human Perception & Performance, 21*, 480–497.

Rio, K. W., Bonneaud, S., & Warren, W. H. (2012). A data-driven model of pedestrian following and emergent crowd behavior. *Proceedings of the 6th International Conference on Pedestrian and Evacuation Dynamics, Zurich, Switzerland* (pp. 1–15).

Rushton, S. K., Harris, J. M., Lloyd, M., & Wann, J. P. (1998). Guidance of locomotion on foot uses perceived target location rather than optic flow. *Current Biology, 8*, 1191–1194.

Stratton, G. (1896). Some preliminary experiments on vision without inversion of the retinal image. *Psychol Review 3*, 611–617.

Sahm, C. S., Creem-Regehr, S. H., Thompson, W. B., & Willemsen, P. (2005). Throwing versus walking as indicators of distance perception in similar real and virtual environments. *ACM Transactions on Applied Perception, 2*, 35–45.

Saunders, J. A., & Durgin, F. H. (2011). Adaptation to conflicting visual and physical heading directions during walking. *Journal of Vision, 11*, 1–10.

Sihvonen, S., Sipilä, S., & Era, P. (2004). Changes in postural balance in frail elderly women during a 4-week visual feedback training: A randomized controlled trial. *Gerontology, 50*(2), 87–95.

Thompson, W. B., Willemsen, P., Gooch, A. A., Creem-Regehr, S. H., Loomis, J. M., & Beall, A. C. (2004). Does the quality of the computer graphics matter when judging distance in visually immersive environments? *Presence: Teleoperators and Virtual Environments, 13*, 560–571.

Trevarthan, C. B. (1968). Two mechanisms of vision in primates. *Psychologische Forschung, 31*, 299–337.

Trillenberg, P., Shelhamer, M., Roberts, D. C., & Zee, D. S. (2003). Cross-axis adaptation of torsional components in the yaw-axis vestibulo-ocular reflex. *Experimental Brain Research, 148*, 158–165.

Turano, K. A., Yu, D., Hao, L., & Hicks, J. C. (2005). Optic-flow and egocentric-direction strategies in walking: Central vs. perhipheral visual field. *Vision Research, 45*, 3117–3132.

Van Peppen, R. P., Kortsmit, M., Lindeman, E., & Kwakkel, G. (2006). Effects of visual feedback therapy on postural control in bilateral standing after stroke: A systematic review. *Journal of Rehabilitation Medicine, 38*(1), 3–9.

Verhoeff, L., Horlings, C., Janssen, L., Bridenbaugh, S., & Allum, J. (2009). Effects of biofeedback on trunk sway during dual tasking in the healthy young and elderly. *Gait & Posture, 30*, 76–81.

Walker, C., Brouwer, B. J., & Culham, E. G. (2000). Use of visual feedback in retraining balance following acute stroke. *Physical Therapy, 80*(9), 886–895.

Wall, C., Wrisley, D., & Statler, K. (2009). Vibrotactile tilt feedback improves dynamic gait index: A fall risk indicator in older adults. *Gait & Posture, 30*, 16–21.

Warren, W. H. (1998). Visually controlled locomotion: 40 years later. *Ecological Psychology, 10*, 177–219.

Warren, W. H. (2008) Optic flow. In: T. D. Albright & R. Masland, Eds. *The senses—a comprehensive reference: Vision II* (Basbaum, A. I., et al., Eds., vol. 2, pp. 219–230). Oxford: Academic Press.

Warren, W. H., & Fajen, B. R. (2008). Behavioral dynamics of visually-guided locomotion. In A. Fuchs & V. Jirsa (Eds.), *Coordination: Neural, behavioral, and social dynamics*. Springer: Heidelberg.

Warren, W. H., Kay, B. A., Zosh, W. D., Duchon, A. P., & Sahuc, S. (2001). Optic flow is used to control human walking. *Nature Neuroscience, 4*, 213–216.

Warren, W. H., Morris, M. W., & Kalish, M. (1988). Perception of translational heading from optical flow. *Journal of Experimental Psychology: Human Perception and Performance, 14*, 646–660.

Wei, M., & Angelaki, D. E. (2001). Cross-axis adaptation of the translational vestibulo-ocular reflex. *Experimental Brain Research, 138*, 304–312.

Willemsen, P., Colton, M. B., Creem-Regehr, S. H., & Thompson, W. B. (2009). The effects of head-mounted display mechanical properties and field of view on distance judgments in virtual environments. *ACM Transactions on Applied Perception, 6*, 8.

Wood, R. (1895). The 'Haunted Swing' illusion. *Psychological Review, 2*(3), 277–278.

Wright, W. G. (2009). Linear vection in virtual environments can be strengthened by discordant inertial input. *Proceedings of the Annual International Conference of the IEEE Engineering in Medicine and Biology Society, 2009*, 1157–1160.

Wright, W. G., Agah, M. R., Darvish, K., & Keshner, E. A. (2013). Head stabilization shows visual and inertial dependence during passive stimulation: Implications for virtual rehabilitation. *IEEE Transactions on Neural Systems and Rehabilitation Engineering, 21*(2), 191–197.

Wright, W. G., DiZio, P., & Lackner, J. R. (2005). Vertical linear self-motion perception during visual and inertial motion: More than weighted summation of sensory inputs. *Journal of Vestibular Research, 15*(4), 185–195.

Wright, W. G., DiZio, P., & Lackner, J. R. (2006). Perceived self-motion in two visual contexts: dissociable mechanisms underlie perception. *Journal of Vestibular Research, 16*, 23–28.

Wright, W. G., & Glasauer, S. (2003). Haptic subjective vertical shows context dependence: task and vision play a role during dynamic tilt stimulation. *The Annals of the New York Academy of Sciences, 1004*, 531–535.

Wright, W. G., & Glasauer, S. (2006). Subjective somatosensory vertical during dynamic tilt is dependent on task, inertial condition, and multisensory concordance. *Experimental Brain Research, 172*(3), 310–321.

Wright, W. G., Schneider, E., & Glasauer, S. (2009). Compensatory manual motor responses while object wielding during combined linear visual and physical roll tilt stimulation. *Experimental Brain Research, 192*(4), 683–694.

Wright, W.G., Schneider, E. (2009). Manual motor control during "virtual" self-motion: Implications for VR rehabilitation. *IEEE Proc ICVR2009* (pp. 166–172).

Xerri, C., Borel, L., Barthelemy, J., & Lacour, M. (1988). Synergistic interactions and functional working range of the visual and vestibular systems in postural control: Neuronal correlates. *Progress in Brain Research, 76*, 193–203.

Yang, Y., Tsai, M., Chuang, T., Sung, W., & Wang, R. (2008). Virtual reality-based training improves community ambulation in individuals with stroke: A randomized controlled trial. *Gait & Posture, 28*, 201–206.

Young, W., Ferguson, S., Brault, S., & Craig, C. (2010). Assessing and training standing balance in older adults: A novel approach using the 'Nintendo Wii' Balance Board. *Gait & Posture, 33*, 303–305.

Chapter 6
Validity of Virtual Reality Environments for Sensorimotor Rehabilitation

Mindy F. Levin, Judith E. Deutsch, Michal Kafri, and Dario G. Liebermann

Objective To describe the fidelity of movements and exercise done in different types of VR environments to those done in physical environments.

6.1 Introduction

Sensorimotor rehabilitation is primarily aimed at improving motor ability so that people can regain their physical independence for the accomplishment of daily life tasks—such as self-care, work, and leisure activities. Following an injury to the central nervous system (CNS) such as stroke, traumatic brain injury, or cerebral

---

M.F. Levin (✉)
School of Physical and Occupational Therapy, McGill University, Montreal, QC, Canada

Centre for Interdisciplinary Research in Rehabilitation, Jewish Rehabilitation Hospital Research Site, 3205 place Alton-Goldbloom, Laval, QC, Canada, H7V 1R2
e-mail: mindy.levin@mcgill.ca

J.E. Deutsch
RiVERS Lab, Department of Rehabilitation and Movement Sciences, Rutger's University, Newark, NJ, USA
e-mail: deutsch@shrp.rutgers.edu

M. Kafri
Department of Physical Therapy, Faculty of Social Welfare & Health Sciences, University of Haifa, Mount Carmel, Haifa, 31905, Israel
e-mail: kafri.michal@gmail.com

D.G. Liebermann
Physical Therapy Department, The Stanley Steyer School of Health Professions, Sackler Faculty of Medicine, Tel Aviv University, P.O.B. 39040, Ramat Aviv—Tel Aviv 69978, Israel
e-mail: dlieberm@post.tau.ac.il

P.L. (Tamar) Weiss et al. (eds.), *Virtual Reality for Physical and Motor Rehabilitation*, Virtual Reality Technologies for Health and Clinical Applications,
DOI 10.1007/978-1-4939-0968-1_6,

palsy, for example, damage to cortical structures and white matter pathways involved in the production of motor output results in sensorimotor impairments such as changes in muscle tone, motor paralysis or weakness, loss of coordination, and reduced muscle and aerobic endurance. In addition to movement, CNS lesions can result in impairments in other body functions that influence the capacity of the individual to gain independence related to cognition and perception. In this chapter, the emphasis is primarily on motor behavior by measuring motor output congruence between physical and virtual environments (VEs). While cognitive and sensory processes are essential for this understanding, they are not emphasized here. It is assumed that the fidelity of virtual to physical world movements is important for rehabilitation that intends to promote the recovery of movement quality.

Despite changes in motor output, patients recover, to a greater or a lesser extent, the ability to perform motor tasks. Improvements or adaptations in motor ability are due to two properties of the nervous system, redundancy and plasticity. Redundancy is reflected in the multiple ways a task can be performed because of the large number of degrees of freedom (joint rotations) available in the biomechanical system (Bernstein, 1967). Instead of having a negative connotation (i.e., too many degrees of freedom, with some having the same function), Latash and his colleagues suggest that the system has an "abundant" number of degrees of freedom, which provides it with the capacity to choose different limb or body configurations to suit changing conditions in the environment (Latash, 2012; Scholz & Schoner, 1999). The second property of the CNS that is involved in motor behavior is plasticity (see Chap. 2). Plasticity is the capacity of the nervous system for reorganization by adapting or forming new neural connections in response to injury, experience, and/or training (Pascual-Leone, Amedi, Fregni, & Merabet, 2005). After CNS injury, the system can take advantage of both redundancy and plasticity to recover lost motor patterns or to adapt to this loss through compensation or substitution (Levin, Kleim, & Wolf, 2009).

While CNS redundancy and plasticity inform the theoretical basis for sensorimotor rehabilitation, repetitive exercise, task specificity, and patient-specific cognitive and emotional factors are used to design rehabilitation interventions. From a physical standpoint, therapists may encourage patients to perform movements using motor patterns similar to those made by individuals without a motor deficit, the so-called typical movement patterns. Therapists can use techniques such as providing active-assisted movement or sensory cueing (e.g., quick stretching, tapping, vibration) to activate specific muscles, verbal instructions or demonstration, and different forms of feedback. This is framed using a patient-centered approach that involves task-specific training (Carr & Shepherd, 1987) accompanied by efforts to reduce motor impairment.

The relevant features of task-specific training include salience, problem solving, and practice in ecologically relevant environments, all of which are provided and enhanced by the use of virtual reality (VR) environments. A challenge to creating practice environments in VR is determining which aspects of the movements made in these environments need to be similar or better than those made in typical physical training environments and how can the capacity of body systems be exploited to adapt and/or learn new motor skills using its inherent redundancy. Several studies have used kinematic and energetic analyses for these comparisons. Production of movement is influenced by the perception of the environment with which we need to interact; that is, in order to move we must perceive and in order to perceive we must move (Michaels & Carello, 1981). This hypothetical action–perception relationship is especially important for limb movements that are influenced by veridical information about the environment for actions of the upper limb such as reaching and grasping (Jeannerod, 1999; Smeets & Brenner, 1999) or of lower limb such as running on uneven terrains (Warren, Young, & Lee, 1986) and landing from a fall (Liebermann & Goodman, 2007).

According to this point of view, the interaction between relative motion with respect to the surrounding objects and the environmental layouts provides a sense of timing and spatial location that leads to appropriate 3D movements particularly during interceptive actions (Gibson, 1979). Strengthening the action–perception interaction may enhance skill acquisition, while poor or erroneous correlation between perception and action is detrimental since it leads to the acquisition of inappropriate motor habits (Gibson & Walk, 1960; Held, 2009) The important question is whether VR can be used to enhance action–perception learning. For this purpose, the following sections address the quality of VR environments and their influence on the production of movement.

6.2 3D Perception and Motor Action

A sense of depth (three-dimensional view) is perceived by stereovision in which the two eyes capture two-dimensional views of the same object from a slightly different perspective. VR setups create an illusion of depth in different ways (see Chap. 4). For upper limb pointing movements, production of a smooth hand path in the workspace requires the CNS to make a sensorimotor transformation of the distance between the start and end hand positions as defined in internal arm joint configuration coordinates (flexion, extension, rotation) and in external visual coordinates of the target position (vertical, horizontal, and depth; x, y, z; Soechting & Flanders, 1993). The shift in hand position can be accomplished by changing the frame of reference of the arm (Feldman, 2011), while the hand path may emerge by continuous changes in the configuration of multiple joints based on specific performance constraints. Failure to correctly perceive the actual coordinates of the to-be-reached object in space leads to errors in performance at several levels. Similarly, for mobility skills, perception of movement when modulated by optic flow can influence movement speed, accuracy, and variability (Gibson, 1958). There is an inverse relationship between optic flow speed and walking speed such that decreases in optic flow result in increases in walking speed (Prokop, Schubert, & Berger, 1997; Schubert, Prokop, Brocke, & Berger, 2005; Varraine, Bonnard, & Pailhous, 2002) and stride length (Prokop et al., 1997; Schubert et al., 2005). Rossignol (1996) explained the modulation of gait speed by optic flow by having visual signals act on central pattern generators, changing the timing or the amplitude of muscle activation in the legs. An alternative explanation is that control of this locomotor activity is based on the perception of speed of self-motion that arises from a combination of body-based and visual senses (De Smet, Malcolm, Lenoir, Segers, & De Clercq, 2009). VR technologies have evolved with the purpose of generating illusions that resemble the 3D physical reality. This is carried out by exploiting the fact that while the eyes are able to sense the visual information, it is actually the "healthy" brain that perceives and processes the spatial information that provide the 3D experience (De Valois, & De Valois, 1980).

Knowledge of sensory and cognitive processes involved in perception is essential to generate a 3D illusion that leads to desired functional movements (Gregory, 1980). However, damage to the CNS may lead to deficits in perception (e.g., inability to see parts of the visual image in patients with spatial neglect), which may further underlie an inability to extract and process salient information to produce appropriate motor actions (e.g., inability to predict events leading to a failure in timing of movements). Most commercial 2D or 3D VR systems developed for entertainment purposes are based on the assumption that the brain of the user is capable of perceiving and interacting with the environment in rapid and appropriate ways. Gaps between the physical and the virtual scenes are filled in by the user who makes assumptions about the continuity of the environment. Under such assumptions, a performer in VR is expected to produce movements or movement surrogates that are similar to those used in the physical world for similar activities. In light of the aforementioned, it is pertinent to ask how valid are movements made in commonly provided 3D environments in users who may be unable to recover missing visual cues. Further, is it possible to use haptic cues to augment or replace visual cues? These are among the questions that should be addressed as a prelude for the implementation of VR in neurorehabilitation.

In this chapter, we consider primarily whether direct or surrogate measures of movement made in VR are valid without a more in-depth analysis of the cognitive and perceptual features of the environments in which they are made. Details about perception and the environment are found in Chap. 4.

6.3 How Does Motor Behavior Need to Be Validated in VR to Determine the Usefulness of Virtual Practice Environments?

Characterization of motor behavior is important to determine how the individual interacts with the VR environment. We define *motor behavior validity* as movements that are made with similar temporal and spatial parameters, muscle activation patterns, and joint forces as those made in a physical environment. There are also surrogate measures of motor behavior including energy expenditure and neural substrates that provide additional sources of validity. In the following sections, motor behavior is described under three categories (Table 6.1). Two categories are related to

Table 6.1 Categories of motor behavior used in VE validation

1. Movement performance	2. Movement quality	3. Surrogate measures of movement
Movement straightness	Range of joint motion	Energy expenditure
Movement smoothness	Inter-joint coordination	Neural correlates
Movement accuracy	Electromyographic signals	
Movement speed		
Movement variability	Forces and torques	

movement production: movement performance and movement quality (Levin et al., 2009). A third category describes surrogate measures of movement. In the *movement performance* category, the parameters of *smoothness*, *speed*, *accuracy*, and variability define how well the end effector (hand or foot) or the whole body arrives at the desired location. A second category, *movement quality*, provides a description of the temporal and spatial aspects of joint ranges of motion and electromyographic (EMG) signals or the *movement patterns* that underlie the endpoint movement. The third category describes surrogate measures or markers of performance beyond those described by kinematics. Some parameters apply more to discrete limb movements (e.g., reaching), and others better describe continuous movements (e.g., walking). Therefore, terminology may vary with the motor behavior studied (e.g., endpoint accuracy for a UL-targeted movement and stride variability for gait).

6.3.1 Performance Level: Movement Straightness

As the arm moves away from the body to reach for objects, the endpoint (hand) follows a relatively straight-line trajectory when moving on a plane (Morasso, 1981). Although it may seem simple to perform, straight-line motion requires a high degree of inter-joint coordination where all joint movements share a common time frame and move in the orchestrated manner. Unlike the endpoint, the limb joints (e.g., shoulder, elbow) follow curved angular trajectories that are related to each other in a nonlinear manner (Hollerbach & Atkeson, 1987). It is the specific relationship between movements of adjacent joints that enables the system to generate the commonly observed straight-line motion of the endpoint. The straight spatial configuration of the endpoint in task space underlies a complex inter-joint coordination that is likely affected by CNS injury (e.g., Archambault, Pigeon, Feldman, & Levin, 1999). Therefore, measures of path deviation from the shortest possible paths (e.g., straight lines in 2D or geodesic paths in 3D) may be used to diagnose motor impairment and to assess upper limb recovery at the performance level. For example, absolute deviation from straight-line trajectories of the hand (i.e., as assessed by the root mean square difference between the observed and the calculated trajectory, RMSD) has been used to compare movements made in healthy and stroke patients performing in VE compared to those performed in physical environments (Liebermann, Berman, Weiss, & Levin, 2012).

6.3.2 Performance Level: Movement Smoothness

Endpoint movements are also characterized by smooth transitions from one point in space to another (Hogan, 1984). This feature is particularly relevant when performing functional motor tasks with the UL such as displacing a cup of tea or performing a graceful pointing movement. Smooth movements start at zero velocity and are generally characterized by symmetric bell-shaped tangential velocity profiles as the limb accelerates and then decelerates to return to zero velocity when an object is approached or movement is terminated. This robust feature of healthy endpoint motion has been observed for planar reaching movements (Flash & Hogan, 1985) as well as for 3D arm movements (Todorov & Jordan, 1998), and it may be unrelated to the trajectory followed to reach for an object (straight, curved, etc.). Parameterization of smoothness has led to several temporal descriptors of normal limb motion associated with the endpoint velocity profile, which describes the evolution of the endpoint path over time. The velocity profile during maximally smooth movement characteristic of healthy individuals is expected to be unimodal and symmetrical, showing a peak velocity at about 50 % of the movement time. The quantification of the number of peaks in the endpoint velocity profile is a temporal measure that has been widely used for the assessment of smoothness of the endpoint path. Fragmentation (characterized by the number of peaks in the endpoint velocity profile) is often increased in movements made by stroke patients (Cirstea & Levin, 2000; Dipietro, Krebs, Fasoli, Volpe, & Hogan, 2009; Rohrer et al., 2002) as well as by Parkinson's disease patients (Dounskaia, Van Gemmert, Leis, & Stelmach, 2009; Inzelberg, Flash, Schechtman, & Korczyn, 1995).

6.3.3 Performance Level: Movement Accuracy

Movement accuracy is defined as a function of movement velocity according to the criteria of Fitts' law (1954). Accordingly, faster movements are associated with a lower chance of ending the movement accurately in a given location in space. Movements are characterized by a linear relationship between the errors in movement accuracy and movement velocity: as movement velocity increases, the error in accuracy increases proportionally. This relationship has been widely investigated, and it is robust under most conditions and in various populations. However, patient populations with UL impairment tend to make slower movements. While Fitts' law would predict higher accuracy with slower reaching movement, the law may not hold under certain clinical conditions. For example, after a stroke, despite slower movements, accuracy is not increased (Cirstea & Levin, 2000).

6.3.4 Movement Quality level

Additional performance measures may be used to assess the quality of movement with respect to the movement elements that contribute to the overall endpoint movement. Movements can be characterized in terms of the number of joints (degrees of freedom, DOFs) involved in the task and the total range of joint rotation of each joint (range of motion, ROM). In addition, the spatiotemporal relationship between movements of different DOFs can be quantified using angle–angle phase plots, cross-correlations, or other methods to describe inter-joint and intra-joint relative timing during reaching (Cirstea, Mitnitski, Feldman, & Levin, 2003) and walking (Daly et al., 2012; Ford, Wagenaar, & Newell, 2007; Krasovsky et al., 2012).

Total forces or inter-joint torques of the endpoint or interactive torques produced between adjacent joints can also be characterized (Dewald & Beer, 2001; Dewald, Pope, Given, Buchanan, & Rymer, 1995). Endpoint forces for the UL and LL are only produced when the limb interacts with an object or a surface (e.g., interactive forces or torques in the UL when painting a wall or using a keyboard) or with the ground (e.g., ground reaction forces during walking). The endpoint (finger, hand, foot) does not produce force in order to move through space, but rather, movement occurs when forces are produced at individual, more proximal joints in an appropriate direction to drive the endpoint towards the desired goal. This factor is important, especially for assessing how the hand interacts in VR (Berman, Liebermann, & McIntyre, 2014) when haptic (tactile/force) feedback is not provided to the user, since the lack of interactive forces affects movement production (Bingham, Bradley, Bailey, & Vinner, 2001; Hibbard & Bradshaw, 2003).

6.3.5 Surrogate Measures of Movement

Body movements and motor behaviors can be characterized not only by kinematics but also by other surrogate measures of movement, including metabolic and physiologic characteristics as well as neural correlates of the movement. Physiologic (e.g., heart rate) and metabolic (e.g., energy expenditure) effects during motor activities are important in neurorehabilitation because they are associated with movement efficiency and have been shown to be altered in neurological populations (Brouwer, Parvataneni, & Olney, 2009, Katzel et al., 2012, Novak & Brouwer, 2012) and during motor learning (Huang, Kram, & Ahmed, 2012). Movements encouraged by VEs designed to simulate life situations are expected to have similar physiologic demands as those made in physical environments. In addition, although sensorimotor rehabilitation traditionally focuses on improving specific aspects of movement, such as performance or movement quality variables, physiologic responses are involved in regaining functional independence. Different forms of rehabilitation, such as treadmill walking and cycling, were suggested to promote cardiovascular fitness by engaging the individual in activities that have relatively high metabolic demands. Varieties of commercial and customized VEs have been developed to promote activity and fitness, and some such as the Xbox Kinect and Nintendo Wii have been adopted for use in rehabilitation of individuals with neurological diseases.

6.4 Validity of UL Movements Made in Virtual Environments

Several studies have addressed the validity of movement kinematics in VEs during movements of the upper and lower limbs. Differences between movements made in physical and virtual environments may be due to the type of VE in which the movement is performed. In this section, kinematic equivalence of movements made in 2D and 3D VEs compared to physical environments is discussed.

6.4.1 Reaching and Grasping Movements in 2D VR

In 2D VR, such as games played on computer screens (interactive virtual gaming, IVG) and certain commercially available VR systems (e.g., video-capture IREX, SeeMe), reaching extent may be influenced by the lack of depth cues. In one of the first studies of kinematic equivalence in VR, Viau, Feldman, McFadyen, and Levin (2004) compared reaching, grasping, transporting, and placing a ball in a 2D virtual environment displayed on a computer screen with no visual depth cues to those made in a physical environment of equivalent dimensions in healthy subjects. For the grasping component of the movement, a virtual hand representation was obtained with a specialized glove that provided both position (strain gauge sensors; Cyberglove, Immersion Corp.) and haptic information about the ball (force-feedback device, Cybergrasp, Immersion Corp.). Arm kinematic data were recorded with an optical motion analysis system (Optotrak, Northern Digital Inc.). Movements for each of the three components (reaching, grasping, and transporting, a ball) were similar in terms of spatial and temporal kinematics in both environments. However, due to the absence of depth cues and tactile feedback at the end of the transporting phase in VR, subjects used more elbow extension and less wrist extension compared to the physical environment. Similarly, Lott, Bisson, Lajoie, McComas, and Sveistrup (2003) found that center of pressure (COP) excursions during a lateral reaching task in a 2D VE viewed on a large screen were larger than those in the physical environment. Larger COP excursions suggested that the range of lateral arm reach was also greater. Viewing the same VE through a head-mounted display (HMD) also resulted in longer arm reaches as well as increased anteroposterior COP sway.

Liebermann et al. (2012) studied the kinematic validity of pointing movements made by healthy subjects and subjects with chronic stroke when viewing targets in a video-capture 2D VR system (IREX, GestureTek Inc.) viewed on a large TV monitor and an equivalent physical environment (Fig. 6.1). Arm and trunk kinematics were

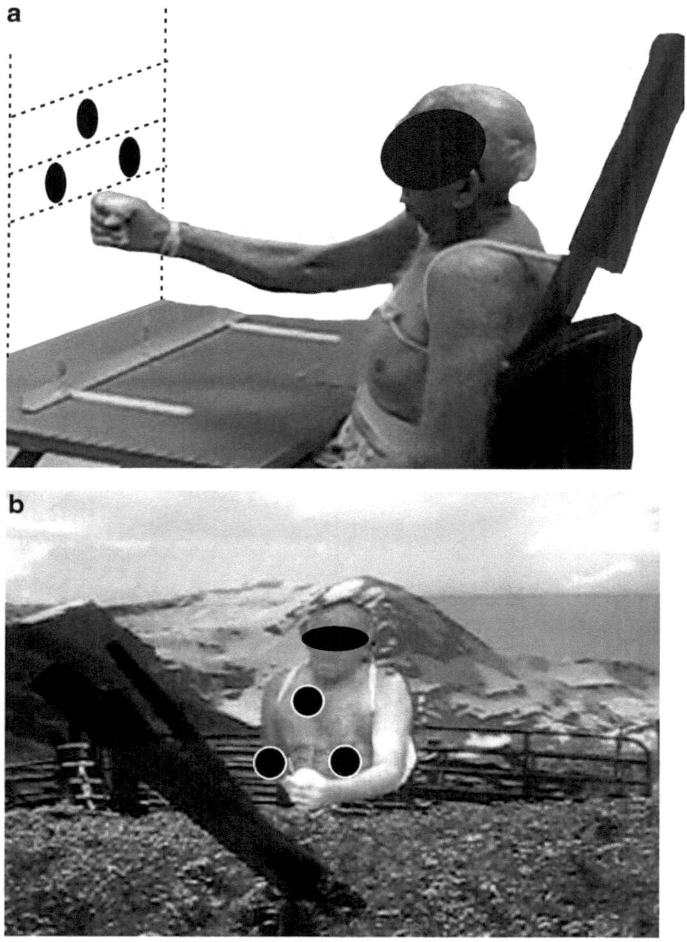

Fig. 6.1 Experimental setup for comparison of reaching in two different environments. (**a**) Physical environment. (**b**) Video-capture 2D virtual reality environment. Targets in each environment were identically calibrated to appear in the same parts of the arm workspace. In the physical environment, the targets were directly observed by the subject. In the virtual environment, the subject saw themselves and the targets in an alpine scene in a television monitor

recorded for reaches made with the right, dominant arm to three targets in the arm workspace. Reaching movements made by both control (healthy, age matched) and stroke subjects were affected by viewing the targets in 2D VR. Movements of the endpoint were slower, hypometric (shorter), shorter, less straight, and less accurate and involved smaller ranges of shoulder and elbow joint excursions for target reaches in VR compared to the physical environment for all subjects (Fig. 6.2). Thus, there was a decrease in the overall movement performance and quality for reaching movements made in 2D VR.

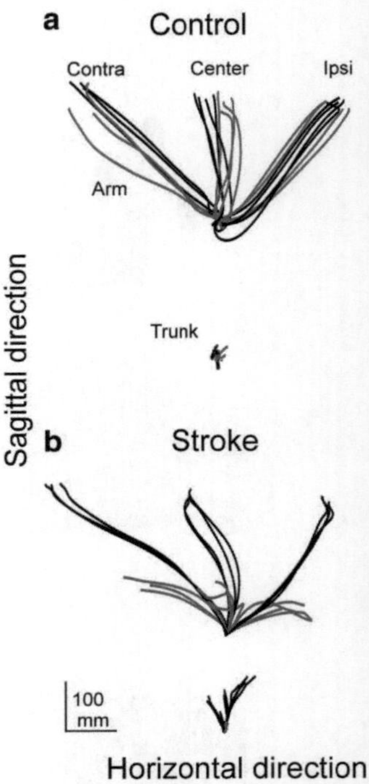

Fig. 6.2 Examples of arm and trunk trajectories for one healthy age-matched control subject (**a**) and one subject with chronic stroke (**b**) reaching for targets located in three parts of the arm workspace (Contra: contralateral target; Center: midline target; Ipsi: ipsilateral target). Movement trajectories are shown for reaches made in the physical (*black lines*) and the video-capture virtual reality environment (*grey lines*). Movements made in the virtual environment were less straight and less accurate in both examples

A possible explanation for the altered movement patterns for reaches made in 2D VR was that subjects did not perceive the depth dimension from the simple 2D cues provided by the environment. Differences in movement patterns between environments were present in both groups, but differences were more marked in the group of stroke subjects and were greater in stroke subjects with more severe motor impairment. The authors concluded that 2D video-capture VR should be used with caution when the goal of the rehabilitation program is to improve the quality of movement patterns of the UL.

6.4.1.1 Kinematics of Movements Made in Game-Like Systems

The kinematic validity of movements recorded with markerless camera-based motion tracking systems is an area of growing interest because of the development of game-like applications for upper and lower limb motor rehabilitation. Several of these systems use the Kinect (Microsoft Xbox) camera that reconstructs the user's gestures using a simplified 15 joint skeleton in real time. The Kinect RGB camera has an 8-bit VGA resolution (640×480 pixels) and a monochrome depth sensor having a VGA resolution of 11 bits that allows 2,048 levels of sensitivity. The approximate resolution of Kinect is 1.3 mm per pixel. Several groups have evaluated the accuracy of movement kinematics recorded with the Kinect camera (Dutta,

2012; Fernandez-Baena, Susın, & Lligadas, 2012; Zhang et al., 2012). Compared to planar joint kinematics recorded with a 24 camera Vicon system, Fernandez-Baena et al. (2012) reported that errors using Kinect camera tracking ranged from 6.8° to 9.0° (7.6–8.5 % of movement amplitude) for movements of the knee and from 7.1° to 13.2° (5.1–16.0 % of movement amplitude) for movements of the shoulder in three planes (sagittal, coronal, and transverse). For the shoulder, the largest errors occurred for movements in the transverse plane. Similarly, Tao, Archambault, and Levin (2013) determined the extent to which Kinect tracking of hand position, elbow angle, and trunk position matched that recorded by an Optotrak motion-tracking system. They used the root mean square difference between Kinect and Optotrak data to estimate Kinect tracking error. For reaching movements, the constant error averaged 6.3 cm and variable error 2.4 cm. These estimates did not take into account larger errors that occurred at extreme lateral positions of the reaching workspace. The mean error for tracking movement of the trunk was 3.9 cm (constant) and 2.5 cm (variable), excluding the farthest and nearest rows where the error jumped to over 12 cm. Elbow angle mean error was 26.7° (constant) and 6.2° (variable). The large constant error for the elbow was likely due to a modeling limitation of the Kinect, which, when corrected for, closely matched Optotrak data. The authors provide recommendations for the camera tracking placement in order to obtain the best motion tracking for upper limb applications. The Kinect camera should be located within a 30×30 cm^2 at a distance of between 1.45 and 1.75 m from the user and at 0.15 m to either the left or the right.

6.4.2 *Reaching Movements in 3D VR and Effect of Display Medium*

UL movements made in 3D VR are reported to be more similar to those made in physical environments than those made in 2D VR. For example, Knaut, Subramanian, McFadyen, Bourbonnais, and Levin (2009) compared the kinematics of pointing movements into different parts of the arm workspace in a physical environment and in fully immersive VE, viewed through a HMD. For healthy subjects, precision and trajectory straightness were higher in the VE when pointing to contralateral targets and movements were slower for all targets in VE. Stroke participants made less accurate and more curved movements in the VE and used less trunk displacement. Elbow/shoulder coordination differed when pointing to the lower ipsilateral target. In a follow-up study, Subramanian, Massie, Malcolm, and Levin (2011) found that in healthy subjects ($n=10$) and subjects with chronic stroke ($n=20$), there were no differences in performance (endpoint trajectory straightness) and movement quality variables (shoulder flexion, shoulder horizontal adduction ranges, and sagittal trunk displacement) between the two media. All subjects, however, made larger errors in the vertical direction using the HMD compared to viewing the VE on a large screen display. Movements in healthy subjects were also less precise in the sagittal direction and slower and used less range of elbow extension for the lower central target when the VR was viewed through the HMD compared to the screen display. The results differed in the stroke group depending on the motor impairment level of the participant. In subjects with mild and moderate-to-severe stroke RMS errors were larger when the environment was viewed through the HMD. The only advantage of using the HMD was that movements were made faster in the stroke subjects compared to those made when the scene was viewed on the screen.

6.4.3 Role of Haptic Feedback for Grasping Movements Made in VR

The question of how the presence or the absence of haptic feedback, especially for hand movements, affects grasping kinematics is an important one in the consideration of VR training environments for UL movements. Wang et al. (2011) compared temporal reaching parameters (movement time, peak velocity, and deceleration) for stationary and moving targets in a 3D VE projected to a large screen and viewed with polarized glasses, but without haptic feedback. Movements were compared to similar movements performed in a physical environment in participants with Parkinson's disease (PD) and healthy subjects. For both groups, reaching movements made in VR were slower and had longer deceleration phases than in the physical environment. However, for moving targets, both healthy and PD subjects were able to increase their movement speed according to the speed of the moving object, indicating that visual movement cues could be used in a similar fashion in the two environments. Similarly, Dvorkin, Shahar, and Weiss (2006) reported that healthy subjects had comparable temporal movement parameters (reaction times, movement time) when responding to moving targets in a physical environment and a 3D VE.

Kinematics of grasping are influenced by the presence or the absence of haptic information in VR. When reaching to grasp stationary objects in a 3D VE without haptic feedback, healthy adults had similar movement times but lower peak velocities compared to a similar task in a physical environment (Kuhlen, Kraiss, & Steffan, 2000). The effect of haptic feedback for reach-to-grasp tasks in a 3D VE was studied by Magdalon and colleagues (2011; Fig. 6.3). Movements to three physical and virtual objects were compared: a cylindrical can, a screwdriver, and a pen (Fig. 6.3b). Haptic feedback was provided by a Cyberglove/Cybergrasp system in VR in ten healthy subjects (eight women, 62.1 ± 8.8 years). Temporal and spatial arm and trunk kinematics were analyzed. Similar hand orientation patterns were used when grasping both physical and virtual objects, except for forearm supination when grasping the can in VR (Fig. 6.3c). Axial and planar joint excursions were similar between environments for grasping the screwdriver in VR. However, overall, movements were slower in the VE compared to those made in the physical environment—relative times to peak hand velocity occurred ~10 % earlier, and relative deceleration times were longer in the VE. Hand aperture was similar between environments for the

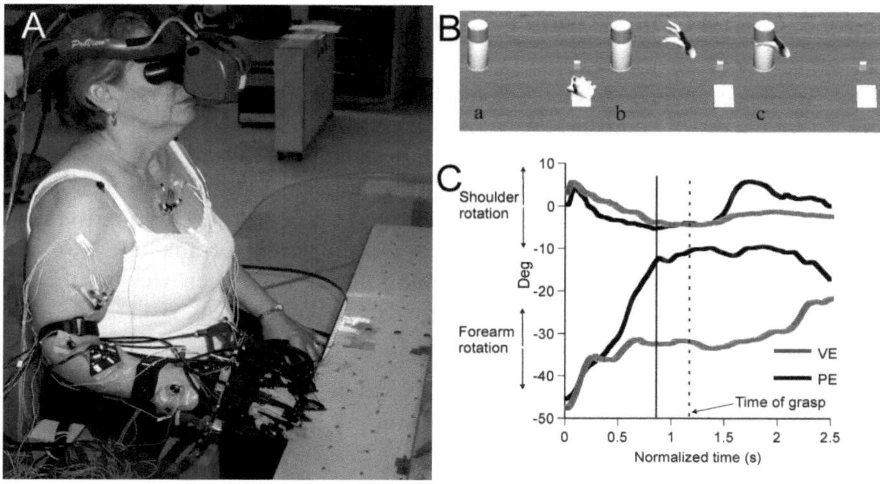

Fig. 6.3 (**a**) Experimental setup used in Magdalon, Michaelsen, Quevedo, and Levin (2011). For reach-to-grasp movements in a virtual environment, subjects viewed a 3D display of three objects via a head-mounted display and received haptic feedback via a Cyberglove/Cybergrasp system. (**b**) View of the reach-to-grasp movement towards a cylindrical can in the virtual environment: a, at start of movement; b, at peak hand aperture; c, at time of grasping. (**c**) Comparison of range of shoulder and forearm rotation during reaching for the cylindrical can in the virtual environment (VE—*grey traces*) and the physical environment (PE—*black traces*). *Solid vertical line*: Time of maximal hand aperture. *Dashed vertical line*: Time of grasping

cylindrical grasp, but apertures were wider for the screwdriver and pen in the VE. Overall, temporal grasping patterns were similar in both environments. Some of the observed differences in kinematics may have been due to the encumbering effect of wearing a haptic glove system on the hand. Compared to movements made in a physical environment without the glove, movements made in this environment while wearing the glove were slower and had wider grip apertures. However, differences in spatial and temporal kinematics of movements made in the 3D VE were greater than those due to wearing the Cyberglove/grasp system. Similar differences in grasping kinematics due to the environment (VR vs. physical environment) and the presence or the absence of haptic information were reported in a group of ten subjects with chronic stroke when grasping movements were done to the same three targets (Magdalon, Levin, Quevedo, & Michaelsen, 2008).

For interceptive actions, movement initiation time, movement time, and the time to intercept a physical or a virtual ball displayed on a 2D white screen were compared in 32 healthy young subjects (Baures, Benguigui, Amorim, & Hecht, 2009). There were only small differences in the timing of the ball interception in the two environments that occurred only in the first series of trials.

6.4.4 Use of Compensatory Movements for Reaching

Three studies evaluated the effect of reaching/grasping movements made in 2D or 3D VR on the use of compensatory movements of the trunk in subjects with stroke. These found that excessive trunk movement was reduced for reaching movements made in a 2D VE viewed on a large screen (Liebermann et al., 2012) or in a 3D VE viewed through an HMD (Knaut et al., 2009) compared to reaching movements made in equivalent physical environments. Compensatory trunk use was also decreased in stroke subjects making reaching movements when viewing the VE through an HMD compared to a large screen (Subramanian et al., 2011).

6.5 Validation of Mobility and Lower Limb Movements

VR systems designed to promote balance and mobility share some motor control requirements with UL movements. Therefore, characterizing movement performance and quality is a relevant approach to establishing the validity of these systems. However, the requirements for mobility do not have the same level of specificity as do those for the UL. The approach to validate mobility and lower limb (LL) movements in VR has been more eclectic. Validation of VR for mobility and walking has taken several forms, which include comparing walking in VR to real-world walking using measures of movement quality such as joint motion, forces, and muscle activation patterns; testing proactive and reactive walking strategies using both movement performance and quality measures; validating walking performance using optic flow manipulations; and indirectly validating movement performance using surrogate measures such as neural substrates of walking and metabolic and physiologic measures during interactive video gaming.

6.5.1 Comparison with Real-World Tasks

Studies of validation of walking, mobility, and balance in VR have taken the form of varying the conditions in VR to determine if the behavior is in the predicted direction. For example, simulating walking on ice may require a walking pattern that has shorter steps, greater hip flexion during the swing phase, and a more vertical ground reaction force to decrease the likelihood of slipping (Deutsch, Lewis, Minsky, Burdea, & Boian, 2007). In another study, Antley and Slater (2011) measured movement quality using the mean number of EMG onsets per second of the erector spinae muscles (at lumbar levels 4 and 5) during walking on a normal floor, a ribbon, and a small balance beam counterbalanced between real-world and 3D cave-like environments. In the VE, the pattern of muscle activation was similar to walking in the physical environment but the magnitude of the EMG signals was lower. Similarly, Hollman, Brey, Robb, Bang, and Kaufman (2006; Hollman, Brey,

Bang, & Kaufman, 2007) characterized movement quality using joint angles and forces and movement performance using a temporal-spatial analysis of variability while walking on an instrumented treadmill with and without a VE. In the 160° curved screen-projected VE, walking occurred in a simulated corridor with colored stripes projected on the walls. Gait was less stable when walking in VR compared to the physical environment as evidenced by increased rates and variability of weight acceptance and push-off (Hollman et al., 2006). Walking performance was also altered as evidenced by reduced stride length, increased step width, and increased variability in stride velocity and step width (Hollman et al., 2007).

6.5.2 Proactive and Reactive Strategies

While locomotion is partially automatic and controlled at lower levels of the nervous system (Pearson & Gordon, 2000), walking behavior requires that the nervous system integrate a complex set of sensory inputs (visual, tactile, proprioceptive, and vestibular) in order for the body to interact with and navigate through diverse environments. The relevance of VR to walking occurs at this higher level of integration.

Walking behavior may be adjusted proactively or reactively (Shumway-Cook & Woollacott, 2012), and both mechanisms have been studied in VR. Using visual perturbations Nyberg et al. (2006) built a 3D model of a marketplace in Umea, Sweden, in which walkers were presented with conditions such as a tilted environment or a sudden snowfall (fed by magnetic trackers viewed through an HMD) that required reactive adjustments in gait. They reported stimulus-specific responses, such as a loss of balance with tilting but not when walking overground and changes in gait speed and stride length associated with slipping in the snowy condition. McAndrew and colleagues (2010) used movement performance and quality measures of the reactive responses of walking to pseudorandom oscillations of the support surface and visual field. Participants walked in a no-perturbation condition and under conditions of anterior-posterior or medial-lateral walking surface perturbations with visual oscillations. The 3D VR Computer Assisted Rehabilitation Environment (CAREN) was projected 300° around the subject from 40° below and 60° above eye level. Relative to no perturbations, participants took shorter and wider steps in the perturbed conditions. Variability of step length, step width, and trunk velocity was greatest in the medio-lateral direction when comparing to walking without perturbations to walking with anteroposterior and medial perturbations (of both the visual and the support surface). The responses to the perturbations were graded based on the intensity and direction of perturbation. This regularity of the response to the pseudorandom perturbations validates the use of VR to study the effects of physical and visual perturbations on locomotor patterns. In a study of proactive responses to a walking stimulus, Cinelli and Patla (2008) compared walking through oscillating doors in the physical world to previous work using the same paradigm by Montagne, Buekers, de Rugy, Camachon, and Laurent (2002; Montagne, Buekers, Camachon, de Rugy, & Laurent, 2003) in a VR walking system (de Rugy, Montagne, Buekers, & Laurent, 2000). The system coupled a treadmill and motion tracking with walking performance on a rear projected 3D VE of doors of different apertures oscillating at different rates presented randomly. They (Cinelli & Patla, 2008) found that young female walkers modulated their walking speed in anticipation of the motion of the doors in both real-world and simulated environments. However, they observed that only in the physical environment participants added a shoulder rotation strategy as they approached the door when they perceived that reducing walking speed alone would not prevent a collision. The perception–action coupling of walking was interpreted to be similar in VR and real-world walking.

6.5.3 Optic Flow

Descending pathways are needed for the initiation and adaptation of walking. The supraspinal regulation of stepping includes (1) activation of the spinal locomotor system to control the overall walking speed, (2) grading of force generation in response to feedback from the limbs, and (3) guiding of stepping direction in response to visual input (Pearson & Gordon, 2000). Therefore, as with UL movement, the role of vision is important for guiding walking and the number of studies that use optic flow manipulations in VR can be considered an indirect form of validation of the use of this technology to study locomotion.

The most common form of validation of walking is an indirect one, in which optic flow is manipulated with the expectation that it will modify walking behavior. Primarily, these manipulations are tested while walking on a treadmill with or without VR. Often, studies include a non-VR condition with inference of validity when behavior changes relative to the non-VR condition. Typically, optic flow is manipulated so that it is neutral, increased, or decreased. Optic flow manipulations have been used to study gait variability during forward and backward walking (Katsavelis, Mukherjee, Decker, & Stergiou, 2010) and as a result of aging (Chou et al., 2009). Using a virtual corridor, Katsavelis and colleagues (2010) found that for forward walking in VR with congruent, fast, slow, or absent optic flow, movement quality variables did not differ with a linear analysis, but did differ when a nonlinear analysis of hip, ankle, and stride variables was performed. In contrast, there was no difference in walking parameters when subjects walked backward under three conditions: no visual cues and forward and backward optic flow. The use of nonlinear measures of walking required longer walking intervals than did the linear measures (20–30 steps compared to 700 steps). It is possible that the understanding of the role of optic flow on walking is changed by the demands of the nonlinear analysis. Namely, there may be some adaptations that are not seen in the shorter studies. This nonlinear method of analysis raises questions about the validation of walking in VR using optic flow under short compared to long walking trials.

6.5.4 Neural Correlates of Movement in VR

Functional neuroimaging studies can serve as another indirect form of validation by identifying similarities between neural networks of walking in VR and physical environments. Mellet and colleagues (2010) demonstrated using fMRI that the neural correlates of recalling images that were learned while navigating in VR were not identical to those recalled by those who walked in a physical environment, even though their performance was similar. Brain regions were activated in common parietal-frontal areas and the parahippocampal gyrus. The individuals who performed the navigation task in VR using a joy stick retained a left-lateralized network that the investigators attributed to tool manipulation and action semantics. It would be interesting to repeat this experiment using the LL as the effector to determine if the dissimilarity between groups may be reduced. Other interesting work on understanding the importance of biological motion identified that the posterior superior temporal sulcus was activated only when the walker approached an avatar that was moving, in contrast to an avatar standing still or inanimate objects. Possibly the study of neural correlates of movement in VR may guide the development of VEs that are highly specific and potentially more effective than those based solely on behavioral outcomes.

6.5.5 Validation of Metabolic and Physiologic Measures of Mobility Activities

Validation of physiologic measures of activities performed in VE refers here to the similarity between the energy expenditure (EE) of the task performed in VR and the same task when performed in a real-life situation. The validation of EE in VR is an active area of research mostly in healthy but also in special populations. The main comparative measures include metabolic equivalents, or calories, for EE and heart rate for the physiologic response. Validity of these measures has been addressed mainly for VR in the form of IVGs, also called active video games (AVGs) when the gaming goal is to promote activity.

The primary aim is to evaluate whether physical activity in VR, usually in the form of a game, can provide physical activity of adequate intensity to promote health, weight control, and cardiovascular fitness. Hence, comparisons are usually done between EE of AVGs and EE of standard modes of physical activity such as walking on a treadmill and cycling. Comparisons show variability between games, with different games having higher, similar, or lower EE as compared with common modes of real-life physical activities. For example, Wii Sports and Fit games have been shown to have EE and physiologic responses similar to treadmill or overground walking at a comfortable speed (Bailey & McInnis, 2011, Graf, Pratt, Hester, & Short, 2009, White, Schofield, & Kilding, 2011). However, since activities performed in VR and in the real-life tasks were different, these studies do not allow validation of EE and HR in the VR.

Comparisons of EE and HR between identical and comparable activities performed in the VE and real life are scarce. Douris, McDonald, Vespi, Kelley, and Herman (2012) compared EE of brisk walking (3.5 mph) on a treadmill with Wii Fit "Free Run," each performed by healthy young adults for 30 min. They found that the physiological response of AVG was significantly higher than standard activity (20 %). However, these two activities are not exactly comparable. While playing "Free Run," participants were allowed to jog, walk, or run, while the standard activity was limited to walking, suggesting that the workload was different. Haddock, Siegel, and Wikin (2009) compared stationary cycling and stationary cycling while playing an interactive video game in healthy children (7–14 years old). Each condition was performed for 20 min, and participants were instructed to "get as much exercise in as possible" and were allowed to self-select the pedaling frequency. Results showed significantly higher EE for cycling in VR (16 %) but no significant difference in HR and rate of perceived exertion between environments. Although significant, the difference in EE was moderate and with minimal clinical significance (addition of 14.5 kcal for the whole session). Warburton et al. (2009) measured EE, HR, and rate of perceived exertion of healthy young adults during traditional cycling and cycling in VR using a stationary bicycle that can be used for either interactive video game exercise or traditional cycling at three workload levels (25, 50, and 75 % of peak power output). Participants were allowed to self-select the pedaling frequency; however, cycling in the VR required cycling at various frequencies to win the game. Therefore, pedaling frequency was significantly higher in the VR. At a constant workload of 25 and 50 %, EE and HR were higher for cycling in the interactive VE, with no difference at a workload level of 75 %. Fitzgerald et al. (2004) tested EE of athletes who were wheelchair users during 19 min of arm-ergometer exercising in VR compared to exercising without VR. No differences were found between environments.

Overall, these studies suggest that EE and physiological responses are higher when the activity is performed in VR. However, it is not clear if those differences have any clinical relevance. It also demonstrates the difficulty of comparing activities when the effort is self-imposed and when the workload cannot be controlled. As demonstrated by Douris et al. (2012) and Warburton et al. (2009), even when the activities are identical, the actual exercise effort may differ.

Findings predominantly apply to populations of children, adolescents, and young adults, who are mostly healthy. However, work characterizing energy expenditure during AVGs has also been reported for people post-stroke (Hurkmans, Ribbers, Streur-Kranenburg, Stam, & van den Berg-Emons, 2011; Kafri, Myslinksi, Gade, & Deutsch, 2013). It is interesting to note that variables, related to the individual, the activity, or the VR characteristics, can modify energy expenditure and affect the association between EE and physiological responses in VR and physical environments. Variables of the individual that were found to modify EE during IVG include the competitiveness of the user (Anderson-Hanley, Snyder, Nimon, & Arciero, 2011), age, and gender (Warburton et al., 2009). Variables related with VR that have been reported to modify EE include the presence of a virtual opponent (avatar) (Anderson-Hanley et al., 2011) and console features such as the type of sensors. Variables related to the activity include the involved muscle groups and type of muscle contraction (Bonetti, Drury, Danoff, & Miller, 2010).

6.6 Conclusion

Since the introduction of VR interfaces into the motor rehabilitation toolkit, considerable work has been done to validate movements made in various environments. However, there is still much work to be done.

To date, studies comparing UL movements made by healthy individuals in VR compared to physical environments have shown that movement performance and quality variables are better when the VR is rendered or viewed in 3D compared to 2D coordinates. This is not surprising given the close interaction between perception and action in movement production. Studies have also shown that VR environments can be chosen to produce desired motor behaviors, such as the reduction of motor compensations made by the trunk when using 2D VR or when viewing the VE through an HMD. More information is needed, however, about the role of haptics and the use of interfaces on the kinematics of reaching and grasping movements produced in 2D and 3D VR.

Compared to the UL, few studies have compared movement performance and quality variables associated with discrete LL movements. Instead most studies have compared walking under different conditions to determine if the behavior occurs in the expected direction. While there is more information about temporal locomotor outcomes, how spatial measures and measures of coordination are affected by VR has received less attention. However, individuals walking in VR with perturbations respond in the expected direction based on models of normal walking. Studies have also focused on the comparison of energy expenditure while exercising in different physical and VR environments as a way of validating VR as an exercise environment.

The potential for VR to enhance sensorimotor recovery is related to the availability of a motivating environment for increasing the frequency of movement and providing salient feedback. However, when improving movement quality is the goal, care should be taken to ensure that movements made in VR are similar in spatial and temporal structure to those which have to be reacquired. This is important since practicing undesired movement may lead to motor compensations because of the inherent redundancy of the nervous system that may ultimately limit the level of motor recovery that can be achieved (Levin et al., 2009; Moon, Alaverdashvili, Cross, & Whishaw, 2009).

References

Anderson-Hanley, C., Snyder, A. L., Nimon, J. P., & Arciero, P. J. (2011). Social facilitation in virtual reality-enhanced exercise: Competitiveness moderates exercise effort of older adults. *Clinical Interventions in Aging, 6*, 275–280.

Antley, A., & Slater, M. (2011). The effect on lower spine muscle activation of walking on a narrow beam in virtual reality. *IEEE Transactions on Visualization and Computer Graphics, 17*(2), 255–259.

Archambault, P., Pigeon, P., Feldman, A. G., & Levin, M. F. (1999). Recruitment and sequencing of different degrees of freedom during pointing movements involving the trunk in healthy and hemiparetic subjects. *Experimental Brain Research, 126*, 55–67.

Bailey, B. W., & McInnis, K. (2011). Energy cost of exergaming: A comparison of the energy cost of 6 forms of exergaming. *Archives of Pediatrics and Adolescent Medicine, 165*(7), 597–602.

Baures, R., Benguigui, N., Amorim, M. A., & Hecht, H. (2009). Intercepting real and simulated falling objects: What is the difference? *Journal of Neuroscience Methods, 184*, 48–53.

Berman, S., Liebermann, D.G., & McIntyre, J. (2014). Constrained motion control on a hemispherical surface: path planning. *Journal of Neurophysiology, 111*(5), 954–968. doi: 10.1152/jn.00132.2013.

Bernstein, N. A. (1967). *The control and regulation of movements*. London: Pergamon Press.

Bingham, G. P., Bradley, A., Bailey, M., & Vinner, R. (2001). Accommodation, occlusion and disparity matching are used to guide reaching: A comparison of actual versus virtual environments. *Journal of Experimental Psychology: Human Perception and Performance, 27*, 1314–1344.

Bonetti, A. J., Drury, D. G., Danoff, J. V., & Miller, T. A. (2010). Comparison of acute exercise responses between conventional video gaming and isometric resistance exergaming. *Journal of Strength and Conditioning Research, 24*(7), 1799–1803.

Brouwer, B., Parvataneni, K., & Olney, S. J. (2009). A comparison of gait biomechanics and metabolic requirements of overground and treadmill walking in people with stroke. *Clinical Biomechanics, 24*(9), 729–734.

Carr, J. H., & Shepherd, R. B. (1987). *Movement science: Foundations for physical therapy in rehabilitation*. Rockville, MD: Aspen Publishers.

Chou, Y. H., Wagenaar, R. C., Saltzman, E., Giphart, J. E., Young, D., Davidsdottir, R., et al. (2009). Effects of optic flow speed and lateral flow asymmetry on locomotion in younger and older adults: A virtual reality study. *Journal of Gerontology, 64*(2), 222–231.

Cinelli, M. E., & Patla, A. E. (2008). Task-specific modulations of locomotor action parameters based on on-line visual information during collision avoidance with moving objects. *Human Movement Science, 27*(3), 513–531.

Cirstea, M. C., & Levin, M. F. (2000). Compensatory strategies for reaching in stroke. *Brain, 123*, 940–953.

Cirstea, C. M., Mitnitski, A. B., Feldman, A. G., & Levin, M. F. (2003). Interjoint coordination dynamics during reaching in stroke patients. *Experimental Brain Research, 151*, 289–300.

Daly, J. J., McCabe, J. P., Gansen, J., Rogers, J., Butler, K., Brenner, I., et al. (2012). Gait Coordination Protocol for recovery of coordinated gait, function, and quality of life following stroke. *Journal of Rehabilitation Research and Development, 49*(8), xix–xxviii.

de Rugy, A., Montagne, G., Buekers, M. J., & Laurent, M. (2000). The study of locomotor pointing in virtual reality: The validation of a test set-up. *Behavior Research Methods, Instruments, and Computing, 32*(4), 515–520.

De Smet, K., Malcolm, P., Lenoir, M., Segers, V., & De Clercq, D. (2009). Effects of optic flow on spontaneous overground walk-to-run transition. *Experimental Brain Research, 193*(4), 501–508.

De Valois, R. L., & De Valois, K. K. (1980). Spatial vision. *Annual Review of Psychology, 31*, 309–341.

Deutsch, J. E., Lewis, J. A., Minsky, A., Burdea, G., & Boian, R. (2007). Realism and gait characteristics of walking in a virtual reality mobility simulator. *Proceeding of the International Society of Posture and Gait Research* (p. 78). Burlington, VT

Dewald, J. P., & Beer, R. F. (2001). Abnormal joint torque patterns in the paretic upper limb of subjects with hemiparesis. *Muscle & Nerve, 24*, 273–283.

Dewald, J. P., Pope, P. S., Given, J. D., Buchanan, T. S., & Rymer, W. Z. (1995). Abnormal muscle coactivation patterns during isometric torque generation at the elbow and shoulder in hemiparetic subjects. *Brain, 118*, 495–510.

Dipietro, L., Krebs, H. I., Fasoli, S. E., Volpe, B. T., & Hogan, N. (2009). Submovement changes characterize generalization of motor recovery after stroke. *Cortex, 45*(3), 318–324.

Dounskaia, N., Van Gemmert, A. W., Leis, B. C., & Stelmach, G. E. (2009). Biased wrist and finger coordination in Parkinsonian patients during performance of graphical tasks. *Neuropsychologia, 47*(12), 2504–2514.

Douris, P. C., McDonald, B., Vespi, F., Kelley, N. C., & Herman, L. (2012). Comparison between Nintendo wii fit aerobics and traditional aerobic exercise in sedentary young adults. *Journal of Strength and Conditioning Research, 26*(4), 1052–1057.

Dutta, T. (2012). Evaluation of the Kinect sensor for 3-D kinematic measurement in the workplace. *Applied Ergonomics, 43*(4), 645–649.

Dvorkin, A. Y., Shahar, M., & Weiss, P. L. (2006). Reaching within video-capture virtual reality: Using virtual reality as a motor control paradigm. *Cyberpsychology and Behavior, 9*(2), 133–136.

Feldman, A. G. (2011). Space and time in the context of equilibrium-point theory. *Wiley Interdisciplinary Reviews: Cognitive Science, 2*, 287–304.

Fernandez-Baena, A., Susın, A., & Lligadas, X. (2012). Biomechanical validation of upper-body and lower-body joint movements of kinect motion capture data for rehabilitation treatments. *Fourth International Conference on Intelligent Networking and Collaborative Systems* (pp. 656–661). IEEE Computer Society. doi:10.1109/iNCoS.2012.66.

Fitts, P. M. (1954). The information capacity of the human motor system in controlling the amplitude of movement. *Journal of Experimental Psychology, 47*, 381–391.

Fitzgerald, S. G., Cooper, R. A., Thorman, T., Cooper, R., Guo, S., & Boninger, M. L. (2004). The game(cycle) exercise system: Comparison with standard ergometry. *Journal of Spinal Cord Medicine, 27*(5), 453–459.

Flash, T., & Hogan, N. (1985). The coordination of arm movements: An experimentally confirmed mathematical model. *Journal of Neuroscience, 5*, 1688–1703.

Ford, M. P., Wagenaar, R. C., & Newell, K. M. (2007). Phase manipulation and walking in stroke. *Journal of Neurologic Physical Therapy, 31*(2), 85–91.

Gibson, J. J. (1958). Visually controlled locomotion and visual orientation in animals. *British Journal of Psychology, 49*(3), 182–194.

Gibson, J. J. (1979). *The ecological approach to visual perception*. Boston, MA: Houghton Mifflin.

Gibson, E. J., & Walk, R. D. (1960). The "visual cliff". *Scientific American, 202*, 67–71.

Graf, D. L., Pratt, L. V., Hester, C. N., & Short, K. R. (2009). Playing active video games increases energy expenditure in children. *Pediatrics, 124*(2), 534–540.

Gregory, R. L. (1980). Perceptions as hypotheses. *Philosophical Transactions of the Royal Society of London, Series B, 290*, 181–197.

Haddock, B. L., Siegel, S. R., & Wikin, L. D. (2009). The addition of a video game to stationary cycling: The impact on energy expenditure in overweight children. *Open Sports Science Journal, 2*, 42–46.

Held, R. (2009). Visual-haptic mapping and the origin of cross-modal identity. *Optometry and Vision Science, 86*(6), 595–598.

Hibbard, P. B., & Bradshaw, M. F. (2003). Reaching for virtual objects: Binocular disparity and the control of prehension. *Experimental Brain Research, 148*, 196–201.

Hogan, N. (1984). An organizing principle for a class of voluntary movements. *Journal of Neuroscience, 4*, 2745–2754.

Hollerbach, J. M., & Atkeson, C. G. (1987). Inferring limb coordination strategies from trajectory kinematics. *Journal of Neuroscience Methods, 21*, 181–194.

Hollman, J. H., Brey, R. H., Bang, T. J., & Kaufman, K. R. (2007). Does walking in a virtual environment induce unstable gait? An examination of vertical ground reaction forces. *Gait & Posture, 26*(2), 289–294.

Hollman, J. H., Brey, R. H., Robb, R. A., Bang, T. J., & Kaufman, K. R. (2006). Spatiotemporal gait deviations in a virtual reality environment. *Gait & Posture, 23*(4), 441–444.

Huang, H. J., Kram, R., & Ahmed, A. A. (2012). Reduction of metabolic cost during motor learning of arm reaching dynamics. *Journal of Neuroscience, 32*(6), 2182–2190.

Hurkmans, H. L., Ribbers, G. M., Streur-Kranenburg, M. F., Stam, H. J., & van den Berg-Emons, R. J. (2011). Energy expenditure in chronic stroke patients playing Wii Sports: A pilot study. *Journal of Neuroengineering and Rehabilitation, 8*, 38.

Inzelberg, R., Flash, T., Schechtman, E., & Korczyn, A. D. (1995). Kinematic properties of upper limb trajectories in idiopathic torsion dystonia. *Journal of Neurology, Neurosurgery and Psychiatry, 58*(3), 312–319.

Jeannerod, M. (1999). Visuomotor channels: Their integration in goal-directed prehension. *Human Movement Science, 18*, 201–218.

Kafri, M., Myslinksi, M. J., Gade, V., & Deutsch, J. E. (2013). Energy expenditure and exercise intensity of interactive video gaming in individuals post-stroke. *Neurorehabilitation and Neural Repair, 28*(1), 56–65.

Katsavelis, D., Mukherjee, M., Decker, L., & Stergiou, N. (2010). The effect of virtual reality on gait variability. *Nonlinear Dynamics, Psychology, and Life Sciences, 14*(3), 239–256.

Katzel, L. I., Ivey, F. M., Sorkin, J. D., Macko, R. F., Smith, B., & Shulman, L. M. (2012). Impaired economy of gait and decreased six-minute walk distance in Parkinson's disease. *Parkinson's Disease,* ID: 241754.

Knaut, L. A., Subramanian, S., McFadyen, B. J., Bourbonnais, D., & Levin, M. F. (2009). Kinematics of pointing movements made in a virtual versus a physical 3D environment in stroke. *Archives of Physical Medicine and Rehabilitation, 90*(5), 793–802.

Krasovsky, T., Banina, M. C., Hacmon, R. R., Feldman, A. G., Lamontagne, A., & Levin, M. F. (2012). Stability of gait and interlimb coordination in older adults. *Journal of Neurophysiology, 107*(9), 2560–2569.

Kuhlen, T., Kraiss, K. E., & Steffan, R. (2000). How VR-based reach-to-grasp experiments can help understand movement organization within the human brain. *Presence, 9*, 350–359.

Latash, M. L. (2012). The bliss (not the problem) of motor abundance (not redundancy). *Experimental Brain Research, 217*, 1–5.

Levin, M. F., Kleim, J. A., & Wolf, S. L. (2009). POINT OF VIEW: Enhancing interdisciplinary perspectives: What do motor "recovery" and "compensation" mean in patients following stroke? *Neurorehabilitation and Neural Repair, 23*(4), 313–319.

Liebermann, D. G., Berman, S., Weiss, P. L., & Levin, M. F. (2012). Kinematics of reaching movements in a 2D virtual environment in adults with and without stroke. *IEEE Transactions on Neural Systems and Rehabilitation Engineering, 20*(6), 778–787.

Liebermann, D. G., & Goodman, D. (2007). Pre- and post-landing effects of falling with and without vision. *Journal of Electromyography and Kinesiology, 17*, 212–227. doi:10.1016/j.jelekin.2006.01.011.

Lott, A., Bisson, E., Lajoie, Y., McComas, J., & Sveistrup, H. (2003). The effect of two types of virtual reality on voluntary center of pressure displacement. *Cyberpsychology and Behavior, 6*(5), 477–485.

Magdalon, E. C., Levin, M. F., Quevedo, A. A. F., & Michaelsen, S. M. (2008). Kinematics of reaching and grasping in a 3D immersive virtual reality environment in patients with hemiparesis. 5th World Conference for NeuroRehabilitation. Brazil. *Neurorehabilitation Neural Repair*, 22(5), ID299.

Magdalon, E. C., Michaelsen, S. M., Quevedo, A. A. F., & Levin, M. F. (2011). Comparison of grasping movements made by healthy subjects in a 3-dimensional immersive virtual versus physical environment. *Acta Psychologica (Amsterdam), 138*(1), 126–134.

McAndrew, P. M., Dingwell, J. B., & Wilken, J. M. (2010). Walking variability during continuous pseudo-random oscillations of the support surface and visual field. *Journal of Biomechanics, 43*(8), 1470–1475.

Mellet, E., Laou, L., Petit, L., Zago, L., Mazoyer, B., & Tzourio-Mazoyer, T. (2010). Impact of the virtual reality on the neural representation of an environment. *Human Brain Mapping, 31*(7), 1065–1075.

Michaels, C., & Carello, C. (1981). *Direct perception*. Englewood, NJ: Prentice Hall.

Montagne, G., Buekers, M., Camachon, C., De Rugy, A., & Laurent, M. (2003). The learning of goal-directed locomotion: A perception-action perspective. *Quarterly Journal of Experimental Psychology A, 56*(3), 551–567.

Montagne, G., Buekers, M., de Rugy, A., Camachon, C., & Laurent, M. (2002). Control of human locomotion under various task constraints. *Experimental Brain Research, 143*(1), 133–136.

Moon, S. K., Alaverdashvili, M., Cross, A. R., & Whishaw, I. Q. (2009). Both compensation and recovery of skilled reaching following small photothrombotic stroke to motor cortex in the rat. *Experimental Neurology, 218*(1), 145–153.

Morasso, P. (1981). Spatial control of arm movements. *Experimental Brain Research, 42*, 223–227.

Novak, A. C., & Brouwer, B. (2012). Strength and aerobic requirements during stair ambulation in persons with chronic stroke and healthy adults. *Archives of Physical Medicine and Rehabilitation, 93*(4), 683–689.

Nyberg, L., Lundin-Olsson, L., Sondell, B., Backman, A., Holmlund, K., Eriksson, S., et al. (2006). Using a virtual reality system to study balance and walking in a virtual outdoor environment: A pilot study. *Cyberpsychology and Behavior, 9*(4), 388–395.

Pascual-Leone, A., Amedi, A., Fregni, F., & Merabet, L. B. (2005). The plastic human brain cortex. *Annual Review of Neuroscience, 28*, 377–401.

Pearson, K., & Gordon, J. (2000). Locomotion. In E. Kandel, J. Schwartz, & T. Jessel (Eds.), *Principles of neural science* (4th ed., pp. 737–755). New York, NY: McGraw-Hill.

Prokop, T., Schubert, M., & Berger, W. (1997). Visual influence on human locomotion. *Experimental Brain Research, 114*, 63–70.

Rohrer, B., Fasoli, S., Krebs, H. I., Hughes, R., Volpe, B., Frontera, W. R., et al. (2002). Movement smoothness changes during stroke recovery. *Journal of Neuroscience, 22*, 8297–8304.

Rossignol, S. (1996). Visuomotor regulation of locomotion. *Canadian Journal of Physiology and Pharmacology, 74*, 418–425.

Scholz, J. P., & Schoner, G. (1999). The uncontrolled manifold concept: Identifying control variables for a functional task. *Experimental Brain Research, 126*(3), 289–306.

Schubert, M., Prokop, T., Brocke, F., & Berger, W. (2005). Visual kinesthesia and locomotion in Parkinson's disease. *Movement Disorders, 20*, 141–150.

Shumway-Cook, A., & Woollacott, M. H. (2012). Control of normal mobility: theory and practical applications. In A. Shumway-Cook & M. H. Woollacott (Eds.), *Motor control* (4th ed., pp. 315–347). Philadelphia, PA: Lippincott Williams and Wilkins.

Smeets, J. B., & Brenner, E. (1999). A new view on grasping. *Motor Control, 3*(3), 237–271.

Soechting, J., & Flanders, M. (1993). Parallel, independent channels for location and orientation in sensorimotor transformations for reaching and grasping. *Journal of Neurophysiology, 70*(3), 1137–1150.

Subramanian, S. K., Massie, C. L., Malcolm, M. P., & Levin, M. F. (2011). Viewing medium affects arm motor performance in 3D virtual environments. *Journal of Neuroengineering and Rehabilitation, 8*, 36.

Tao, G., Archambault, P. S., & Levin, M. F. (2013, August). Evaluation of Kinect skeletal tracking in a virtual reality rehabilitation system for upper limb hemiparesis. *International Conference of Virtual Rehabilitation, Philadelphia*.

Todorov, E., & Jordan, M. (1998). Smoothness maximization along a predefined path accurately predicts the speed profiles of complex arm movements. *Journal of Neurophysiology, 80*(2), 696–714.

Varraine, X. E., Bonnard, M., & Pailhous, J. (2002). Interaction between different sensory cues in the control of human gait. *Experimental Brain Research, 142*(3), 374–384.

Viau, A., Feldman, A. G., McFadyen, B. J., & Levin, M. F. (2004). Reaching in reality and virtual reality: A comparison of movement kinematics in healthy subjects and in adults with hemiparesis. *Journal of Neuroengineering and Rehabilitation, 1*, 1–11.

Wang, C.-Y., Hwang, W.-J., Fang, J.-J., Sheu, C.-F., Leong, I.-F., & Ma, H.-I. (2011). Comparison of virtual reality versus physical reality on movement characteristics of persons with Parkinson's Disease: Effects of moving targets. *Archives of Physical Medicine and Rehabilitation, 92*, 1238–1245.

Warburton, D. E., Sarkany, D., Johnson, M., Rhodes, R. E., Whitford, W., Esch, B. T., et al. (2009). Metabolic requirements of interactive video game cycling. *Medicine and Science in Sports and Exercise, 41*(4), 920–926.

Warren, W. H., Jr., Young, D. S., & Lee, D. N. (1986). Visual control of step length during running over irregular terrain. *Journal of Experimental Psychology: Human Perception and Performance, 12*(3), 259–266.

White, K., Schofield, G., & Kilding, A. E. (2011). Energy expended by boys playing active video games. *Journal of Science and Medicine in Sport, 14*(2), 130–134.

Zhang, M., Koenig, S., Requejo, P., Somboon, N., Sawchuk, A. A., Chang, C. -Y., et al. (2012, May). Towards pervasive physical rehabilitation using Microsoft Kinect. In: *International Conference on Pervasive Computing Technologies for Healthcare (Pervasive-Health), San Diego, CA, USA*.

Chapter 7
Rehabilitation Applications Using Virtual Reality for Persons with Residual Impairments Following Stroke

Alma S. Merians and Gerard G. Fluet

Objective To describe current clinical evidence for the effectiveness of VR applications on upper limb recovery in individuals who have had a stroke.

7.1 Introduction

According to the World Health Organization, 15 million people worldwide suffer a stroke each year, leaving 5 million survivors permanently disabled. In most developed countries, the incidence of stroke is declining due to control of hypertension and cardiovascular disease. However, the overall rate of stroke remains high due to the aging of the population http://www.strokecenter.org/patients/about-stroke/stroke-statistics/. People post-stroke exhibit paresis of the upper and lower extremities. This consists of a group of coexisting sensorimotor impairments such as weakness, spasticity, decreased ability to isolate movements, diminished range of motion, as well as higher order cognitive and motor planning functions. When a person with paresis uses their upper extremity (UE) for purposeful movement, the paretic movements differ from normal movements in that they are slower, less accurate, have delayed or reduced force, and are uncoordinated in terms of magnitude and timing of the movement (Sathian et al., 2011). People post-stroke are often unable to perform actions, tasks, and activities needed for self-care, home management, employment, and social activities. Therefore, rehabilitation of movement dysfunction is confronted with multiple and complex challenges.

This chapter focuses on VR interventions for the UE of people post-stroke. Existing physical and occupational therapy interventions are the foundation for

A.S. Merians (✉) • G.G. Fluet
Department of Rehabilitation and Movement Science, Rutgers University,
65 Bergen Street, Newark, NJ 07107, USA
e-mail: alma.merians@shrp.rutgers.edu; fluet179@comcast.net

P.L. (Tamar) Weiss et al. (eds.), *Virtual Reality for Physical and Motor Rehabilitation*, Virtual Reality Technologies for Health and Clinical Applications,
DOI 10.1007/978-1-4939-0968-1_7,

treatment of the residual movement dysfunction exhibited by people after a stroke. Currently, the management of these interventions within the patient/client relationship usually follows the framework developed by the World Health Organization ICF model, a disability classification for use in health and health-related sectors. In general, the classification describes three levels of human function, at (1) the body level, (2) the whole person level, and (3) the level of the whole person in a social context. More specifically, disability at the body level refers to impairments to body function and structure (physiological functions and anatomical parts), at the whole person level to limitations in activity (execution of a task or action by an individual) and at the social context level to participation in a life situation (Jette, 2006; World Health Organization, 2002). (http://www.who.int/classifications/icf/training/icfbeginnersguide.pdf.)

In the clinical environment, therapeutic interventions are designed to address problems in each of these three areas of function. The construction of virtual environments used to rehabilitate motor deficits has progressed from simple two-dimensional visual experiences to more complex three-dimensional gaming and functional environments that are integrated with haptics, electromyography, and fMRI. These complex environments are being designed to address the multiple sensorimotor impairments that remain a pervasive problem for patients with motor dysfunction post-stroke with recent studies demonstrating evidence of the potential for these VR-based interventions to benefit patients with disordered movement due to neurological dysfunction. Known neurophysiological and behavioral benefits of movement observation (Buccino, Solodkin, & Small, 2006; Celnik et al., 2006), imagery (Butler, Blanton, Rowe, & Wolf, 2006), repetitive massed practice and imitation therapies (Gaggioli, Meneghini, Morganti, Alcaniz, & Riva, 2006) used to facilitate voluntary production of movement can be easily incorporated into a virtual environment (see Chap. 3). This allows the clinician to use sensory stimulation through VR as a tool to facilitate targeted brain networks, such as the motor areas, critical for neural and functional recovery. The potential for functional recovery can be optimized by tapping into a number of neurophysiological processes that occur after a brain lesion, such as enhanced potential for neuroplastic changes early in the recovery phase and stimulation of sensorimotor areas that may otherwise undergo deterioration due to disuse (see Chap. 2).

If repetition and skill learning are important for motor learning and recovery of function after stroke what does VR technology add over and above real-world task practice? What can training within an interactive virtual environment contribute to skill learning and improved motor control in people who have had a stroke? Are these technological interventions able to model and incorporate accepted rehabilitation practices? Is there a relationship between the elements of practice and sensory input available through interventions delivered within virtual environments and the clinical therapeutic interventions designed to address the areas of dysfunction described by the ICF model (body function/structure, activity, or participation)? These are important and timely concerns. In this chapter we summarize the published outcomes of UE rehabilitation studies utilizing the ICF model as a framework and then explore the motor learning principles used in physical and occupational therapy interventions such as (1) intensity and dosing of interventions, (2) knowledge of results and knowledge of performance, (3) adaptive scaling of task difficulty, (4) visual and auditory feedback, and (5) attentional focus, describing how each of these approaches have been utilized in VR simulations and interventions, specifically with respect to recovery from stroke. The chapter concludes with a case study that explores how to effectively use VR/robotic technology for an individualized treatment intervention. The intervention follows a patient/client management model that reflects the clinical decision making process and demonstrates the implementation and manipulation of several of the principles discussed in this chapter.

7.2 VR Interventions Within the ICF Framework

The ICF model describes three levels of function, all of which can be negatively impacted by a cerebrovascular accident. Body level impairments result in activity limitations and subsequent participation restrictions. Virtual environments can be used to intervene at all three of these levels of function. For more than a decade, simple environments used to provide feedback and expand the motivation of persons performing exercises designed to correct intrinsic aspects of active movement such as range of motion and strength have been used in the rehabilitation of people who have had a stroke (Holden, 2005; Sveistrup, 2004). Controlled trials of systems described in these reviews have demonstrated comparable (Piron, Turolla, Agostini, Zucconi, Cortese, et al., 2009) or larger (Piron, Turolla, Agostini, Zucconi, Ventura, et al., 2009; Yavuzer, Senel, Atay, & Stam, 2008) improvements in active range of motion strength than traditional therapy. A systematic review of these studies described a significantly larger effect on measurements of UE impairment when comparing virtually simulated repetitive task practice (RTP) to dose-matched programs of traditional therapy (Laver, George, Thomas, Deutsch, & Crotty, 2011). Other impairment-level interventions have combined simple, non- or semi-immersive virtual environments with robots to add interaction forces allowing participants to train grip strength (Merians, Poizner, Boian, Burdea, & Adamovich, 2006), shoulder strength (Adamovich, Fluet, Merians, Mathai, & Qiu, 2009), shoulder–elbow disassociation (Acosta, Dewald, & Dewald, 2011; Volpe et al., 2008), and finger disassociation (Stein, Bishop, Gillen, & Helbok, 2011). These studies were all uncontrolled pilot studies with the exception of Volpe et al., who compared their intervention to a time-matched dose of occupational therapy, finding no difference in adaptation to these two regimens. Because body function level impairments often contribute to activity limitations and participation restrictions, several uncontrolled pilot studies have used activity level simulations and have demonstrated improvements at the activity level (Boian et al., 2002; Piron et al., 2003, 2005). One study comparing a program of virtual reality based RTP and a time-matched program of traditional occupational therapy demonstrated no significant difference between activity level outcomes for the two interventions (Yavuzer et al., 2008). Saposnik et al. (2010) compared a program of game-based UE rehabilitation activities presented in VR with a program of game based Recreational Therapy. The rehabilitation activity subjects demonstrated larger improvement measured at the participation level than the Recreation Therapy group.

Some more recent interventions performed at the body function level are investigating how VR affects recovery at the neural level and have used specific feedback manipulations to upregulate hypoactive areas of the brain caused by damage due to stroke (Adamovich, Fluet, Mathai, et al., 2009; Adamovich, Fluet, Merians, et al., 2009; Adamovich, Fluet, Tunik, & Merians, 2009; Merians, Tunik, & Adamovich, 2009). The study of rehabilitation activities incorporating these manipulations and their ability to make longer term modifications in properties of brain networks are being initiated. The negative impact of a stroke on UE function seems to extend beyond the sum of individual impairments. A particularly discouraging study describes a lack of improvements in activity limitations related to hemiparetic upper extremities despite amelioration of impairments including strength and range of motion (Dromerick et al., 2006). This lack of improvement may be secondary to the complex, varied, and interdependent nature of normal UE function and may require interventions and practice at the activity level. Simulations in virtual environments have now progressed from simple target reaching activities to more complex activity level interventions. Examples of simulations that have been developed at the activity level include, cleaning a stove top, grocery shopping, playing basketball (Housman, Scott, & Reinkensmeyer, 2009) placing cups on a haptically rendered shelf, or hammering a haptically rendered nail (Merians et al., 2011). These systems expand the ability of therapists to provide repetitive task practice interventions that are more time, resource and manpower efficient than traditionally presented programs of rehabilitation (Adamovich, Fluet, Tunik, et al., 2009), allowing for the performance of large volumes of practice using complex movement activities required to elicit neuroplastic adaptations (Birkenmeier, Prager, & Lang, 2010). Multiple studies of virtually simulated repetitive task practice (RTP) demonstrate activity-level improvements using standardized measurements of UE function (Saposnik & Levin, 2011). It is interesting to note that two studies of virtually simulated RTP demonstrated large treatment effects compared to controls in untrained ADL ability (Piron et al., 2007; Piron, Turolla, Agostini, Zucconi, Ventura, et al., 2009). Another study comparing the effects of virtually simulated RTP on grip strength demonstrated comparable effects with those of a program of traditionally presented rehabilitation activities that included strength training (Housman et al., 2009). In addition, two other uncontrolled studies of virtually facilitated RTP, which did not directly train strength also describe improvements in grip strength (Broeren, Rydmark, Bjorkdahl, & Sunnerhagen, 2007; Connelly et al., 2010).

A smaller group of studies has examined interventions designed to limit the impact of participation restrictions. To date these interventions have consisted of training activities related to the use of power wheelchairs, the use of simulations to train persons with stroke to use hand controls to drive automobiles (Archambault, Chong, Sorrento, Routhier, & Boissy, 2011; Erren-Wolters, van Dijk, de Kort, Izerman, & Jannink, 2007) and navigating through a series of activities required to use the public train system (Lam, Man, Tam, & Weiss, 2006). Allowing subjects to trial these activities and or train during the earlier stages of recovery is significantly expanded because of the safety of practicing these activities in virtual environments. Another group of virtual rehabilitation activities have been designed to address the sensory processing and cognitive demands of participation in activities such as shopping (Rand, Katz, & Weiss, 2009). Virtual environments offer multiple advantages for rehabilitation at the participation level by allowing subjects to practice these functions safely and repeatedly, including elimination of the time demands associated with transportation to and from shopping centers, decreasing the burden of supervision of these activities and the ability to grade the complexity of the sensory presentations that participants are required to manage with great precision.

7.3 VR as a Tool to Provide Intensive Intervention Dosing

One of the difficulties in designing rehabilitation programs congruent with the literature supporting repetitive task practice is the labor-intensive nature of these interventions. Difficulties in the provision of adequate training volumes for persons with stroke are well documented (Lang, Macdonald, & Gnip, 2007). Typical rehabilitation programs do not provide enough repetitions to elicit neuroplasticity. In a study of 36 outpatient therapy sessions for persons with strokes, Lang, Macdonald, et al. (2007) observed that subjects performed an average of 27 repetitions of functional activities during these sessions. This volume of intervention stands in stark contrast to training volumes of 500–600 repetitions of tasks performed by animal subjects in stroke rehabilitation studies (Lang, Macdonald, et al., 2007) and the 600–800 repetitions of activity per hour (Housman et al., 2009; Krebs et al., 2008; Lum, Burgar, & Shor, 2004) reported in virtual rehabilitation and robotic studies. Dose of treatment can be described in terms of number of repetitions per session or total hours of intervention. A 2011 review by Saposnik and Levin indicated that the duration of VR sessions in most of the 12 studies included in their review was 1 h with a range of 30 min to 2.5 h, with total number of sessions ranging between 6 and 30. However, they did not indicate the average number of repetitions performed. The impact of the total volume of activity performed during UE rehabilitation interventions and its impact on outcomes is not completely clear. One meta-analysis has identified a minimum of 16 h of non-automated training as being necessary to improve ADL function in persons with stroke (Kwakkel et al., 2004). A Cochrane Report (Laver et al., 2011), based on 19 studies found that interventions providing less than 15 h of practice had a non-significant effect but interventions providing more than 15 h of practice showed a moderate effect on ADL outcomes. There seems to be a rate of diminishing returns subsequent to training after approximately 20 h of UE training have been performed (Fig. 7.1). Studies by Saposnik & Levin (2011), Fischer et al. (2007) and Merians et al. (2010) demonstrate a correlation between intervention time and outcome. This effect does not seem to continue when training times increase beyond 23 h. Studies by Wolf et al. (2006) and Lo et al. (2009) that use considerably longer periods of training do not demonstrate

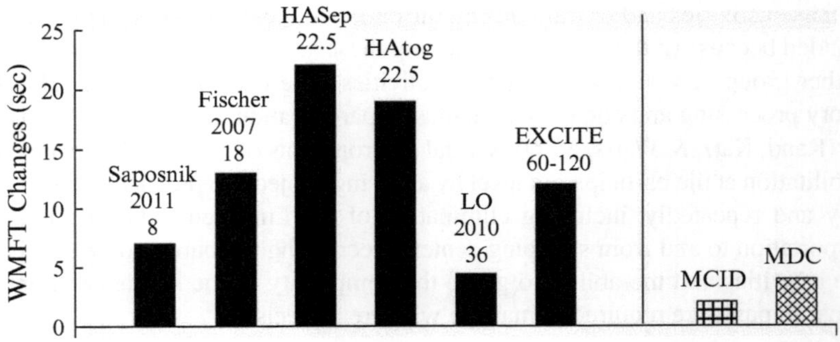

Fig. 7.1 *Left panel* indicates Wolf Motor Function Test (WMFT) outcomes based upon number of hours of repetitive task practice in both virtual and real-world environments. *Right panel* indicates published Minimal Clinical Important Difference (MCID) and Minimal Detectable Change (MCD) for the WMFT

substantially better outcomes. While the studies presented in Fig. 7.1 did not consider a perfectly homogenous group of subjects—subjects in the Saposnik study were in the acute phase of recovery and also received concurrent inpatient rehabilitation, and the subjects in Lo et al. (2009) had a greater level of upper extremity impairment—the argument that more training time will always produce better outcomes is clearly not supported and that the consideration of other factors to explain differences in outcome must continue to be entertained.

7.4 Manipulation of Elements in VR to Facilitate Motor Skill Development

7.4.1 Activity Scaling

A skilled movement is characterized by consistency, stability, flexibility, and adaptability. These features are achieved through practice-dependent changes in kinematic and force errors (Krakauer, 2006). With practice, one progresses through the stages of skill acquisition, eventually achieving a movement that is autonomous with fewer errors. Evidence suggests that repetitive practice resulting in "actual motor skill acquisition, or motor learning" may be a more potent stimulus for "driving representational plasticity in the primary motor cortex," than the simple repetition of activities that are well within the movement capabilities of a subject (Plautz, Milliken, & Nudo, 2000; Remple, Bruneau, VandenBerg, Goertzen, & Kleim, 2001). Thus activity scaling is a critical issue related to neuroplasticity when considering the need for continuous skill development. In some virtual environments, movement characteristics may be similar to those for movements made in the physical environment (see Chap. 5). Such virtual environments may be particularly well-suited to the systematic scaling of movements and activities. The intensity of practice (time and/or number of repetitions), the visual,

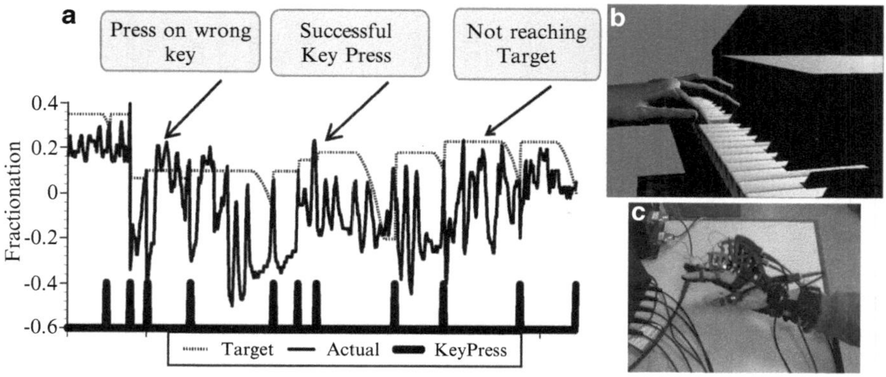

Fig. 7.2 (**a**) Representative example of the adaptive algorithm used in the Virtual Piano simulation showing the adjustable fractionation target based on an individual subject's actual ability to isolate their finger movements at each attempted key press. The *dotted line* indicates the target fractionation, the *thin line* is the actual fractionation and the *thick line* indicates when the key is successfully pressed. The *left section* shows the scenario when the subject reaches the target fractionation but the finger is not aligned with the correct key. The *center section* indicates a successful key press. The *right section* shows the scenario when the subject fails to reach the target fractionation and the target is lowered. (**b**) Screenshot of the Virtual Piano simulation. (**c**) The Cybergrasp used with patient MP

auditory, and haptic feedback presented, the speed and range and force of the movement required to interact with task-related objects can all be manipulated to drive movement reeducation and skill development. In addition, kinematic and kinetic data on subjects' performance and learning history are available to provide definitive measurable data regarding the changes in motor behavior. Virtual workspaces, target sizes, and activity speeds and forces can be increased in minute gradients allowing for an infinite range of difficulty for any task. This provides an opportunity for persons with stroke to develop and refine skills steadily throughout a rehabilitation session. Physical fatigue during large volume training sessions also presents challenges to persons with strokes. Motor fatigue can be easily addressed in VR training through VE modifications (Fluet et al., 2012).

It has been proposed that a favorable learning experience occurs when the task in neither too difficult nor too easy (Cameirao, Badia, Oller, & Verschure, 2010; Jack et al., 2001). In the Cameirao study, a reaching task in which moving spheres moved toward the participant who had to intercept them, the speed of the moving spheres, the interval between the appearance of the spheres and the horizontal spread of the spheres could all be manipulated based upon patient success rate. In this study the difficulty was increased by 10 % when the participant intercepted more than 70 % of the spheres and was decreased when less than 50 % of the spheres were intercepted (Cameirao et al., 2010). In a study of robotically facilitated UE training in virtual environments, task difficulty was manipulated over the 2-week training period through the use of online algorithms and changes in the dimensions of the workspace (Merians et al., 2011). A Virtual Piano simulation (Fig. 7.2b and Table 7.1) consisting of a complete virtual piano that played the appropriate notes as they were pressed by

Table 7.1 Describes each simulation, the performance measure used to track progress, and the approach to increasing the intensity of the activity

Virtual reality simulation	Impairment	Game	Strategies	Metric
Space pong 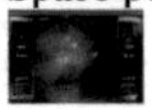	Decreased finger extension modulation	Subject plays a pong type game against the computer. Subject moves the paddle to the right by opening their fingers and to the left by closing them.	Decrease proportion of subject movement (finger extension) to paddle movement if accuracy does not improve with practice. Increase proportion when accuracy increases.	Accuracy
Hammer 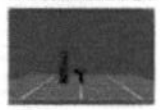	Decreased shoulder stabilization	Subject reaches for a target peg and hammers it into the floor by flexing and extending his fingers. Hammer only hits the target when it is in target area.	Decrease the size of the target as time to hammer pegs decreases.	End point deviation Time to hammer pegs
Hammer 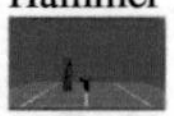	Decreased shoulder–elbow isolation	Subject hammers peg into the floor by pronating his forearm. Robot holds hammer stable over the target peg.	Decrease proportion of subject movement (pronation) to hammer movement as time to hammer pegs decreases.	Peak pronation range of motion Time to hammer pegs
Piano 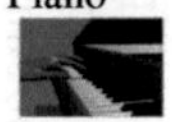	Decreased finger individuation	Subject plays scales and simple songs. Each key is cued and the finger to press it designated.	Algorithm sets fractionation target based on performance. Utilize CyberGrasp™ to teach movement pattern if subject does not respond to algorithm.	Fractionation Time to press keys
Cups 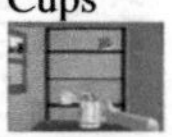	Decreased shoulder–trunk isolation	Subject attaches virtual hand to virtual mugs and places them on virtual shelves in a 3D workspace.	Increase volume of workspace as time to place cups on shelf decreases. Recalibrate workspace weekly.	Time to place nine cups on shelf Reaching trajectory length
Reach-touch 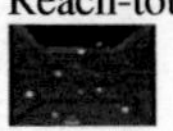	Decreased shoulder AROM	Subject moves cursor to touch ten targets in a 3D workspace.	Increase size of workspace as duration decreases. Recalibrate workspace weekly.	Time to touch ten targets Trajectory length

the virtual fingers while the subject was wearing a CyberGlove, was designed to help improve the ability of subjects post-stroke to move each finger in isolation (fractionation). Fractionation was calculated as the difference in the amount of flexion in the metacarpophalangeal (MCP) joint between the cued finger and the most flexed non-cued finger. An adaptive algorithm used to shape fractionation required more isolated finger flexion to elicit a key press as participants succeeded and less fractionation if their performance diminished. Initial target fractionation was calculated based on each subject's actual fractionation. If the actual fractionation reached 90 % of target fractionation, the next initial target fractionation was increased by 8 % of the previous target fractionation If not, the next initial target fractionation was decreased by 10 % of the previous target fractionation. Figure 7.2a shows an example of the variation in the adjustable fractionation target based on an individual subject's actual ability to isolate their finger movements at each attempted key press. The dotted line indicates the target fractionation, the thin line is the actual fractionation and the thick line indicates when the key is successfully pressed. The left section of Fig. 7.2a shows the scenario when the subject reaches the target fractionation but the finger is not aligned with the correct key, the middle section shows a successful key press and the right section shows the scenario when the subject fails to reach the target fractionation and the target is lowered. In an uncontrolled pilot study, that trained ten subjects who had a stroke, the subjects performed the piano simulation described above for 30 min/day for 8 days in a 2-week period. At posttest the subjects significantly improved in fractionation showing on average a 39 % change pre-post training. There was also a significant improvement in the time to complete the task after training, showing a 19 % change without a subsequent change in accuracy, indicating that the subjects were able to do the task faster while maintaining their accuracy. This is thought to be consistent with motor learning (Krakauer, 2006). Further, it is interesting to note that in this study, the largest improvements demonstrated with the Virtual Piano were for finger fractionation. Subjects made larger improvements in fractionation than speed or accuracy that were not shaped with an algorithm or reinforced with feedback (Merians et al., 2011).

In an arm transport simulation in which the goal of the activity was to improve forward, sideways and overhead reaching ability, subjects reached to touch a series of ten targets placed randomly throughout the workspace. To adapt to the range of arm motion of each subject, the Reach-Touch simulation workspace size was calibrated for each subject on the first day of each training week according to their available range of motion in a single reach. To prevent fatigue and keep the game at a reasonably challenging level, training began at 60 % of the calibrated workspace volume, and gradually increased to a consistent 100 % of the volume at the end of the week. Figure 7.3 shows a graphic representation the change in workspace volume for one subject. Workspace size of day 3 and day 4 were 60 % and 80 % of the calibration range of the first week. Workspace size of day 5, day 7, and day 8 were 60 %, 70 %, and 90 % of the increased calibration range of the second week. The workspace volume gradually and continuously expanded throughout the training period. Another example of workspace modification is the Cup Placing simulation (Table 7.1).

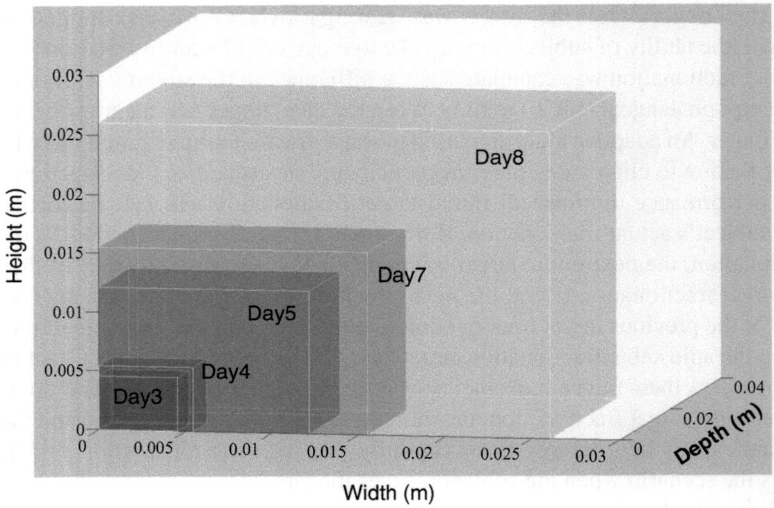

Fig. 7.3 Graphic representation of the changes in the three-dimensional workspace of a subject on training days 3, 4, 5, 7, and 8. The workspace gradually and continually expanded in height, width, and depth throughout the training

The shelf height on which the cups were placed was calibrated at the beginning of each week of the training, and the cups were placed further away and higher as the training proceeded (Merians et al., 2011).

7.4.2 Augmented Feedback

In addition to activity scaling, VR environments use both visual and auditory sensory input in the form of Knowledge of Results (KR) and Knowledge of Performance (KP) both for clarification of task parameters and for motivation. Simulations can provide immediate visual or faded KR in the form of scoring and timing incentives (e.g., number of successful repetitions, number of warriors eliminated, number of space ships destroyed in a set time limit) or when task performance scores exceed a predetermined limit (Piron, Turolla, Agostini, Zucconi, Cortese, et al., 2009; Weiss & Katz, 2004). Summary feedback is often given as a score after a group of trials. The IREX system is a video-capture system that captures the whole body movement of the user and immerses it into the virtual environment where they can interact with on-screen images and objects. This visual illusion is designed to enhance the sense of "presence" for the patient. In a study of ten patients using simulations in which reaching, lifting and grasping motions were performed, faded KR and KP feedback were provided that included error rate, speed, direction, joint position, and resistive force (Jang et al., 2005) Auditory feedback can be provided through music that impels continuous activity such as in Pong Games as well as through the inherent nature of the activity as found in the Virtual Piano Trainer that uses well known melodies (Adamovich, Fluet, Mathai, Qiu, Merians et al., 2009; Subramanian, Lourenco, Chilingaryan, Sveistrup, & Levin, 2013). KP has been used by both Holden (2005) and Piron, Turolla, Agostini, Zucconi, Cortese, et al. (2009). In an example of one type of KP used in a virtual reaching task, the patient moves a real object and sees a display of both their own trajectory and the trajectory of the "virtual teacher," thereby providing the subject with ongoing knowledge of their reaching hand path (Holden, Dyar & Dayan-Cimadoro, 2007).

7.4.3 Attentional Focus

Another factor to consider is that VR simulations structure the attentional focus of the subject. It has been shown in people with and without disabilities that the learning of a motor task is more effective when attention is focused on externally rather than on internally based instructions (Wulf, Landers, Lewthwaite, & Tollner, 2009; Wulf, McNevin, Fuchs, Ritter, & Toole, 2000). In many VR simulations, practice is directed to achieve action goals rather than performing specific movements. The instructions for the game, the feedback provided and the inherent structure of the simulations direct the attention of the player to the task to be achieved. In other words, the focus of attention is on the effect of one's movements rather than on the movement itself (Merians et al., 2011). VR can be a particularly effective tool for the rehabilitation of another type of attentional deficit, persons with unilateral spatial neglect secondary to stroke. The performance of large volumes of scanning or motor tasks directed into the impaired hemi-space is required to ameliorate the functional limitations and reduce subsequent activity limitations and participation restrictions. Virtually simulated activities are ideal for this type of training because the position and density of targets can be manipulated easily with precision (Tsirlin, Dupierrix, Chokron, Coquillart, & Ohlmann, 2009) and the activities can be presented in formats that are more engaging and entertaining, facilitating long periods of training (Smith, Hebert, & Reid, 2007). An example of this approach was implemented by Smith et al. (2007) who had subjects play computer games using a camera based VR system. Subjects played games requiring attention and movement of their upper extremities into their neglected hemi-space. Subjects improved in motor and sensory tasks subsequent to training and also reported improvements in their ability to perform activities of daily living. Another study examining the rehabilitation of persons with unilateral spatial neglect highlights one of the unique features of virtual environments that have also been used in other areas of rehabilitation—the ability to alter the visual feedback provided to participants. Glover and Castiello (2006) had subjects with stroke reach toward virtual targets located in their neglected space. The visual representation of the workspace was shrunk and translated into their intact visual hemispace. After practicing for several sessions with this translation, subjects were able to reach toward targets in their impaired space with decreased errors and were able to better attend to targets in their impaired hemispace during a non-motor transfer test, providing possible evidence of a "re-mapping" of the neglected hemi-space. The use of 3D VR has been suggested as a possible assessment tool to map out the full dimensions of the spatial deficit of a patient (Dvorkin, Bogey, Harvey, & Patton, 2006).

7.5 Commercially Available VR Exercise Systems

Many clinical settings have begun to use commercially available off-the-shelf, low-cost gaming systems that can be displayed on a standard TV monitor (e.g., the Wii (Nintendo; Redmond), EyeToy, PlayStation2, (Sony Computer Entertainment; Tokyo, Japan); and the Xbox Kinect, (Microsoft). These commercial applications include motivating environments, some of which are more functional (serving meals, cooking activities) but most use competitive gaming activities (tennis, boxing, soccer, baseball, bowling, golf). For a full review of the design, activity levels and energy expenditure associated with these systems see (Taylor, McCormick, Shawis, Impson, & Griffin, 2011). In a randomized controlled trial of 20 patients post stroke, all subjects received 1 h of conventional physical and occupational therapy but the 10 subjects in the EyeToy group received an additional 30 min of game playing. At posttest and at follow-up, the EyeToy group showed significantly more improvement in UE motor function as measured by the FIM (Functional Independence Measure) than the control group. No changes in the motor recovery of the paretic limb were found as measured by Brunnstrom arm and hand stages (Yavuzer, Senel, Atay, & Stam, 2008). Most research VR systems are extremely expensive and complex. This makes the commercial gaming systems attractive for rehabilitation. However, there are many unanswered questions related to their use. Are the changes reported by therapists and reported in the literature related to increased activity by the participants or importantly are there actual changes in motor recovery and in movement kinematics? Currently the commercial systems cannot provide kinematic data, nor can they be modified for individual patient impairment levels.

7.6 Integration of Vision and Haptics in VR

A newer generation of virtual environments incorporates tactile information and interaction forces into what had been an essentially visual experience. Traditional visual and auditory VE presentations are being interfaced with robots of varying complexity to provide haptic feedback that (1) adds physical task parameters, (2) enriches the sensory experience, and (3) provides global forces such as gravity that result in neuromuscular and biomechanical interactions with the VE that simulate real-world movement more accurately than visual only VEs. Haptic feedback gives cues on manipulated object weight, inertia, and solidity. Haptic interfaces allow users to touch, feel, and manipulate objects during VR simulations thus contributing to increased simulation realism. Haptic feedback can be used to add the perception of contact to skills like placing a cup on a shelf, hammering a peg (Merians, Tunik, Fluet, Qiu, & Adamovich, 2008), or kicking a soccer ball. Lam et al. (2008) describe a system that uses vibratory disks to simulate the feeling of impact between the foot and the object when kicking a soccer ball. The authors reported a greater degree of skill learning in a group of healthy subjects training with visual and haptic feedback than a group of subjects practicing with visual feedback alone (Lam et al., 2008). As previously described "virtual tutor trajectories" (Holden, Dyar, & Dayan-Cimadoro, 2007; Piron et al., 2005) have been used in subjects with hemiparesis due to stroke to model the appropriate movement path. Alternatively, collisions with haptically rendered objects can also be used to teach normal movement trajectories such as the action required to place an object on a shelf or navigating a space ship through space (Adamovich, Fluet, Tunik, et al., 2009). Using haptically rendered obstacles to indirectly shape trajectories may decrease the effects of the explicit cognitive processes associated with presenting a model, such as an "ideal" trajectory into what is usually an implicit process (Boyd & Winstein, 2006). Investigation into this potential advantage is necessary because of the significant increases in cost associated with adding haptic effects to virtual rehabilitation applications.

Haptic environments can also exert global forces on the user such as increased resistance, antigravity support or viscous stabilization forces. Anti-gravity and viscous stabilization allow persons with force generation impairments to perform reaching and object manipulation tasks in 3D space. These activities invoke muscular force synergies that are comparable to those exerted in real-world movements. Several authors employ these concepts in VR simulations designed to train reaching, grasping, and lifting. Wolbrecht, Chan, Reinkensmeyer, and Bobrow (2008) used a haptic robotic interface to provide anti-gravity assistance to subjects with chronic hemiparesis secondary to stroke as they performed reaching movements in virtual environments. In a single session, single group study, the as need assistance improved their reaching kinematics so they resembled more normal reaching patterns. Many important activities of daily living require interaction with tools to achieve movement goals like feeding and grooming. In the physical world, object manipulation produces an interaction between the user and the object that is unique (e.g., torques exerted on the wrist by the interaction between the subject's hand and a knife and a cutting surface). Haptics can simulate the interaction forces produced by tools in virtual environments. The left panel of Fig. 7.4 shows the changes in the reaching trajectory when the lifting force shown generated during the reaching movement (right panel Fig. 7.4) is modified by manipulating the load of the cup to be lifted onto the shelf. See description of cup simulation in Table 7.1. Lambercy et al. (2007) described a haptic knob that can be used to simulate rotational forces using a set of objects that vary in size and shape allowing for customization based on therapeutic goals. Haptic forces can also be synchronized with visual feedback to improve the sense of presence of the user in the virtual environment. In two small studies involving healthy subjects, this feedback combination was found to be more effective for skill learning than visual only feedback in healthy subjects (Huang, Gillespie, & Kuo, 2007; Singapogu, Sander, Burg, & Cobb, 2008).

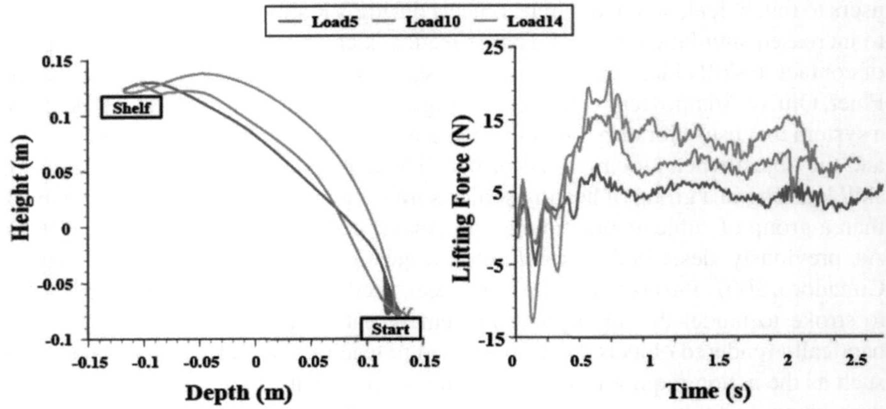

Fig. 7.4 *Left panel* shows the trajectory used to transport a haptic cup and place it on a shelf at three different haptic "weights" of the cup. Heaviest load is top line medium load is *middle line* lightest load is *bottom line*. *Right panel* shows how the force generated during the reaching movement, is modified based on the load of the cup to be lifted. To maintain the appropriate trajectory the force generated increases as the load on the cup increases. Force necessary to lift heaviest load represented by *top line*, medium load represented by *middle line*, lightest load generated by lowest line

7.7 Conclusions

The literature describing the efficacy of virtually simulated UE rehabilitation activities summarized in this chapter make a clear case for the effectiveness of this approach to treatment. The ability of simulated rehabilitation activities to address many of the requirements of motor learning and neuroplasticity in persons with a wide range of abilities seems to be central to this effectiveness. Virtually simulated rehabilitation treatments are inherently safe, time efficient and flexible, allowing for large volumes of training to be presented at appropriate levels of difficulty in a time efficient manner. Augmented feedback in the form of either KP or KR is known to enhance motor skill learning in normal adults (Lee, White, & Carnahan, 1990), in older healthy populations (Swanson & Lee, 1992) and in individuals post stroke (Winstein, Merians, & Sullivan, 1999) and Chap. 3. Both KR and KP can easily and systematically be delivered with specificity and predetermined frequency within virtual environments. Importantly it appears that VR interventions can be modeled on the clinical therapeutic framework described by the ICF model at the body function/structure level, as an activity based task or to enhance participation within social contexts.

Several areas of study are indicated to continue the development of this treatment approach for persons with stroke. The first would be to expand the study of virtual interventions to include persons in the acute phase of recovery. Further studies of the neural effects of VR sensory manipulations are needed. Future studies should include visuomotor discordance as a promising tool to enhance neuroplasticity. One of the examples described in the literature is mirror visual stimulation of the lesioned hemisphere controlled by the non-paretic hand in persons with no active movement of their hemiplegic upper extremities (Ramachandran & Altschuler, 2009; Tunik & Adamovich, 2009). Continued study of the manipulation of task difficulty using online algorithms is another area of study unique to simulated rehabilitation activities that should be pursued as well as the manipulation of the ratio of active patient movement to avatar movement. Two competing approaches to these manipulations use smaller avatar movements compared to subjects' movement to make them work harder in order to facilitate increased activity in the motor cortex, or large avatar movements compared to patient movement to allow patients with very little active movement to perform purposeful movements with their paretic upper extremity (Bagce, Saleh, Adamovich, & Tunik, 2011). An important next step toward translating the work done by researchers into clinical practice will be to design interventions that leverage the flexibility of virtually simulated environments. These interventions should be designed specifically for the impairment, activity, or participation level of the patient utilizing the patient management model. This chapter concludes with a case study that describes just such an intervention. The intervention includes task parameter scaling and gain scaling into a personalized rehabilitation program designed for an individual patient by a physical therapist utilizing the patient management model to inform decision making.

7.8 Case Study

Virtual environments have been used to facilitate the intensity and volume requirements of repetitive task practice in several studies (for recent reviews, see Henderson, Korner-Bitensky, & Levin, 2007; Laver et al., 2011; Merians et al., 2008; Saposnik & Levin, 2011). One of the strengths of virtually simulated rehabilitation systems is their ability to tailor activities to the unique motor abilities and rehabilitation goals of participants (Adamovich, Fluet, Tunik, et al., 2009). This case study will present a rehabilitation intervention customized to match the goals and clinical presentation of a gentleman with UE hemiparesis secondary to a chronic stroke. Detailed descriptions of the responses of the subject during the intervention and the modification of the intervention made by the therapist will be presented to demonstrate the ability of the technology to facilitate clinical practice.

7.8.1 Case Description: History and Systems Review

MP is an 85-year-old man with left hemiparesis secondary to an intracerebral hemorrhage and craniotomy 5 years prior to the interventions described in this case. Past medical history included an atrophic right kidney, recurrent urinary tract infections and several bouts of pneumonia and paroxysmal atrial fibrillation. Surgical history includes a permanent pacemaker placement, an abdominal aortic aneurysm repair and radical prostatectomy. Eleven years prior to this intervention,

MP suffered a fall and incomplete spinal cord injury and a subsequent C3–C8 laminectomy and decompression from which he recovered from completely. Rehabilitation history following the stroke included 16 weeks of inpatient rehabilitation, 9 months of outpatient physical therapy (PT) and occupational therapy (OT), and 4 years of home therapy combining PT and OT that focused on ambulation, balance, transfers, sensory integration, and upper extremity function. MP performs bed mobility, transfers, grooming and feeding with supervision. He requires moderate assistance for toileting and upper body dressing and maximum assistance for lower body dressing. MP uses a power wheelchair for mobility but is able to walk up to 150 ft with contact guard using a cane. MP actively participates in his extended family and is on the board of several nonprofit organizations. His goals included improved use of the impaired upper extremity during transfers and dressing and improved use of the UE during eating, grooming, and computer activities.

7.8.2 Initial Examination and Outcome Measurements

A screening examination included active movements of his UE against gravity and several functional grasping movements to establish that MP had the motor ability necessary to participate in our study. This examination identified partially isolated, partial range of motion movement against gravity at all joints of the UE as well as gross and fine motor coordination impairments. Initial baseline data collection was performed prior to 4 weeks of biweekly home PT/OT sessions that were typical of the therapy performed by MP over the previous 18 months. A second data collection session immediately followed this period of home training and preceded a month of robotically facilitated training. A third data collection session was performed 4 days after completion of the robotically facilitated training period. To evaluate UE impairment at the body structure/function level we used the Upper Extremity Fugl-Meyer Assessment (FM) (Fugl-Meyer, Jaasko, Leyman, Olsson, & Steglind, 1975) and the Reach-to-Grasp test (RTG), a kinematic analysis of untrained UE movement (Schettino et al., 2006). The Wolf Motor Function Test (WMFT) (Wolf et al., 2005), the Jebsen Test of Hand Function (JTHF) (Jebsen, Taylor, Trieschmann, Trotter, & Howard, 1969), and the Nine Hole Peg Test (9HPT) (Mathiowetz, Volland, Kashman, & Weber, 1985) were used to test for changes at the activity level. This combination was chosen in order to capture change in the ability to perform gross and fine motor movements. During the initial examination, we noticed that MP had difficulty flexing his trunk during reaching. We added the Modified Functional Reach Test (MFR) (Katz-Leurer, Fisher, Neeb, Schwartz, & Carmeli, 2009) to track changes in this skill. Changes at the activity level were also tested outside the laboratory by collecting UE accelerometer data for 24 h immediately after each testing session. Measurements included the ratio of impaired to unimpaired UE vertical plane activity, total vertical plane activity (Lang, Macdonald, 2007; Lang, Wagner et al., 2007; Uswatte et al., 2005), and total roll plane activity. Roll plane motion was chosen because pronation movements are associated with

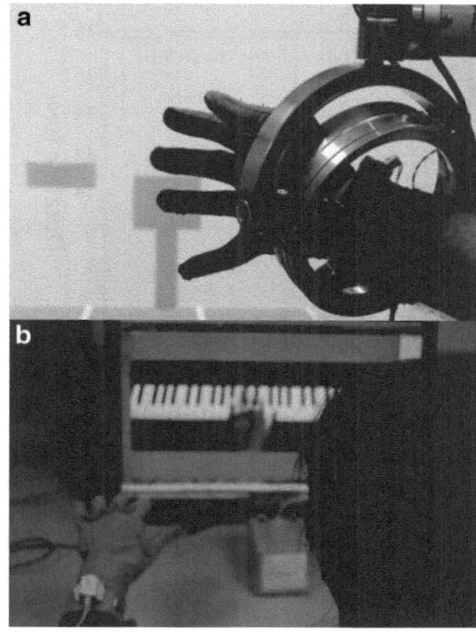

Fig. 7.5 (**a**) NJIT RAVR system. (**b**) NJIT Trackglove system

neurological recovery and tend to be associated with purposeful UE movement (Fan & He, 2006; Fan, He, & Tillery, 2006). MP completed the hand, mobility, activities of daily living, and social participation subscales of the Stroke Impact Scale (SIS; Duncan et al., 1999) to assess changes at the participation level.

7.8.3 Intervention

The VR intervention consisted of 12, 60 to 90 min sessions of training over 4 weeks with two virtual rehabilitation systems, the NJIT-RAVR system (Fig. 7.5a) and the NJIT TrackGlove system (Fig. 7.5b), which are described in detail elsewhere (Adamovich, Fluet, Mathai, et al., 2009; Adamovich, Fluet, Merians, et al., 2009; Merians et al., 2008). MP performed six simulated rehabilitation activities in each of 12 sessions.

7.8.3.1 Simulations

A brief description of each simulation, the therapeutic goals it was designed to address, the performance measure designed to track progress and the approach to increasing the intensity of the activity are described in Table 7.1. A discussion of the configuration and application of each simulation follows. MP had difficulty manipulating small objects due to an inability to flex fingers individually. The Virtual Piano

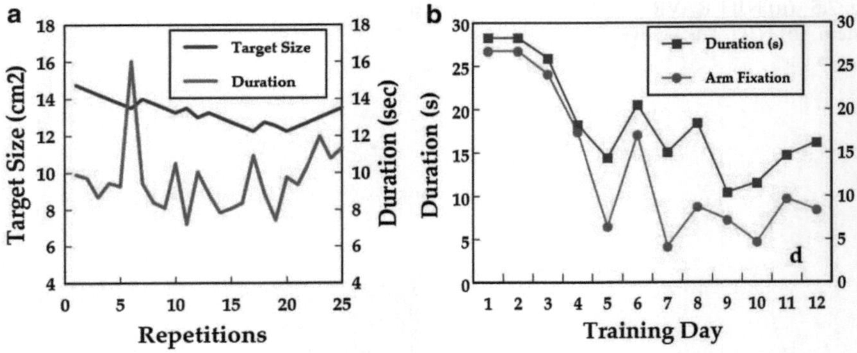

Fig. 7.6 (**a**) A representative example of 25 repetitions of MP performing the Hammer simulation in dynamic mode. The size of the peg to be hammered (*top line*) increases when the subject required more than 12 s to perform the task (*bottom line*) and decreased when he was able to hammer the peg in less than 12 s. (**b**) Average time to hammer a peg on each training day (*squares*) and average distance between peg and hammer during hammering (*circles*). This distance decreased as training progressed demonstrating improvements in MP's ability to stabilize his upper extremity during hammering

trainer simulation (Fig. 7.2 and Table 7.1) was used to address this impairment. MP played scales and drills with his hand in a stationary position and attempted simple songs with his hand moving across the entire keyboard. The program controlling the simulation measured the difference between the angle of the finger cued to press a key and the average of the non-cued fingers. When a predetermined difference between these two measurements was exceeded, the key was pressed. The algorithm previously described under "Activity Scaling" controlled the target difference. The Space Pong simulation (Table 7.1) addressed the difficulty controlling the aperture of the hand during grasping activities. MP played the Space Pong game using opening and closing of his hand to control the paddle. The Hammer simulation in dynamic mode (Table 7.1) was used to address difficulties with the manipulation of objects that were far from his body. MP reached to targets in a virtual space and hammered them using repetitive finger extension movements. We used an algorithm that increased target size, effectively decreasing proximal shoulder stabilization demands, when MP hammered targets slowly and decreased target size, increasing stabilization demands, when MP hammered targets quickly (Fig. 7.6a, b). We utilized the same hammer simulation in static mode to train a repetitive pronation movement in varying degrees of elbow extension and shoulder flexion (Table 7.1). MP demonstrated synergistic extension of his trunk during shoulder flexion making large excursion forward reaches difficult for him. We approached this impairment using two different simulations. The Reach-Touch simulation trained shoulder active range of motion with the trunk kept stationary (Table 7.1) and we used the Cup Reaching simulation to address shoulder elevation combined with active trunk movement (Table 7.1). During training with this simulation, MP attached his hand to a virtual cup near his body, reached forward and placed it in one of nine spaces on a virtual

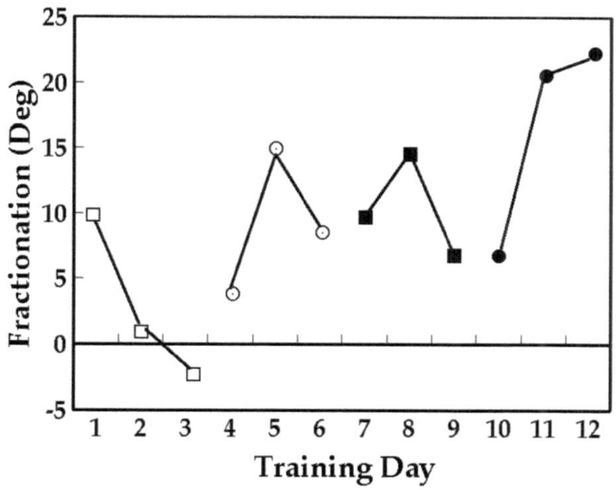

Fig. 7.7 Shows changes in MP's ability to isolate individual fingers during the training. These are the daily fractionation scores during the Virtual PIano simulation. The first 3 days (*open squares*) and the last 3 days (*open circles*) are performed without the Cybergrasp. Training days 4 through 6 (*solid squares*) are performed using the Cybergrasp 100 % of the time during the training session. Training days 7 through 9 (*solid circles*) are performed using the Cybergrasp for the first 5 min of each session

shelf. We set the height, width and distance of the shelves based on the maximal reaching distance of MP's arm which we measured weekly, with MP's trunk moving freely. We encouraged him to flex at the trunk to increase his forward reaching distance.

7.8.4 Responses and Modifications to Intervention

MP made little progress in the ability to flex his fingers during the Virtual Piano Trainer simulation performance as evidenced by his first three daily fractionation scores. We added the CyberGrasp™ (Fig. 7.2c), an exoskeleton robot, to assist MP in maintaining extension of the non-cued fingers while allowing flexion of the cued finger. Figure 7.7 shows the changes in MP's ability to isolate individual fingers (fractionation) during the training. MP used the CyberGrasp™ on training days 4 through 6 (Fig. 7.7 open circles). During training days 7 through 9 (Fig. 7.7 solid squares), MP used the CyberGrasp™ during the first 5 min of Virtual Piano trainer practice, and finished the 15-min block without the CyberGrasp™. He did not use the CyberGrasp™ at all during the final week (Fig. 7.7 solid circles). MP had difficulty performing the Space Pong simulation as evidenced by very low accuracy scores, due to an all-or-nothing quality of his hand opening. After week 1, we

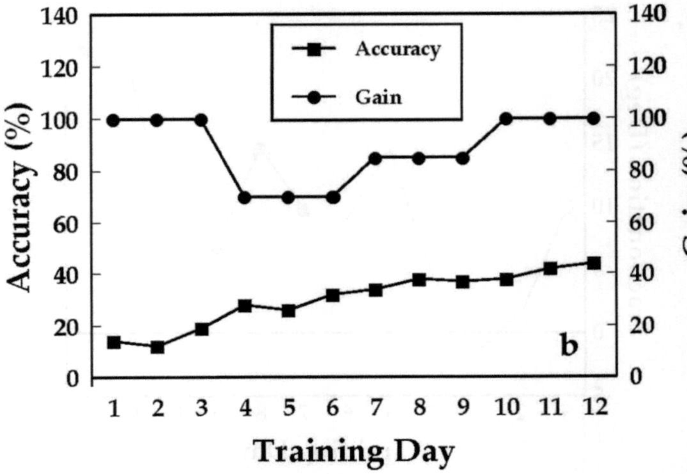

Fig. 7.8 Average accuracy scores for each training day demonstrated by MP during the Space Pong simulation (*circles*). Changes in the ratio of MP's finger movement and movement of the pong paddle (*squares*). This ratio was manipulated to allow MP to learn to more effectively control the opening and closing of his hand and play the game with a reasonable level of success

decreased the gain (Fig. 7.8 circles) from movement to virtual movement by 30 % which increased the amount of finger movement required to produce the paddle movement. This allowed MP to control his paddle accurately using the movement strategy available to him. The gain was increased by 15 % for training days 6 through 9 and back to 100 % for training days 10 through 12 as MP's accuracy scores increased (Fig. 7.8 squares). MP did not make significant improvements in his ability to pronate his forearm with his shoulder flexed and elbow extended during the use of the Hammer simulation in fixed mode (Table 7.1). We modified the relationship between the active pronation movement and the hammer swinging movement in an attempt to stimulate progress during this activity but none of these manipulations resulted in consistent increase in pronation excursion. MP made steady improvements in proximal stabilization while performing the Hammer finger extension simulation in dynamic mode during the first 2 weeks of the trial and maintained them in weeks 3 and 4. MP made small steady improvements in the time to touch all ten targets in the Reach-Touch simulation despite a steadily increasing workspace. In addition, the excursion of his forward reaching movement improved during performance of the Cup Reaching simulation while decreasing the movement time required to perform the activity. Prior to calibrating the workspace on training day 10, the PT managing the trial encouraged MP to challenge himself during the calibration process. This resulted in a much larger increase in reach excursion accomplished with a combination of trunk flexion and shoulder elevation. MP was able to use this strategy during the rest of the training period.

7.8.5 Outcomes

MP demonstrated no change in UEFMA after the month of home PT/OT (pretest 1 to pretest 2) and then a four-point improvement in the UEFMA after the month of robotically facilitated training (posttest). MP's improvements in UE activity measures were impressive as well. He made a small, 5 s improvement in JTHF time after the month of home therapy and an additional 35 s of improvement after the robotic intervention. MP demonstrated a 3 s decline in WMFT during his period of home training but a robust 44-s improvement subsequent to robotic training that greatly exceeds the published minimal clinical important difference of 2.7 s (Lin et al., 2009). There was no improvement in the NHPT following home training and a 14 s improvement following the VR training program. MFR distance increased 2 in. following home training and 10 in. following robotic training utilizing the strategy MP developed during the last week of training using the cup reaching simulation. MP also demonstrated improvements in all three 24-h activity measurements. Active vertical plane movement increased 1,538 s (26 min) which is consistent with those demonstrated during an acute rehabilitation stay (Lang, Macdonald, et al., 2007; Lang, Wagner, et al., 2007). Roll plane movement increased 789 s (13 min). Impaired arm movement to unimpaired arm movement ratio increased from 41 to 51 %, which is consistent with changes measured in a constraint induced movement therapy study of subjects post stroke (Uswatte et al., 2005). MP demonstrated an improvement of seven points on the hand scale of the SIS, eight points in the ADL scale and six points in the social participation scale. His caregivers confirmed MP's reports of increased use of his hand and arm during several activities of daily living.

7.8.6 Discussion

This case study presents the use of six VR simulations (four of them integrated with haptic robots) for the clinical management of a gentleman with hemiparesis due to chronic stroke. As in customary care, the intervention was specifically tailored for the patient and modified over time based upon the responses of the subject. The control systems governing the robotic interactions with the subject as well as the feedback presented by the VR simulations were adapted to address his specific impairments and functional limitations. Modifications in approach to training were made in four of the six simulations (Piano Trainer, Space Pong, Hammer Training, and Cup Reach) based on therapist observation. This resulted in dramatic improvements in performance in three of the four modified simulations, as well as robust improvements at the body structure/function, activity, and participation levels. The training protocols described in a large majority of the investigations of rehabilitation robotics involve set protocols that do not vary significantly based on subject response. While highly standardized protocols are valuable in determining specific changes elicited by specific interventions, there is also a possibility that they result in an underestimation of the potential benefits of this technology as they fail to address the specific impairments of a heterogeneous patient population or leverage the flexibility of virtual environments as rehabilitation platforms.

References

Acosta, A. M., Dewald, H. A., & Dewald, J. P. (2011). Pilot study to test effectiveness of video game on reaching performance in stroke. *Journal of Rehabilitation Research and Development, 48*(4), 431–444.

Adamovich, S. V., Fluet, G. G., Mathai, A., Qiu, Q., Lewis, J., & Merians, A. S. (2009). Design of a complex virtual reality simulation to train finger motion for persons with hemiparesis: A proof of concept study. *Journal of Neuroengineering and Rehabilitation, 6*, 28.

Adamovich, S. V., Fluet, G. G., Merians, A. S., Mathai, A., & Qiu, Q. (2009). Incorporating haptic effects into three-dimensional virtual environments to train the hemiparetic upper extremity. *IEEE Transactions on Neural Systems and Rehabilitation Engineering, 17*(5), 512–520.

Adamovich, S., Fluet, G. G., Tunik, E., & Merians, A. S. (2009). Sensorimotor training in virtual reality: A review. *NeuroRehabilitation, 25*(1), 29–44.

Archambault, P. S., Chong, J. N. F., Sorrento, G., Routhier, F., & Boissy, P. (2011). *Comparison of powered wheelchair driving performance in a real and in a simulated environment*. Paper presented at the International Conference on Virtual Rehabilitation (ICVR), 2011, Zurich.

Bagce, H. F., Saleh, S., Adamovich, S. V., & Tunik, E. (2011). Visuomotor discordance in virtual reality: Effects on online motor control. *Proceedings of the IEEE Engineering Medicine and Biological Society (EMBS)*, 2011, Boston (pp. 7262–7265).

Birkenmeier, R. L., Prager, E. M., & Lang, C. E. (2010). Translating animal doses of task-specific training to people with chronic stroke in 1-hour therapy sessions: A proof-of-concept study. *Neurorehabilitation and Neural Repair, 24*(7), 620–635.

Boian, R., Sharma, A., Han, C., Merians, A., Burdea, G., Adamovich, S., et al. (2002). Virtual reality-based post-stroke hand rehabilitation. *Studies in Health Technology and Informatics, 85*, 64–70.

Boyd, L., & Winstein, C. (2006). Explicit information interferes with implicit motor learning of both continuous and discrete movement tasks after stroke. *Journal of Neurologic Physical Therapy, 30*(2), 46–57.

Broeren, J., Rydmark, M., Bjorkdahl, A., & Sunnerhagen, K. S. (2007). Assessment and training in a 3-dimensional virtual environment with haptics: A report on 5 cases of motor rehabilitation in the chronic stage after stroke. *Neurorehabilitation and Neural Repair, 21*(2), 180–189.

Buccino, G., Solodkin, A., & Small, S. L. (2006). Functions of the mirror neuron system: Implications for neurorehabilitation. *Cognitive and Behavioral Neurology, 19*(1), 55–63.

Butler, A., Blanton, S., Rowe, V., & Wolf, S. (2006). Attempting to improve function and quality of life using the FTM Protocol: Case report. *Journal of Neurological Physical Therapy, 30*(3), 148–156.

Cameirao, M. S., Badia, S. B., Oller, E. D., & Verschure, P. F. (2010). Neurorehabilitation using the virtual reality based Rehabilitation Gaming System: Methodology, design, psychometrics, usability and validation. *Journal of Neuroengineering and Rehabilitation, 7*, 48.

Celnik, P., Stefan, K., Hummel, F., Duque, J., Classen, J., & Cohen, L. G. (2006). Encoding a motor memory in the older adult by action observation. *NeuroImage, 29*(2), 677–684.

Connelly, L., Jia, Y., Toro, M. L., Stoykov, M. E., Kenyon, R. V., & Kamper, D. G. (2010). A pneumatic glove and immersive virtual reality environment for hand rehabilitative training after stroke. *IEEE Transactions on Neural Systems and Rehabilitation Engineering, 18*(5), 551–559.

Dromerick, A. W., Lang, C. E., Birkenmeier, R., Hahn, M. G., Sahrmann, S. A., & Edwards, D. F. (2006). Relationships between upper-limb functional limitation and self-reported disability 3 months after stroke. *Journal of Rehabilitation Research and Development, 43*(3), 401–408.

Duncan, P. W., Wallace, D., Lai, S. M., Johnson, D., Embretson, S., & Laster, L. J. (1999). The stroke impact scale version 2.0. Evaluation of reliability, validity, and sensitivity to change. *Stroke, 30*(10), 2131–2140.

Dvorkin, A. Y., Bogey, R. A., Harvey, R. L., & Patton, J. L. (2006). Mapping the neglected space: Gradients of detection revealed by virtual reality. *Neurorehabilitation and Neural Repair, 26*(2), 120–131.

Erren-Wolters, C. V., van Dijk, H., de Kort, A. C., Izerman, M. J., & Jannink, M. J. (2007). Virtual reality for mobility devices: Training applications and clinical results: A review. *International Journal of Rehabilitation Research, 30*(2), 91–96.

Fan, J., & He, J. (2006). Motor cortical encoding of hand orientation in a 3-D reach-to-grasp task. *Proceedings of IEEE Engineering in Medicine and Biology Society (EMBS), 2006*(1), 5472–5475.

Fan, J., He, J., & Tillery, S. I. (2006). Control of hand orientation and arm movement during reach and grasp. *Experimental Brain Research, 171*(3), 283–296.

Fischer, H. C., Stubblefield, K., Kline, T., Luo, X., Kenyon, R. V., & Kamper, D. G. (2007). Hand rehabilitation following stroke: A pilot study of assisted finger extension training in a virtual environment. *Topics in Stroke Rehabilitation, 14*(1), 1–12.

Fluet, G. G., Merians, A. S., Qiu, Q., Lafond, I., Saleh, S., Ruano, V., et al. (2012). Robots integrated with virtual reality simulations for customized motor training in a person with upper extremity hemiparesis: A case study. *Journal of Neurologic Physical Therapy, 36*(2), 79–86.

Fugl-Meyer, A. R., Jaasko, L., Leyman, I., Olsson, S., & Steglind, S. (1975). The post-stroke hemiplegic patient. 1. A method for evaluation of physical performance. *Scandinavian Journal of Rehabilitation Medicine, 7*(1), 13–31.

Gaggioli, A., Meneghini, A., Morganti, F., Alcaniz, M., & Riva, G. (2006). A strategy for computer-assisted mental practice in stroke rehabilitation. *Neurorehabilitation and Neural Repair, 20*(4), 503–507.

Glover, S., & Castiello, U. (2006). Recovering space in unilateral neglect: A neurological dissociation revealed by virtual reality. *Journal of Cognitive Neuroscience, 18*(5), 833–843.

Henderson, A., Korner-Bitensky, N., & Levin, M. (2007). Virtual reality in stroke rehabilitation: A systematic review of its effectiveness for upper limb motor recovery. *Topics in Stroke Rehabilitation, 14*(2), 52–61.

Holden, M. K. (2005). Virtual environments for motor rehabilitation: Review. *Cyberpsychology and Behavior, 8*(3), 187–211.

Holden, M. K., Dyar, T. A., & Dayan-Cimadoro, L. (2007). Telerehabilitation using a virtual environment improves upper extremity function in patients with stroke. *IEEE Transactions on Neural Systems and Rehabilitation Engineering, 15*(1), 36–42.

Housman, S. J., Scott, K. M., & Reinkensmeyer, D. J. (2009). A randomized controlled trial of gravity-supported, computer-enhanced arm exercise for individuals with severe hemiparesis. *Neurorehabilitation and Neural Repair, 23*(5), 505–514.

Huang, F. C., Gillespie, R. B., & Kuo, A. D. (2007). Visual and haptic feedback contribute to tuning and online control during object manipulation. *Journal of Motor Behavior, 39*(3), 179–193.

Jack, D., Boian, R., Merians, A. S., Tremaine, M., Burdea, G. C., Adamovich, S. V., et al. (2001). Virtual reality-enhanced stroke rehabilitation. *IEEE Transactions on Neural Systems and Rehabilitation Engineering, 9*(3), 308–318.

Jang, S. H., You, S. H., Hallett, M., Cho, Y. W., Park, C. M., Cho, S. H., et al. (2005). Cortical reorganization and associated functional motor recovery after virtual reality in patients with chronic stroke: An experimenter-blind preliminary study. *Archives of Physical Medicine and Rehabilitation, 86*(11), 2218–2223.

Jebsen, R. H., Taylor, N., Trieschmann, R. B., Trotter, M. J., & Howard, L. A. (1969). An objective and standardized test of hand function. *Archives of Physical Medicine and Rehabilitation, 50*(6), 311–319.

Jette, A. M. (2006). Toward a common language for function, disability, and health. *Physical Therapy, 86*(5), 726–734.

Katz-Leurer, M., Fisher, I., Neeb, M., Schwartz, I., & Carmeli, E. (2009). Reliability and validity of the modified functional reach test at the sub-acute stage post-stroke. *Disability and Rehabilitation, 31*(3), 243–248.

Krakauer, J. W. (2006). Motor learning: Its relevance to stroke recovery and neurorehabilitation. *Current Opinion in Neurology, 19*(1), 84–90.

Krebs, H. I., Mernoff, S., Fasoli, S. E., Hughes, R., Stein, J., & Hogan, N. (2008). A comparison of functional and impairment-based robotic training in severe to moderate chronic stroke: A pilot study. *NeuroRehabilitation, 23*(1), 81–87.

Kwakkel, G., van Peppen, R., Wagenaar, R. C., Wood-Dauphinee, S., Richards, C., Ashburn, A., et al. (2004). Effects of augmented exercise therapy time after stroke: A meta-analysis. *Stroke, 35*(11), 2529–2539.

Lam, P., Hebert, D., Boger, J., Lacheray, H., Gardner, D., Apkarian, J., et al. (2008). A haptic-robotic platform for upper-limb reaching stroke therapy: Preliminary design and evaluation results. *Journal of Neuroengineering and Rehabilitation, 5*, 15.

Lam, Y. S., Man, D. W., Tam, S. F., & Weiss, P. L. (2006). Virtual reality training for stroke rehabilitation. *NeuroRehabilitation, 21*(3), 245–253.

Lambercy, O., Dovat, L., Gassert, R., Burdet, E., Teo, C. L., & Milner, T. (2007). A haptic knob for rehabilitation of hand function. *IEEE Transactions on Neural Systems and Rehabilitation Engineering, 15*(3), 356–366.

Lang, C., Macdonald, J., & Gnip, C. (2007). Counting repetitions: An observational study of outpatient therapy for people with hemiparesis post-stroke. *Journal of Neurological Physical Therapy, 31*(1), 3–11.

Lang, C. E., Wagner, J. M., Edwards, D. F., & Dromerick, A. W. (2007). Upper extremity use in people with hemiparesis in the first few weeks after stroke. *Journal of Neurological Physical Therapy, 31*(2), 56–63.

Laver, K. E., George, S., Thomas, S., Deutsch, J. E., & Crotty, M. (2011). Virtual reality for stroke rehabilitation. *Cochrane Database of Systematic Reviews, 9*, CD008349.

Lee, T. D., White, M. A., & Carnahan, H. (1990). On the role of knowledge of results in motor learning: Exploring the guidance hypothesis. *Journal of Motor Behavior, 22*(2), 191–208.

Lin, K. C., Hsieh, Y. W., Wu, C. Y., Chen, C. L., Jang, Y., & Liu, J. S. (2009). Minimal detectable change and clinically important difference of the Wolf Motor Function Test in stroke patients. *Neurorehabilitation and Neural Repair, 23*(5), 429–434.

Lo, A. C., Guarino, P., Krebs, H. I., Volpe, B. T., Bever, C. T., Duncan, P. W., et al. (2009). Multicenter randomized trial of robot-assisted rehabilitation for chronic stroke: Methods and entry characteristics for VA ROBOTICS. *Neurorehabilitation and Neural Repair, 23*(8), 775–783.

Lum, P. S., Burgar, C. G., & Shor, P. C. (2004). Evidence for improved muscle activation patterns after retraining of reaching movements with the MIME robotic system in subjects with post-stroke hemiparesis. *IEEE Transactions on Neural Systems and Rehabilitation Engineering, 12*(2), 186–194.

Mathiowetz, V., Volland, G., Kashman, N., & Weber, K. (1985). Adult norms for the 9 hole peg test of manual dexterity. *American Journal of Occupational Therapy, 39*(6), 386–391.

Merians, A., Fluet, G. G., Qiu, Q., Saleh, S., Lafond, I., & Adamovich, S. V. (2010). *Integrated arm and hand training using robotics and virtual reality simulations*. Paper presented at the 8th Annual International Conference on Disability, Virtual Reality and Associated Technologies, Vina del Mar/Valaparaiso, Chile.

Merians, A. S., Fluet, G. G., Qiu, Q., Saleh, S., Lafond, I., Davidow, A., et al. (2011). Robotically facilitated virtual rehabilitation of arm transport integrated with finger movement in persons with hemiparesis. *Journal of Neuroengineering and Rehabilitation, 8*, 27.

Merians, A. S., Poizner, H., Boian, R., Burdea, G., & Adamovich, S. (2006). Sensorimotor training in a virtual reality environment: Does it improve functional recovery poststroke? *Neurorehabilitation and Neural Repair, 20*(2), 252–267.

Merians, A. S., Tunik, E., & Adamovich, S. V. (2009). Virtual reality to maximize function for hand and arm rehabilitation: Exploration of neural mechanisms. *Studies in Health Technology and Informatics, 145*, 109–125.

Merians, A. S., Tunik, E., Fluet, G. G., Qiu, Q., & Adamovich, S. V. (2008). Innovative approaches to the rehabilitation of upper extremity hemiparesis using virtual environments. *European Journal of Physical and Rehabilitation Medicine, 45*(1), 123–133.

Piron, L., Tombolini, P., Turolla, A., Zucconi, C., Agostini, M., Dam, M., et al. (2007). *Reinforced feedback in virtual environment facilitates the arm motor recovery in patients after a recent stroke*. Paper presented at the International Conference on Virtual Rehabilitation (ICVR), 2007, Beijing.

Piron, L., Tonin, P., Atzori, A. M., Zucconi, C., Massaro, C., Trivello, E., et al. (2003). The augmented-feedback rehabilitation technique facilitates the arm motor recovery in patients after a recent stroke. *Studies in Health Technology and Informatics, 94*, 265–267.

Piron, L., Tonin, P., Piccione, F., Iaia, V., Trevello, E., & Dam, M. (2005). Virtual environment training for arm motor rehabilitation. *Presence, 16*(6), 732–740.

Piron, L., Turolla, A., Agostini, M., Zucconi, C., Cortese, F., Zampolini, M., et al. (2009). Exercises for paretic upper limb after stroke: A combined virtual-reality and telemedicine approach. *Journal of Rehabilitation Medicine, 41*(12), 1016–1102.

Piron, L., Turolla, A., Agostini, M., Zucconi, C. S., Ventura, L., Tonin, P., et al. (2009). Motor learning principles for rehabilitation: A pilot randomized controlled study in poststroke patients. *Neurorehabilitation and Neural Repair, 24*(6), 501–508.

Plautz, E. J., Milliken, G. W., & Nudo, R. J. (2000). Effects of repetitive motor training on movement representations in adult squirrel monkeys: Role of use versus learning. *Neurobiology of Learning and Memory, 74*(1), 27–55.

Ramachandran, V. S., & Altschuler, E. L. (2009). The use of visual feedback, in particular mirror visual feedback, in restoring brain function. *Brain, 132*(Pt 7), 1693–1710.

Rand, D., Katz, N., & Weiss, P. L. (2009). Intervention using the VMall for improving motor and functional ability of the upper extremity in post stroke participants. *European Journal of Physical and Rehabilitation Medicine, 45*(1), 113–121.

Remple, M. S., Bruneau, R. M., VandenBerg, P. M., Goertzen, C., & Kleim, J. A. (2001). Sensitivity of cortical movement representations to motor experience: Evidence that skill learning but not strength training induces cortical reorganization. *Behavioral and Brain Research, 123*(2), 133–141.

Saposnik, G., & Levin, M. (2011). Virtual reality in stroke rehabilitation: A meta-analysis and implications for clinicians. *Stroke, 42*(5), 1380–1386.

Saposnik, G., Teasell, R., Mamdani, M., Hall, J., McIlroy, W., Cheung, D., et al. (2010). Effectiveness of virtual reality using Wii gaming technology in stroke rehabilitation: A pilot randomized clinical trial and proof of principle. *Stroke, 41*(7), 1477–1484.

Sathian, K., Buxbaum, L. J., Cohen, L. G., Krakauer, J. W., Lang, C. E., Corbetta, M., et al. (2011). Neurological principles and rehabilitation of action disorders: Common clinical deficits. *Neurorehabilitation and Neural Repair, 25*(5 Suppl), 21S–32S.

Schettino, L. F., Adamovich, S. V., Hening, W., Tunik, E., Sage, J., & Poizner, H. (2006). Hand preshaping in Parkinson's disease: Effects of visual feedback and medication state. *Experimental Brain Research, 168*(1–2), 186–202.

Singapogu, R. B., Sander, S. T., Burg, T. C., & Cobb, W. S. (2008). Comparative study of haptic training versus visual training for kinesthetic navigation tasks. *Studies in Health Technology and Informatics, 132*, 469–471.

Smith, J., Hebert, D., & Reid, D. (2007). Exploring the effects of virtual reality on unilateral neglect caused by stroke: Four case studies. *Technology and Disability, 19*(1), 29–40.

Stein, J., Bishop, L., Gillen, G., & Helbok, R. (2011). *A pilot study of robotic-assisted exercise for hand weakness after stroke*. Paper presented at the IEEE International Conference on Rehabilitation Robotics (ICORR), Zurich.

Subramanian, S. K., Lourenco, C. B., Chilingaryan, G., Sveistrup, H., & Levin, M. F. (2013). Arm motor recovery using a virtual reality intervention in chronic stroke: Randomized control trial. *Neurorehabilitation and Neural Repair, 27*(1), 13–23.

Sveistrup, H. (2004). Motor rehabilitation using virtual reality. *Journal of Neuroengineering and Rehabilitation, 1*(1), 10.

Swanson, L. R., & Lee, T. D. (1992). Effects of aging and schedules of knowledge of results on motor learning. *Journal of Gerontology, 47*(6), 406–411.

Taylor, M. J., McCormick, D., Shawis, T., Impson, R., & Griffin, M. (2011). Activity-promoting gaming systems in exercise and rehabilitation. *Journal of Rehabitational Research and Development, 48*(10), 1171–1186.

Tsirlin, I., Dupierrix, E., Chokron, S., Coquillart, S., & Ohlmann, T. (2009). Uses of virtual reality for diagnosis, rehabilitation and study of unilateral spatial neglect: Review and analysis. *Cyberpsychology and Behavior, 12*(2), 175–181.

Tunik, E., & Adamovich, S. V. (2009). Remapping in the ipsilesional motor cortex after VR-based training: A pilot fMRI study. *Proceedings of IEEE Engineering in Medicine and Biology Society (EMBS)*, 2009, Minneapolis (pp. 1139–1142).

Uswatte, G., Foo, W., Olmstead, H., Lopez, K., Holand, A., & Simms, L. B. (2005). Ambulatory monitoring of arm movement using accelerometry: An objective measure of upper-extremity rehabilitation in persons with chronic stroke. *Archives of Physical Medicine and Rehabilitation, 86*(7), 1498–1501.

Volpe, B. T., Lynch, D., Rykman-Berland, A., Ferraro, M., Galgano, M., Hogan, N., et al. (2008). Intensive sensorimotor arm training mediated by therapist or robot improves hemiparesis in patients with chronic stroke. *Neurorehabilitation and Neural Repair, 22*(3), 305–310.

Weiss, P. L., & Katz, N. (2004). The potential of virtual reality for rehabilitation. *Journal of Rehabilitation Research and Development, 41*(5), vii–x.

Winstein, C. J., Merians, A. S., & Sullivan, K. J. (1999). Motor learning after unilateral brain damage. *Neuropsychologia, 37*(8), 975–987.

Wolbrecht, E. T., Chan, V., Reinkensmeyer, D. J., & Bobrow, J. E. (2008). Optimizing compliant, model-based robotic assistance to promote neurorehabilitation. *IEEE Transactions on Neural Systems and Rehabilitation Engineering, 16*(3), 286–297.

Wolf, S. L., Thompson, P. A., Morris, D. M., Rose, D. K., Winstein, C. J., Taub, E., et al. (2005). The EXCITE trial: Attributes of the Wolf Motor Function Test in patients with subacute stroke. *Neurorehabilitation and Neural Repair, 19*(3), 194–205.

Wolf, S., Winstein, C., Miller, J., Taub, E., Uswatte, G., Morris, D., et al. (2006). Effect of constraint-induced movement therapy on upper extremity function 3 to 9 months after stroke. *JAMA, 296*, 2095–2104.

World Health Organization. (2002). *Towards a common language for functioning, disability and health (ICF)*. Geneva. Retrieved January 5, 2013 from http://www.who.int/classifications/icf/training/icfbeginnersguide.pdf

Wulf, G., Landers, M., Lewthwaite, R., & Tollner, T. (2009). External focus instructions reduce postural instability in individuals with Parkinson disease. *Physical Therapy, 89*(2), 162–168.

Wulf, G., McNevin, N. H., Fuchs, T., Ritter, F., & Toole, T. (2000). Attentional focus in complex skill learning. *Research Quarterly for Exercise and Sport, 71*(3), 229–239.

Yavuzer, G., Senel, A., Atay, M. B., & Stam, H. J. (2008). "Playstation eyetoy games" improve upper extremity-related motor functioning in subacute stroke: A randomized controlled clinical trial. *European Journal of Physical and Rehabilitation Medicine, 44*(3), 237–244.

Chapter 8
Virtual Reality Augmented Training for Improving Walking and Reducing Fall Risk in Patients with Neurodegenerative Disease

Anat Mirelman, Judith E. Deutsch, and Jeffrey M. Hausdorff

Objective To present a review of VR augmented training for improving walking and reducing fall risk in patients with neurodegenerative disease.

8.1 Neurodegenerative Diseases

Neurodegeneration is the umbrella term for the progressive loss of structure or function of neurons or neuronal death. Neurodegeneration can be found in all levels of neuronal circuitry ranging from molecular to systemic. Neurodegeneration in essence is part of the normal process of aging. With aging, neurons gradually lose function and white matter lesions start to appear. However the term is most often associated with pathological processes known as neurodegenerative diseases including diseases such as Parkinson's disease (PD) and Alzheimer's disease (AD)

A. Mirelman (✉)
Movement Disorders Unit, Department of Neurology,
Tel-Aviv Sourasky Medical Center, Tel-Aviv, Israel
e-mail: anatmi@tlvmc.gov.il

J.E. Deutsch
RiVERS Lab, Department of Rehabilitation and Movement Science,
Rutgers Biomedical and Health Sciences, 65 Bergen Street SSB 723,
Newark, NJ 07101, USA
e-mail: deutsch@shrp.rutgers.edu

J.M. Hausdorff
Movement Disorders Unit, Department of Neurology,
Tel-Aviv Sourasky Medical Center, Tel-Aviv, Israel

Department of Physical Therapy, Sackler Faculty of Medicine,
Tel-Aviv University, Tel-Aviv, Israel

Harvard Medical School, Boston, MA, USA
e-mail: jhausdor@tlvmc.gov.il

P.L. (Tamar) Weiss et al. (eds.), *Virtual Reality for Physical and Motor Rehabilitation*, Virtual Reality Technologies for Health and Clinical Applications,
DOI 10.1007/978-1-4939-0968-1_8,

(Bredesen, Rao, & Mehlen, 2006) which in a sense could be considered "rapid aging diseases." In fact, the greatest risk factor for neurodegenerative diseases is aging, with neurons gradually losing more function as the disease progresses with age and with the involvement of extended brain regions and networks that affect different modalities resulting in motor and cognitive deficits (Bredesen et al., 2006; Lin & Beal, 2006).

Many common features exist among different neurodegenerative diseases such as atypical protein assemblies and induced cell death. However, the brain regions that are involved differ between the diseases and therefore lead to different initial symptoms and pathologies (Bredesen et al., 2006; Rubinsztein, 2006). For example, AD is characterized by loss of neurons and synapses in the cerebral cortex and certain subcortical regions while PD is characterized by the death of dopamine-generating cells in the basal ganglia. Nevertheless, as the disease progresses, multiple brain regions may be involved and symptoms are highly variable. Affected systems include motor, cognitive function, autonomic, and affective function. Motor and physical deficits include muscle weakness, loss of range, changes in posture, and reduced aerobic capacity which have a direct impact on balance, gait, and mobility (Schenkman & Butler, 1989). Autonomic function includes urinary and bowl control as well as cardiac denervation (Goldstein, 2003). Cognitive and affective deficits include reduced attention and impaired executive function which affect task planning, dual tasking, sensory integration, judgment, and reasoning (van Iersel, Kessels, Bloem, Verbeek, & Olde Rikkert, 2008; Yogev-Seligmann, Hausdorff, & Giladi, 2008) and behavioral changes that involve depression, loss of motivation and initiation, and increased anxiety.

In this chapter, we briefly discuss the common impairments in gait that are fundamental to neurodegenerative diseases and provide examples from studies on aging, PD, a classical neurodegenerative disease, and multiple sclerosis (MS), an inflammatory progressive disease that involves neuronal loss. Factors that contribute to problems in mobility will be presented along with current treatment approaches. The review of these topics will lead to the rationale and potential advantages of virtual reality-based methods for improving walking and mobility in patients with neurodegenerative disease.

8.2 Gait Impairments and Falls in Neurodegenerative Conditions

Gait impairments and falls are ubiquitous among the general older adult population and among patients with common neurological diseases. Approximately 30 % of community-dwelling elderly over the age of 65 fall at least once a year, and 6 % of these falls result in fractures (Blake et al., 1988; Tinetti, Speechley, & Ginter, 1988).

These figures are even higher in populations with pathologies such as PD, with an annual incidence of 60–80 % (Tinetti et al., 1988; Wood, Bilclough, Bowron, & Walker, 2002), at least twice that of the general elderly population. The impact of falls is severe. Falls often lead to institutionalization and loss of functional independence, disability, depression, and social isolation (Rubenstein & Josephson, 2006). Given the significance of falls on quality of life and functional independence, the careful assessment of the mechanisms that underlie the reasons for falls is needed prior to considering the appropriate therapeutic interventions.

With aging, elderly individuals generally walk more slowly, with shorter strides, decreased arm swing, and longer double-limb support times (Morris, Huxham, McGinley, & Iansek, 2001; Morris, Iansek, Matyas, & Summers, 1994). Fear of falling, a cautious gait (Ashburn, Stack, Pickering, & Ward, 2001; Legters, 2002), gait unsteadiness, or inconsistency and dysrhythmicity of stepping have also been closely associated with decreased mobility and an increased risk of falls in the elderly and are recognized mediators of fall risk (Hausdorff et al., 2001; Hausdorff & Yogev, 2006).

Commonly observed gait changes in individuals with PD also include small shuffling steps and spatial and temporal asymmetry (Morris, Iansek, Matyas, & Summers, 1996; Morris et al., 2001) as well as start hesitation, difficulty in maneuvering through tight or occluded spaces (Bloem, Hausdorff, Visser, & Giladi, 2004; Gray & Hildebrand, 2000), and a loss of consistency in one's ability to produce a steady gait rhythm, which in turn produces stride-to-stride variability (Baltadjieva, Giladi, Gruendlinger, Peretz, & Hausdorff, 2006; Hausdorff, Cudkowicz, Firtion, Wei, & Goldberger, 1998). In PD, reports on the effects of cueing support the idea that impairment of internal clocking mechanisms results in disruption of the normal motor programming. It seems that the "internal cueing" needed to perform automatic, sequential movements (Baltadjieva et al., 2006; Schaafsma et al., 2003) is the principal determinant of the increased gait variability in PD, while force production issues are important, but secondary (Baltadjieva et al., 2006). In support of this hypothesis, it is noted that stride variability improves, to some degree, in response to dopamine treatment (Schaafsma et al., 2003) and in response to external cueing (Rubenstein, Giladi, & Hausdorff, 2002; Thaut et al., 1996).

In MS, common symptoms include paresis, sensory impairment, spasticity, balance deficits, and fatigue (O'Sullivan, 1984). These impairments often lead to gait disturbances and difficulty walking. Approximately 50 % of individuals with MS will require assistance and/or an assistive device to ambulate short distances within 15 years of onset of the disease (Weinshenker, 1994), and between 50 and 60 % of people with MS identify fatigue as the worst symptom that they experience (Fisk, Pontefract, Ritvo, Archibald, & Murray, 1994; Freal, Kraft, & Coryell, 1984), which in turn severely affects functional walking endurance and independence.

8.3 Obstacle Negotiation and Dual Tasking: Two Key Elements to Functional Independence

8.3.1 Obstacle Negotiation

The alterations in gait that commonly occur in aging and neurodegenerative disease may be further challenged in complex everyday, walking environments that require obstacle negotiation. These challenges further increase the risk of falls in these populations. Obstacle crossing is a daily activity that involves tasks such as going up a curb or stepping over a crack in the ground or a branch. A decline in obstacle crossing performance with advancing age has been implicated in the high incidence of trips and stumbles in older adults (Overstall, Exton-Smith, Imms, & Johnson, 1977; Tinetti et al., 1988). In patients with PD, obstacle avoidance (Robinson et al., 2005) and dual or multitasking situations (Brown & Brockmole, 2010) have been implicated as the foremost extrinsic (environmental) risk factors for falls. The majority of trips arise from errors in foot contact with ground-based obstacles during obstacle negotiation (Fingerhut, Cox, & Warner, 1998). Compared to healthy young adults, older adults walk more slowly during obstacle crossing (Chapman & Hollands, 2007; Lowrey, Watson, & Vallis, 2007) with smaller steps (Chen, Ashton-Miller, Alexander, & Schultz, 1994; Lowrey et al., 2007) and land dangerously closer to the obstacle with their lead limb after crossing (Galna, Murphy, & Morris, 2010; Lowrey et al., 2007), increasing the risk of falls. Vitorio, Pieruccini-Faria, Stella, Gobbi, and Gobbi (2010) compared obstacle crossing between patients with mild-to-moderate PD and age-matched older adults and found that during the approach phase, people with PD demonstrated even shorter stride length and greater stride duration than controls. For the crossing phase, people with PD demonstrated shorter step length over the obstacle and a shorter distance from the lead limb foot to the obstacle both before and after crossing.

Age-related deficits in vision, proprioception, visual-spatial orientation, cognition, and attention can also negatively impact postural stability and lower limb kinematics when crossing obstacles (Lord, Smith, & Menant, 2010; Menant, St George, Fitzpatrick, & Lord, 2010). Indeed, obstacle negotiation is attentionally demanding and thus relies heavily on the availability of ample cognitive resources due to the need for motor planning and visually dependent gait regulation (Brown, McKenzie, & Doan, 2005). In fact, in situations when attention is divided, older people negotiate obstacles even more slowly and contact more obstacles (Menant et al., 2010). With neurodegeneration, motor and cognitive abilities deteriorate and the ability to negotiate obstacles depreciates even further (Vitorio et al., 2010).

8.3.2 Executive Function, Attention, and Dual Tasking

Diminished cognitive function, specifically executive function (EF) and attention, negatively affects gait and postural stability in older adults, in individuals with PD, and in patients with MS (Adams & Parsons, 2003; Woollacott & Shumway-Cook, 2002). EF refers to a variety of higher cognitive processes including initiation of goal-directed

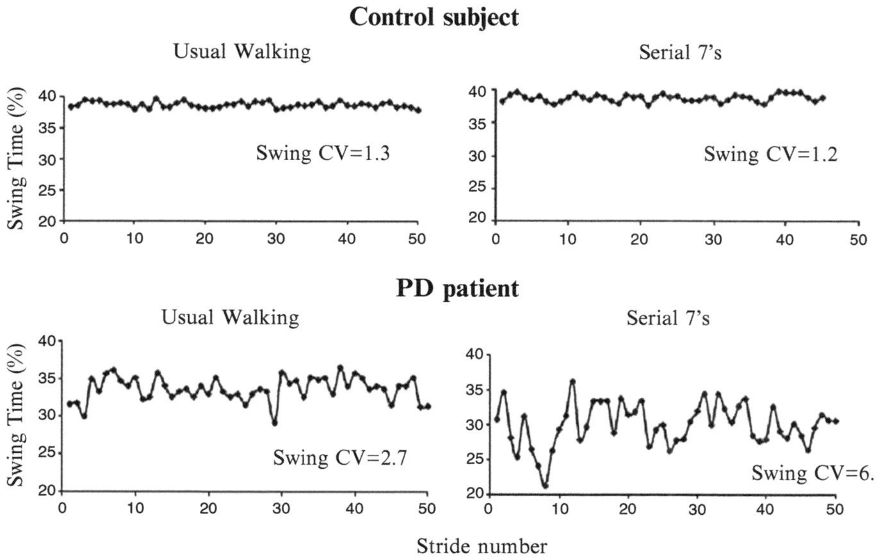

Fig. 8.1 Example of swing time series in a patient with PD and a control under usual walking conditions and when performing a dual task (serial 7 subtractions). Variability increases during dual tasking in the subject with PD, but not in the control subject. Adapted from Yogev et al. (2005)

behavior, intention of action, planning, working memory, and attention (Fuster, 1999). Attention is driven in part by sensory perception and refers to the selection of a preferred stimulus for a particular action while ignoring or rejecting the irrelevant (D'Esposito, Ballard, Zarahn, & Aguirre, 2000; Jueptner, Frith, Brooks, Frackowiak, & Passingham, 1997; Passingham, 1996; Rowe et al., 2002; Yogev et al., 2005). Lezak (1995) divided EF into four major components: volition, planning, purposive action, and effective performance (action monitoring). Others also explicitly include cognitive inhibition as an EF component (Stuss & Alexander, 2000; Yogev-Seligmann et al., 2008). Impairment of one or more of these EF components may impact one's ability to walk efficiently and safely. Poor self-awareness of limitations, an aspect of volition, might result in an increased risk of falling (van Iersel et al., 2008). Impaired planning skills can lead to getting lost, choices that produce inefficient pathways or unnecessary effort to arrive at a destination, and collisions with obstacles.

Healthy young adults pay little attention to their gait when they walk in simple, unobstructed environments. However when encountering complex environments such as uneven surfaces, negotiating obstacles, diminished visibility, or crowded places their walking becomes slower. This also occurs when young adults are asked to walk and perform another task simultaneously (i.e., dual task, DT) (Beauchet et al., 2003; Ebersbach et al., 1999; Gage, Sleik, Polych, McKenzie, & Brown, 2003; Yogev, Plotnik, Peretz, Giladi, & Hausdorff, 2006). Healthy older adults and, to a greater extent, patient populations (e.g., patients with PD or MS) not only slow down, increasing double-limb support on the ground, but also become less stable (i.e., increased gait variability) (Bond & Morris, 2000; Hausdorff, Balash, & Giladi, 2003; Sheridan, Solomont, Kowall, & Hausdorff, 2003; Yogev et al., 2005) (see Fig. 8.1).

The simultaneous performance of two or more tasks often creates a conflict and a need to determine which of the tasks receives priority, especially when information processing is limited (Pashler, 1994). Bloem et al. (Bloem, Boers, Cramer, Westendorp, & Gerschlager, 2001; Bloem, van Vugt, & Beckley, 2001) reported that young adults and healthy elderly spontaneously prioritize gait stability over success on the "secondary," cognitive task, when no specific prioritization instructions or allocation of attention is given. This "posture first strategy" makes sense from an ecologic perspective as it helps to prevent loss of balance. Interestingly, with aging, this prioritization is not as efficient increasing the "cost" of performing a secondary task and thus increasing the risk of falls. Further, several studies have shown that DT during gait in patients with PD results in a slower walk, with shorter strides, and much higher "DT" decrement than that seen in controls (Bloem, Valkenburg, Slabbekoorn, & Willemsen, 2001; Bond & Morris, 2000; Hausdorff et al., 2003; Lundin-Olsson, Nyberg, & Gustafson, 1997; Yogev et al., 2006).

8.4 Cognitive Deficits and Their Contribution to Gait Problems and Fall Risk

In the past decade, many studies have contributed to the body of knowledge on the importance of cognitive function in walking. Gait is no longer considered to be an automatic, biomechanical task; instead, the role of cognitive function is increasingly recognized (Alexander & Hausdorff, 2008; Yogev-Seligmann et al., 2008). Cognitive impairments are common in neurodegenerative diseases even in the early stages of the disease, and they tend to further deteriorate as the disease progresses. In the following paragraph, we briefly summarize the evidence indicating that impaired cognitive function is related to gait disturbances in specific neurodegenerative conditions. This relationship is important because it helps to define the requirements for optimal interventions, as described further below.

8.4.1 Parkinson's Disease

Cognitive impairment is a well-recognized non-motor feature of PD. About 15–40 % of patients with PD suffer some degree of cognitive impairment (Muslimovic, Post, Speelman, & Schmand, 2005). The main feature of cognitive decline associated with PD is impairment of EF. Deficits in EF can already be detected shortly after motor symptoms appear (Aarsland, Bronnick, Larsen, Tysnes, & Alves, 2009). EF is traditionally associated with the frontal lobes and related brain networks. The area of the prefrontal lobe and, in particular, the dorsolateral prefrontal cortex (DLPFC, Brodmann's area 9) and the cingulate cortex (e.g., the anterior cingulate: ACC, Brodmann's areas 24, 32) have been related to the cognitive aspects of EF

(Lezak, 1995; Stuss & Alexander, 2000; Yogev-Seligmann et al., 2008). In general, the anterior parts of the frontal lobes are involved with aspects of self-regulation, such as inhibition and self-awareness, whereas the dorsal parts are involved with reasoning processes.

In PD, cognitive deterioration also manifests as a profound difficulty in motor planning, resulting in both slowness of initiating motor action, slowed generation of ideas and plans, and reduced performance on tasks that involve attentional processes. This becomes especially apparent during DT activities. As noted above, studies have shown that DT during gait in patients with PD causes patients to walk slower, with shorter strides, and much higher "DT" decrement than that seen in controls (Bloem, Valkenburg, et al., 2001; Bond & Morris, 2000; Hausdorff et al., 2003; Lundin-Olsson et al., 1997; Lundin-Olsson, Nyberg, & Gustafson, 1998). In fact, several studies demonstrated a relationship between attention abilities, gait, and fall risk in PD (Deane et al., 2002; Hausdorff et al., 2003, 2006; Yogev et al., 2006).

8.4.2 Multiple Sclerosis

The neuropathology of MS is characterized by multifocal inflammatory demyelination and neuroaxonal injury (Tomassini et al., 2012). The prevalence of cognitive impairments in persons with MS is high, with estimates ranging from 43 to 65 % (Peyser, Rao, LaRocca, & Kaplan, 1990; Rao et al., 1991). Processing speed, attention, EF, learning, and memory are common areas of cognition affected by MS (Arnett et al., 1997; Calabrese, 2006; Drew, Tippett, Starkey, & Isler, 2008). While these common cognitive impairments have been identified in MS, it is important to underscore that the pattern of cognitive decline in each patient with MS is variable and unpredictable (Larocca, 2011).

A recent review concluded that the changes in postural control underlying gait impairments and fall risk in MS are primarily due to slowed somatosensory conduction and impaired central integration of information (Cameron & Lord, 2010). Some of these main predictors appear to be related to the cognitive capacities of sustained attention, processing speed, and EF. In addition, patients with a clinically isolated syndrome and a diagnosis of possible MS had greater decrements in speed and gait stability during cognitive tasks than healthy controls, suggesting that there may be cognitive difficulties interfering with parameters of gait even during the earliest stages of the disease (Kalron, Dvir, & Achiron, 2010). Using a DT paradigm, Benedict et al. also showed that patients with MS had greater decrements in walking speed than healthy controls (Benedict et al., 2011; Benedict & Zivadinov, 2011). Interestingly, the degree of the decrement was related to fatigue, measures of general cognitive function, and self-reported cognitive errors rather than measures of overall disability, and processing speed and EF were also found to be significant predictors of lower and upper motor function in patients with MS (Benedict et al., 2011; Benedict & Zivadinov, 2011).

D'Orio et al. (2012) investigated the associations between cognitive functions, walking speed, and falls in patients with MS. They found that after controlling for age, gender, and disease severity, slower processing speed and IQ predicted slower gait speed, while poorer verbal memory predicted increased frequency of falls. Thus, the authors concluded that specific cognitive functions are meaningfully related to mobility limitations in patients with MS and that risk assessment for gait decline and falls should include cognitive assessment in patients with MS (D'Orio et al., 2012).

8.4.3 *Older Adults*

Age-associated changes in cognitive function are well documented. Memory may be the most widely reported complaint; however, EF and attentional deficits are also evident. The frontal lobes are apparently highly susceptible to age-associated changes (Craik & Grady, 2002; Dorfman, 1998). These include lesions of diffused white matter, which might affect fronto-striatal circuits and cause, among other things, impairment in EF (Buckner, 2004). Neuropsychological studies demonstrated impaired EF in generally healthy elderly subjects. This includes difficulties in problem solving that requires flexible thinking and cognitive shifting, impaired response inhibition, and impaired creative thinking (Dorfman, 1998). These impairments place older adults at a heightened risk of falling when they attempt to perform two or more tasks simultaneously, even if the tasks are otherwise considered to be automatic or demand minimal attention (Marsh & Geel, 2000). When performing dual tasks, reaction time becomes significantly longer in older adults, gait velocity is reduced, and stride length variability and stride time increase (van Iersel et al., 2008). These effects are even larger among elderly fallers than in the general elderly population (Herman, Mirelman, Giladi, Schweiger, & Hausdorff, 2010; Montero-Odasso et al., 2009; Yogev-Seligmann et al., 2008).

In a prospective study that investigated 201 healthy older adults who were free from falls in the year prior to baseline testing, Herman et al. (2010) showed that worse EF scores at baseline were associated with falls that occurred during the 2-year follow-up (Herman et al., 2010) (see Fig. 8.2). In an extension to this study, EF and gait variability during DT were still the strongest predictors of falls during 5 years of follow-up, reenforcing the importance of evaluating cognitive function as part of the assessment of fall risk and impaired mobility in the elderly.

8.5 Physical and Motor Rehabilitation in Neurodegenerative Diseases

To understand the advantages of training mobility in virtual reality, we first briefly summarize the current "state of the art" in mobility rehabilitation. Given the progressive decline in neurodegenerative pathology and aging of the brain areas

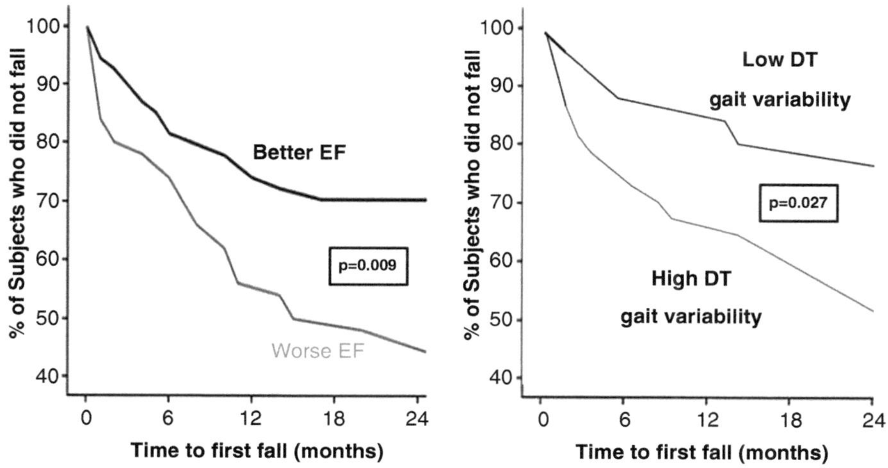

Fig. 8.2 Survival curves illustrating the percent of participants who did not fall (the *y*-axes) as a function of time and executive function group (*left*) or DT gait variability (*right*). Participants with worse EF (*lowest quartile*) or increased DT gait variability were more likely to become fallers and recurrent fallers sooner than those with better EF or DT gait (*upper quartile*). Adapted from Herman et al.

responsible for learning, it was previously thought that training could not elicit long-term effects in these patient populations; therefore management was based on compensation and prevention rather than rehabilitation. Recent evidence suggests, however, that this is not the case (Graybiel, 2005; Herman, Giladi, & Hausdorff, 2009; Wu & Hallett, 2005). Several key features for successful motor learning have been identified: learning sessions should be intensive (Guadagnoli, Leis, Van Gemmert, & Stelmach, 2002; Jobges et al., 2004), focus on a single desired outcome, and involve extensive feedback. Interventions following these principles have provided new evidence on impressive training effects as well as retention effects after training even in the face of neurodegeneration (Abbruzzese, Trompetto, & Marinelli, 2009; Mirelman et al., 2010; Rochester et al., 2010; Verghese et al., 2002).

Physical therapy (PT) is often prescribed for older adults and patients with PD in order to maximize function and minimize secondary complications. PT is delivered through movement rehabilitation within the context of education and support for the whole person (Deane et al., 2001). Although there are presently no widely accepted, standardized guidelines for treatment (Graybiel, 2005), PT covers different treatment techniques. Recommended interventions include strengthening, fitness training and active and functional task exercises using "strategy training," where the person is taught how to best utilize his/her ability in order to overcome difficulties, and cueing strategies to enhance gait (Graybiel, 2005). Still, recent meta-analyses concluded that there is little evidence to support or refute the use of PT for patients with PD, in part because of methodological flaws in published studies (Deane et al., 2001; Ellis et al., 2005; Graybiel, 2005; Rubenstein et al., 2002).

8.5.1 Cueing

Sensory cueing has been used extensively as a form of "strategy training" to improve function in PD. One explanation for this phenomenon suggests that "tricks" (cues) are effective because they activate the pre-motor cortical system either by bypassing the basal ganglia or by better focusing the cortico-basal ganglia–thalamo–cortical motor loop in relation to other psychomotor or associative loops (Lowenthal et al., 2004). For example, training with rhythmic auditory stimulation (RAS) demonstrated that patients with PD were able to match their cadence to a beat that was set at 10 % faster than their baseline values, significantly improving their velocity and stride length (Dam et al., 1996; Lowenthal et al., 2004). Walking while hearing RAS improves the rhythmicity of gait in a sense that provides an external rhythm by which a person can improve his/her gait. Patients who underwent gait training combined with auditory cueing improved significantly, as compared to patients who received only conventional PT (Marchese, Diverio, Zucchi, Lentino, & Abbruzzese, 2000; Van Wegen et al., 2006). Some studies also showed long-term effects (at least 6 weeks) after training. Similar findings were observed after training with visual and somatosensory cues, although significant long-term effects were not observed (Nieuwboer et al., 2007). Despite the promising evidence of cueing, therapy based on cueing does not address everyday tasks that challenge mobility such as dual-task activities or obstacle avoidance.

8.5.2 The Treadmill as a Pacemaker and a Rehabilitation Tool

Several studies suggested that training with a treadmill (TT) can enhance overground routine walking in patients with a variety of neurological diseases. Perhaps the most obvious relief is seen in stroke patients and in patients with spinal cord injuries (Laufer, Dickstein, Chefez, & Marcovitz, 2001). A handful of studies have also examined the effects of TT on the gait of PD patients (Herman, Giladi, Gurevich, & Hausdorff, 2005; Miyai et al., 2000, 2002) and MS (Benedetti et al., 2009; Pilutti et al., 2011). Training with TT and BWS improved physical and mental subscales and provided beneficial effects on quality of life and potentially reduced fatigue in patients with MS (Benedetti et al., 2009; Pilutti et al., 2011). The mechanism by which TT improves gait in PD is not yet clear. TT may activate neuronal circuits that mediate central pattern generators (Muir & Steeves, 1997) or enhance motor learning by reinforcing the synaptic connections in the spinal cord level or triggering reorganization of neural networks (Mathiowetz & Haugen, 1994). Walking on a moving walkway may also inherently provide external cueing, mediated through proprioceptive and vestibular receptors (Holden, 2005).

Results from recent studies support the efficacy and long-term carryover effects of TT on gait and balance with some reduction in fear of falling in patients with PD (Kurtais, Kutlay, Tur, Gok, & Akbostanci, 2008; Toole, Maitland, Warren, Hubmann,

& Panton, 2005). Retention of TT training effects was reported along with carryover effects on QOL (Herman, Giladi, Gruendlinger, & Hausdorff, 2007). In fact, TT has become widely available and is often prescribed to promote mobility, exercise, and physical activity, even in nursing home facilities. Although TT is apparently beneficial in improving usual walking in patients with PD, TT alone apparently does not generate improvements in dual-tasking abilities or lead to a reduction in fall risk. This lack of an effect on dual tasking and fall risk likely stems from the fact that TT focuses exclusively on usual walking, essentially ignoring the more complex, attention-demanding situations that are common in daily activity and community ambulation.

8.5.3 Multifactorial Interventions

The complex symptoms in neurodegenerative conditions that lead to mobility decline and an increased fall risk highlight the need for multifactorial interventions (Gillespie et al., 2009; Kannus, Sievanen, Palvanen, Jarvinen, & Parkkari, 2005). Earlier reviews suggested that multifactorial interventions may be among the most effective, and the American Geriatrics Society and British Geriatrics Society recommended this approach as a primary treatment strategy in their guideline for prevention of falls (2011). Exercise groups have become a widely accepted approach as a rehabilitation technique for the elderly and patients with neurodegenerative disease. Typically, group exercise programs are held two or three times per week for an hour and are supervised by physical therapists or trained exercise instructors. The programs include a combination of exercises to improve flexibility, strength, and balance and some level of aerobic conditioning. Within the exercise category, there is some evidence for the effectiveness of three different approaches in reducing both rate of falls and risk of falling while improving mobility: multiple component group exercise, Tai Chi as a group exercise, and individually prescribed multiple component exercise carried out at home (Gillespie et al., 2009). Although one RCT demonstrated significant effects of Tai Chi on fall frequency in PD (Li et al., 2012), the effects on fall risk generally tend to be small and the reported changes are focused on motor aspects with limited long-term retention (Gillespie et al., 2009; Goodwin, Richards, Taylor, Taylor, & Campbell, 2008; Kannus et al., 2005).

Weerdesteyn et al. (2006) demonstrated that a 5-week exercise program that trained dual-task gait and a highly structured and complex obstacle negotiation task leads to a dramatic reduction in the number of falls reported in the trained group (46 %), as compared to the control group of older adults. Similarly, Yogev-Seligmann, Giladi, Brozgol, and Hausdorff (2012) demonstrated that DT costs during walking respond to training in patients with PD. These findings suggest that appropriate training of DT could be effective in improving the ability to both divide attention and improve stability while walking in complex situations. Because most walking takes place in these more challenging conditions, the potential influence on functional ambulation and fall risk cannot be underscored.

8.6 Evidence for the Added Benefits of VR Augmented Training in Neurodegenerative Disease

Mahoney (2010) suggested that in order for rehabilitation interventions to be successful in improving mobility and reducing the risk of falls, they need to address three major constructs: (1) content: training should be intensive, be focused on the key impairment, and become progressively more rigorous; (2) fit the target population; and (3) intervention process: delivery of the intervention should maximize uptake and include mechanisms to maximize motor learning and induce a behavioural change. The motor learning literature dictates that with proper training, older adults and even patients with various motor disorders or cognitive deficits can improve their functional ability, even in the presence of ongoing disease and motor dysfunction (Schwenk, Zieschang, Oster, & Hauer, 2010; Shumway-Cook, Woollacott, Kerns, & Baldwin, 1997; Winstein, 1990).

These key elements can be easily achieved using VR systems making VR, at least theoretically, a useful tool for intervention in neurodegenerative conditions. The impetus for using VR is that the technology may enable individualized repetitive practice of motor function, graded in accordance to the needs and level of ability of the person while engaging in and stimulating cognitive processes. At the same time, VR provides feedback about performance that may assist with learning new motor strategies of movement. The realism of the virtual environments permits individuals to safely explore their environments independently, increasing their sense of autonomy and independence in directing their own therapeutic experience. Participants with different disorders and motor impairments report that these training sessions are typically quite enjoyable and motivating allowing for higher intensity of training in short duration protocols with relatively low patient burden (de Bruin, Dorflinger, Reith, & Murer, 2010; Deutsch & Mirelman, 2007; Fung, Richards, Malouin, McFadyen, & Lamontagne, 2006; Holden, 2005; Keshner & Weiss, 2007). With advances in technology, VR systems have become affordable and more portable allowing for easy use. The use of VR in the literature varies widely. In the following section, we describe the evidence found in the literature on VR interventions for improving gait and mobility and reducing the risk of falls in patients with PD and MS and in older adults.

8.6.1 Parkinson's Disease

VR has been used with subjects with PD as an evaluation tool for cognitive and executive function assessments. EF difficulties in planning were easily detected (Klinger, Chemin, Lebreton, & Marie, 2006). Subjects with PD demonstrated the ability to learn new paradigms of movement, but at a slower pace and with more difficulties in movement corrections (Albani et al., 2002; Messier et al., 2007) compared to control participants.

Only a handful of studies have investigated the use of VR for studying gait in PD. Studies include investigating navigation abilities in PD as well as training gait and performance using VR. Davidsdottir, Wagenaar, Young, and Cronin-Golomb (2008) examined the impact of optic flow and egocentric coordinates on navigation during walking in patients with PD. Thirty-one patients with PD (Hoehn and Yahr II–IV) and 18 healthy age-matched controls participated in the study. The researchers used a head-mounted display to project a virtual environment (VE) consisting of a virtual hallway, composed of two sidewalls of white random dots on a black background, with a black floor and ceiling devoid of texture. Participants walked overground at a speed of 0.8 m/s while observing a virtual scene with varied optic flow speeds. Veering was assessed as the change in gait during the trials using a motion capture system. The results showed that parietal-mediated perception of visual space is affected in PD including perception of optic flow speed and egocentric midline coordinates. Side of motor-symptom onset and gender affected spatial performance (with women more affected than men). The walking assessment demonstrated that visual input affected veering, which corresponded to the shifting of the egocentric midline rather than to abnormal perception of optic flow speed. These findings are in line with previous studies reporting impaired navigational abilities in PD patients as seen on the route-walking test (Bowen, Hoehn, & Yahr, 1972) and in indirect measurements of visuospatial neuropsychological tests (Bowen et al., 1972; Heikkila, Turkka, Korpelainen, Kallanranta, & Summala, 1998; Radford, Lincoln, & Lennox, 2004), further suggesting that cognitive and visual-spatial dysfunction, rather than motor impairments per se, can contribute to difficulties in navigation.

To address the motor and cognitive deficits that commonly contribute to fall risk, Mirelman et al. (2010) developed a VR system based on an obstacle navigation task. Twenty patients with PD (H&Y II–III), walked on a treadmill, while wearing a safety harness, three times a week for 6 weeks. The virtual scene consisted of an outdoor environment of a boardwalk on which virtual obstacles were placed at random intervals. Participants walked in the VE negotiating obstacles and tried to avid stepping on them by stepping over them. Using a camera for motion capture which tracked the movement of the feet, the patient's movements were inserted into the VR simulation and projected on the wall in front of the treadmill via a large projector (Fig. 8.3). Visual and auditory feedbacks were provided by the VR simulation upon error (stepping or hitting an obstacle) and at the end of each walk in the form of knowledge of results. After 6 weeks of training, comfortable gait speed significantly improved, as did stride length, gait variability, and overground obstacle negotiation. The DT decrement (cost of dual tasking on gait as compared to single task) became smaller (i.e., better), and there was evidence of improved task planning and set shifting, i.e., cognitive function measured using neuropsychological standardized tests. Increased gait speeds under all conditions (comfortable, fast, DT, and 6-min walk) were not only maintained at follow-up but also continued to improve 4 weeks later at the time of follow-up, suggesting that the training generated a positive feedback loop that modified behavior and overall mobility (perhaps a result of motor learning) (Mirelman et al., 2010). DT walking abilities were significantly improved after TT+VR, much more than that seen among subjects who trained only with treadmill, without VR.

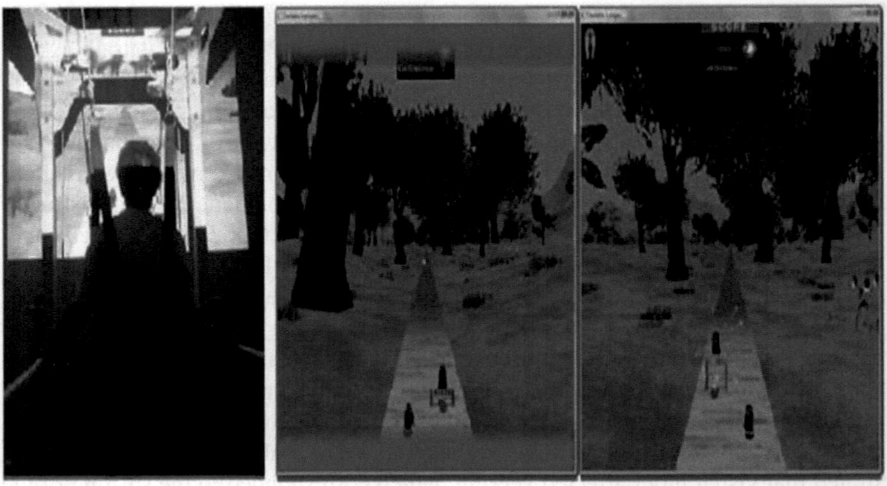

Fig. 8.3 The VR simulation consists of a boardwalk with obstacles. On the *left*, a patient trains on a treadmill while viewing the virtual environment. *Center* and *right*: Different types of challenges and feedback provided. Mirelman et al. (2010)

Recently two groups independently started to look at VR as a tool for characterization of freezing of gait (FOG). FOG is a common episodic gait disorder in PD which occurs most often in conflict situations such as gait initiation, turns, crowded places, and narrow pathways. FOG has been associated with deficits in bilateral coordination, EF, and emotional state (Nutt et al., 2011; Plotnik, Giladi, & Hausdorff, 2009; Plotnik & Hausdorff, 2008). Using VR to study and elucidate the mechanism of FOG enables to subject patients to different FOG-inducing situations in a safe environment. Park et al. described in a methodology paper the development of a virtual reality (VR)-based body weight-supported treadmill interface (BWSTI) designed and applied to investigate FOG. The VR-based BWSTI was tested with three patients with PD who were known to have FOG. Visual stimuli that might cause FOG were shown to them, while the speed adaptation controller adjusted treadmill speed to follow the subjects' own preferred speed. Two of the three subjects demonstrated FOG during the treadmill walking. Shine, Ward, Naismith, Pearson, and Lewis (2011) reported a case study in which a VR simulation was used to investigate walking under dual-tasking conditions using fMRI. The participant was instructed to simulate walking by pressing two pedals while concurrently performing cognitive tasks such as the stroop test or following simple commands on a screen. The results showed distinct activation patterns during "walking," "dual-task walking," and episodes of freezing. Patients with FOG exhibited delayed motor responses (Gilat et al., 2013; Matar, Shine, Naismith, & Lewis, 2013; Shine et al., 2012), impaired sequencing (Matar et al., 2013), and a specific decrease in neural activation in the anterior insula, ventral striatum, and subthalamic nucleus (STN) (Shine, Matar, et al. 2013; Shine, Naismith, et al. 2013) demonstrating a distinct control of gait. Together these studies highlight the potential utility of VR in elucidating the underlying neural correlates of the freezing phenomenon in PD. The relatively large number of studies that used VR to assess FOG may be related to the unique susceptibility of FOG to cognitive, emotional, and sensory stimulation which can easily be manipulated using VR and is more challenging to reproduce overground (Mirelman, Maidan, & Deutsch, 2013).

8.6.2 *Multiple Sclerosis*

Very few studies have looked at the use of VR for treatment of MS-related gait disorders. Fulk (2005) described the results of a locomotor training using both a body weight support (BWS) with a treadmill (TM) and overground walking as well as a VR-based balance intervention to improve walking ability, balance, and endurance for a 48-year-old female with MS. The intervention was provided twice weekly for 12 weeks and after which the patient showed improved gait speed, endurance, and balance. These improvements were sustained for at least 2 months post-intervention.

Baram and Miller used a portable visual-feedback VR apparatus consisting of stereoscopic glasses to provide visual cues of a virtual tiled floor in a checkerboard arrangement, responding dynamically to the patient's own motion, much like a real floor, fixed in space. In their first study (Baram & Miller, 2006), 16 patients with cerebellar ataxia due to MS participated in a single evaluation session consisting of four training bouts. In general, subjects with moderate-to-severe gait impairments showed an average online improvement (while walking with the device) of 13.46 % in their walking speed, while patients whose baseline walking speed was above the median walking speed of the group improved their speed by 1.47 %. In a follow-up study (Baram & Miller, 2010), 10 patients trained with a simulation that provided cues of transverse lines while 11 patients trained with virtual checkerboard tiles, both provided by a wearable virtual reality device. Following 20-min training with the device and 10-min rest, performance without the device was measured again and compared to the baseline performance. The group training with the transverse tiles showed significantly better immediate results in walking speed and stride length overground as compared to the control group; however, long-term training effects were not assessed and therefore the transfer and retention of this training to "real-world" environment are yet to be studied.

8.6.3 *Older Adults*

Reports on the use of VR for training of balance, gait, and fall risk among older adults are also scarce. The use of VR for older adults has been primarily used for balance training and cognitive training or to improve upper extremity function (Cherniack, 2010; de Bruin, Schoene, Pichierri, & Smith, 2010). Pichierri, Wolf, Murer, and de Bruin (2011) recently reviewed nine studies that used computerized interventions such as VR or gaming for training of older adults, but only two of those investigated forms of mobility. de Bruin, Dorflinger, et al. (2010) studied the transfer effects on gait characteristics of elderly who executed a traditional progressive physical balance and resistance training with integrated computer game of dancing (Dance Dance Revolution). The task of the dancing game consisted of stepping on arrows on a dance pad. Results indicated a positive effect of the computer game dancing training on relative DT costs of walking, e.g., stride time and step length. The more traditional physical training consisting of fitness and balance exercises showed no transfer effects to DT cost-related gait characteristics.

In another study looking at perceptual adaptation (Buccello-Stout et al., 2008), 16 adults, aged 66–81 years, were randomized to one of the two groups. Both groups first completed six trials of walking an obstacle course. Participants then trained twice a week for 4 weeks. In the training, the control group walked on a treadmill for 20 min while viewing a static visual scene and the experimental group walked on a treadmill for 20 min while viewing a rotating visual scene that provided a perceptual-motor mismatch. Following training, both groups were tested again on the obstacle course. The group trained with the rotating visual scene performed faster on the obstacle course and had fewer penalties than those who received a static visual scene, and training effects were retained for at least 4 weeks. Exposure to perceptual-motor mismatch induced information processing and provided a motor–cognitive training that resulted in an adaptive training effect that improved balance and gait in this group of older adults.

Recently, Mirelman et al.(2011) conducted a pilot study among five elderly idiopathic fallers who trained using the same TT+VR protocol as described above (in the study with patients with PD) (Mirelman et al., 2011). The purpose of the study was to examine the effects of training with VR on the frequency of falls measured over a period of 6 months. Five elderly females (mean age 78.2±5.3 years), with a history of more than two falls in the 6 months prior to the study and who were otherwise healthy, participated in the study. Subjects walked on a treadmill while negotiating virtual obstacles three times a week for 6 weeks. After 6 weeks, improvements in gait speed and stride length were observed under usual, DT, and obstacle negotiation conditions. Additional very promising results include improvements in endurance and functional abilities and a marked decrease (improvement) in the DT cost. Frequency of falls in this small pilot study decreased by 73 % compared to the fall rate 6 months before the intervention. This very exciting finding suggests that perhaps using VR for motor–cognitive training in the elderly could lead to enhanced usual walking performance and major improvements in the ability to allocate attention to simultaneous tasks, and subjects learn to walk safely when negotiating obstacles. Conceivably these gains could then potentially reduce fall risk and fall rate in this population.

8.7 Future Directions

Patients with neurodegenerative disease suffer from deficits in motor and cognitive function that lead to an increased risk of falls. Until recently, therapeutic options for this population consisted of maintaining function and preventing deterioration.

In the past decade there has been a shift in the understanding that even in the face of neurodegeneration, learning and plasticity can be achieved and hence treatment should be targeted towards improving function. However still, current therapeutic options do not fully address the multifactorial motor and cognitive deficits associated with neurodegeneration in an optimal fashion. The advances in technology, affordability, and accessibility have opened the door for assessing whether VR could be used for the geriatric population and for those with neurodegenerative diseases. There are only a small number of studies using VR for training gait and reducing falls in this population; however the evidence is encouraging demonstrating that VR is likely helpful for addressing impairments among a diverse group of older adults. However, large-scale randomized controlled trials are needed to provide evidence-based results for reducing fall frequency. In addition, many questions remain about optimal dosing, retention, and the utility of VR for achieving motor learning in the presence of neurodegenerative disease. The existing studies should provide a springboard for exciting future work.

References

Aarsland, D., Bronnick, K., Larsen, J. P., Tysnes, O. B., & Alves, G. (2009). Cognitive impairment in incident, untreated Parkinson disease: The Norwegian ParkWest study. *Neurology, 72*(13), 1121–1126.

Abbruzzese, G., Trompetto, C., & Marinelli, L. (2009). The rationale for motor learning in Parkinson's disease. *European Journal of Physical and Rehabilitation Medicine, 45*(2), 209–214.

Adams, R., & Parsons, O. (2003). *Neuropsychology for clinical practice: Etiology, assessment, and treatment of common neurologic disorders*. Washington, DC: American Psychological Association.

Albani, G., Pignatti, R., Bertella, L., Priano, L., Semenza, C., Molinari, E., et al. (2002). Common daily activities in the virtual environment: A preliminary study in parkinsonian patients. *Neurological Sciences, 23*(Suppl. 2), S49–S50.

Alexander, N. B., & Hausdorff, J. M. (2008). Linking thinking, walking, and falling. *Journals of Gerontology. Series A, Biological Sciences and Medical Sciences, 63*(12), 1325–1328.

Arnett, P. A., Rao, S. M., Grafman, J., Bernardin, L., Luchetta, T., Binder, J. R., et al. (1997). Executive functions in multiple sclerosis: An analysis of temporal ordering, semantic encoding, and planning abilities. *Neuropsychology, 11*(4), 535–544.

Ashburn, A., Stack, E., Pickering, R. M., & Ward, C. D. (2001). A community-dwelling sample of people with Parkinson's disease: Characteristics of fallers and non-fallers. *Age and Ageing, 30*(1), 47–52.

Baltadjieva, R., Giladi, N., Gruendlinger, L., Peretz, C., & Hausdorff, J. M. (2006). Marked alterations in the gait timing and rhythmicity of patients with de novo Parkinson's disease. *European Journal of Neuroscience, 24*(6), 1815–1820.

Baram, Y., & Miller, A. (2006). Virtual reality cues for improvement of gait in patients with multiple sclerosis. *Neurology, 66*(2), 178–181.

Baram, Y., & Miller, A. (2010). Glide-symmetric locomotion reinforcement in patients with multiple sclerosis by visual feedback. *Disability and Rehabilitation. Assistive Technology, 5*(5), 323–326.

Beauchet, O., Kressig, R. W., Najafi, B., Aminian, K., Dubost, V., & Mourey, F. (2003). Age-related decline of gait control under a dual-task condition. *Journal of American Geriatrics Society, 51*(8), 1187–1188.

Benedetti, M. G., Gasparroni, V., Stecchi, S., Zilioli, R., Straudi, S., & Piperno, R. (2009). Treadmill exercise in early multiple sclerosis: A case series study. *European Journal of Physical and Rehabilitation Medicine, 45*(1), 53–59.

Benedict, R. H., Holtzer, R., Motl, R. W., Foley, F. W., Kaur, S., Hojnacki, D., et al. (2011). Upper and lower extremity motor function and cognitive impairment in multiple sclerosis. *Journal of the International Neuropsychological Society, 17*(4), 643–653.

Benedict, R. H., & Zivadinov, R. (2011). Risk factors for and management of cognitive dysfunction in multiple sclerosis. *Nature Reviews. Neurology, 7*(6), 332–342.

Blake, A. J., Morgan, K., Bendall, M. J., Dallosso, H., Ebrahim, S. B., Arie, T. H., et al. (1988). Falls by elderly people at home: Prevalence and associated factors. *Age and Ageing, 17*(6), 365–372.

Bloem, B. R., Boers, I., Cramer, M., Westendorp, R. G., & Gerschlager, W. (2001). Falls in the elderly. I. Identification of risk factors. *Wiener Klinische Wochenschrift, 113*(10), 352–362.

Bloem, B. R., Hausdorff, J. M., Visser, J. E., & Giladi, N. (2004). Falls and freezing of gait in Parkinson's disease: A review of two interconnected, episodic phenomena. *Movement Disorders, 19*(8), 871–884.

Bloem, B. R., Valkenburg, V. V., Slabbekoorn, M., & Willemsen, M. D. (2001). The multiple tasks test: Development and normal strategies. *Gait & Posture, 14*(3), 191–202.

Bloem, B. R., van Vugt, J. P., & Beckley, D. J. (2001). Postural instability and falls in Parkinson's disease. *Advances in Neurology, 87*, 209–223.

Bond, J. M., & Morris, M. (2000). Goal-directed secondary motor tasks: Their effects on gait in subjects with Parkinson disease. *Archives of Physical Medicine and Rehabilitation, 81*(1), 110–116.

Bowen, F. P., Hoehn, M. M., & Yahr, M. D. (1972). Parkinsonism: Alterations in spatial orientation as determined by a route-walking test. *Neuropsychologia, 10*(3), 355–361.

Bredesen, D. E., Rao, R. V., & Mehlen, P. (2006). Cell death in the nervous system. *Nature, 443*(7113), 796–802.

Brown, L. A., & Brockmole, J. R. (2010). The role of attention in binding visual features in working memory: Evidence from cognitive ageing. *The Quarterly Journal of Experimental Psychology, 63*(10), 2067–2079.

Brown, L. A., McKenzie, N. C., & Doan, J. B. (2005). Age-dependent differences in the attentional demands of obstacle negotiation. *Journals of Gerontology. Series A, Biological Sciences and Medical Sciences, 60*(7), 924–927.

Buccello-Stout, R. R., Bloomberg, J. J., Cohen, H. S., Whorton, E. B., Weaver, G. D., & Cromwell, R. L. (2008). Effects of sensorimotor adaptation training on functional mobility in older adults. *Journals of Gerontology. Series B, Psychological Sciences and Social Sciences, 63*(5), 295–300.

Buckner, R. L. (2004). Memory and executive function in aging and AD: Multiple factors that cause decline and reserve factors that compensate. *Neuron, 44*(1), 195–208.

Calabrese, P. (2006). Neuropsychology of multiple sclerosis—An overview. *Journal of Neurology, 253*(Suppl. 1), I10–I15.

Cameron, M. H., & Lord, S. (2010). Postural control in multiple sclerosis: Implications for fall prevention. *Current Neurology and Neuroscience Reports, 10*(5), 407–412.

Chapman, G. J., & Hollands, M. A. (2007). Evidence that older adult fallers prioritise the planning of future stepping actions over the accurate execution of ongoing steps during complex locomotor tasks. *Gait & Posture, 26*(1), 59–67.

Chen, H. C., Ashton-Miller, J. A., Alexander, N. B., & Schultz, A. B. (1994). Effects of age and available response time on ability to step over an obstacle. *Journal of Gerontology, 49*(5), M227–M233.

Cherniack, E. P. (2010). Not just fun and games: Applications of virtual reality in the identification and rehabilitation of cognitive disorders of the elderly. *Disability and Rehabilitation. Assistive Technology, 6*(4), 283–289.

Craik, F. I. M., & Grady, C. L. (2002). Aging, memory and frontal lobe functioning. In D. T. Stuss & R. T. Knight (Eds.), *Principles of frontal lobe function* (pp. 528–540). New York, NY: Oxford University Press.

Dam, M., Tonin, P., Casson, S., Bracco, F., Piron, L., Pizzolato, G., et al. (1996). Effects of conventional and sensory-enhanced physiotherapy on disability of Parkinson's disease patients. *Advances in Neurology, 69*, 551–555.

Davidsdottir, S., Wagenaar, R., Young, D., & Cronin-Golomb, A. (2008). Impact of optic flow perception and egocentric coordinates on veering in Parkinson's disease. *Brain, 131*(Pt 11), 2882–2893.

de Bruin, E., Dorflinger, M., Reith, A., & Murer, K. (2010). The effect of dance dance revolution gaming compared to conventional physical training on dual task walking costs in elderly. *Parkinsonism & Related Disorders, 16*, s59.

de Bruin, E. D., Schoene, D., Pichierri, G., & Smith, S. T. (2010). Use of virtual reality technique for the training of motor control in the elderly. Some theoretical considerations. *Zeitschrift für Gerontologie und Geriatrie, 43*(4), 229–234.

Deane, K. H., Ellis-Hill, C., Jones, D., Whurr, R., Ben Shlomo, Y., Playford, E. D., et al. (2002). Systematic review of paramedical therapies for Parkinson's disease. *Movement Disorders, 17*(5), 984–991.

Deane, K. H., Jones, D., Ellis-Hill, C., Clarke, C. E., Playford, E. D., & Ben Shlomo, Y. (2001). A comparison of physiotherapy techniques for patients with Parkinson's disease. *Cochrane Database of Systematic Reviews, 1*, CD002815.

D'Esposito, M., Ballard, D., Zarahn, E., & Aguirre, G. K. (2000). The role of prefrontal cortex in sensory memory and motor preparation: An event-related fMRI study. *NeuroImage, 11*(5 Pt 1), 400–408.

Deutsch, J. E., & Mirelman, A. (2007). Virtual reality-based approaches to enable walking for people poststroke. *Topics in Stroke Rehabilitation, 14*(6), 45–53.

Dorfman, J. (1998). Problem solving, inhibition and frontal lobe function. In N. Raz (Ed.), *The other side of the error team: Aging and development as model systems in cognitive neuroscience* (pp. 395–448). Amsterdam, The Netherlands: Elsevier Science.

D'Orio, V. L., Foley, F. W., Armentano, F., Picone, M. A., Kim, S., & Holtzer, R. (2012). Cognitive and motor functioning in patients with multiple sclerosis: Neuropsychological predictors of walking speed and falls. *Journal of the Neurological Sciences, 316*(1–2), 42–46.

Drew, M., Tippett, L. J., Starkey, N. J., & Isler, R. B. (2008). Executive dysfunction and cognitive impairment in a large community-based sample with multiple sclerosis from New Zealand: A descriptive study. *Archives of Clinical Neuropsychology, 23*(1), 1–19.

Ebersbach, G., Heijmenberg, M., Kindermann, L., Trottenberg, T., Wissel, J., & Poewe, W. (1999). Interference of rhythmic constraint on gait in healthy subjects and patients with early Parkinson's disease: Evidence for impaired locomotor pattern generation in early Parkinson's disease. *Movement Disorders, 14*(4), 619–625.

Ellis, T., de Goede, C. J., Feldman, R. G., Wolters, E. C., Kwakkel, G., & Wagenaar, R. C. (2005). Efficacy of a physical therapy program in patients with Parkinson's disease: A randomized controlled trial. *Archives of Physical Medicine and Rehabilitation, 86*(4), 626–632.

Fingerhut, L. A., Cox, C. S., & Warner, M. (1998). International comparative analysis of injury mortality. Findings from the ICE on injury statistics. International Collaborative Effort on Injury Statistics. *Advance Data, 303*, 1–20.

Fisk, J. D., Pontefract, A., Ritvo, P. G., Archibald, C. J., & Murray, T. J. (1994). The impact of fatigue on patients with multiple sclerosis. *Canadian Journal of Neurological Sciences, 21*(1), 9–14.

Freal, J. E., Kraft, G. H., & Coryell, J. K. (1984). Symptomatic fatigue in multiple sclerosis. *Archives of Physical Medicine and Rehabilitation, 65*(3), 135–138.

Fulk, G. D. (2005). Locomotor training and virtual reality-based balance training for an individual with multiple sclerosis: A case report. *Journal of Neurologic Physical Therapy, 29*(1), 34–42.

Fung, J., Richards, C. L., Malouin, F., McFadyen, B. J., & Lamontagne, A. (2006). A treadmill and motion coupled virtual reality system for gait training post-stroke. *Cyberpsychology & Behavior, 9*(2), 157–162.

Fuster, J. M. (1999). Synopsis of function and dysfunction of the frontal lobe. *Acta Psychiatrica Scandinavica, Supplement, 395*, 51–57.

Gage, W. H., Sleik, R. J., Polych, M. A., McKenzie, N. C., & Brown, L. A. (2003). The allocation of attention during locomotion is altered by anxiety. *Experimental Brain Research, 150*(3), 385–394.

Galna, B., Murphy, A. T., & Morris, M. E. (2010). Obstacle crossing in people with Parkinson's disease: Foot clearance and spatiotemporal deficits. *Human Movement Science, 29*(5), 843–852.

Gilat, M., Shine, J. M., Bolitho, S. J., Matar, E., Kamsma, Y. P. T., Naismith, S. L., et al. (2013). Variability of stepping during a virtual reality paradigm in Parkinson's disease patients with and without freezing of gait. *PLoS One, 8*(6), e66718.

Gillespie, L. D., Robertson, M. C., Gillespie, W. J., Lamb, S. E., Gates, S., Cumming, R. G., et al. (2009). Interventions for preventing falls in older people living in the community. *Cochrane Database of Systematic Reviews, 2*, CD007146.

Goldstein, D. S. (2003). Dysautonomia in Parkinson's disease: Neurocardiological abnormalities. *Lancet Neurology, 2*(11), 669–676.

Goodwin, V. A., Richards, S. H., Taylor, R. S., Taylor, A. H., & Campbell, J. L. (2008). The effectiveness of exercise interventions for people with Parkinson's disease: A systematic review and meta-analysis. *Movement Disorders, 23*(5), 631–640.

Gray, P., & Hildebrand, K. (2000). Fall risk factors in Parkinson's disease. *Journal of Neuroscience Nursing, 32*(4), 222–228.

Graybiel, A. M. (2005). The basal ganglia: Learning new tricks and loving it. *Current Opinion in Neurobiology, 15*(6), 638–644.

Guadagnoli, M. A., Leis, B., Van Gemmert, A. W., & Stelmach, G. E. (2002). The relationship between knowledge of results and motor learning in Parkinsonian patients. *Parkinsonism & Related Disorders, 9*(2), 89–95.

Hausdorff, J. M., Balash, J., & Giladi, N. (2003). Effects of cognitive challenge on gait variability in patients with Parkinson's disease. *Journal of Geriatric Psychiatry and Neurology, 16*(1), 53–58.

Hausdorff, J. M., Cudkowicz, M. E., Firtion, R., Wei, J. Y., & Goldberger, A. L. (1998). Gait variability and basal ganglia disorders: Stride-to-stride variations of gait cycle timing in Parkinson's disease and Huntington's disease. *Movement Disorders, 13*(3), 428–437.

Hausdorff, J. M., Doniger, G. M., Springer, S., Yogev, G., Giladi, N., & Simon, E. S. (2006). A common cognitive profile in elderly fallers and in patients with Parkinson's disease: The prominence of impaired executive function and attention. *Experimental Aging Research, 32*(4), 411–429.

Hausdorff, J. M., Nelson, M. E., Kaliton, D., Layne, J. E., Bernstein, M. J., Nuernberger, A., et al. (2001). Etiology and modification of gait instability in older adults: A randomized controlled trial of exercise. *Journal of Applied Physiology, 90*(6), 2117–2129.

Hausdorff, J. M., & Yogev, G. (2006). Cognitive function may be important for fall injury prevention trials. *Journal of the American Geriatrics Society, 54*(5), 865–866.

Heikkila, V. M., Turkka, J., Korpelainen, J., Kallanranta, T., & Summala, H. (1998). Decreased driving ability in people with Parkinson's disease. *Journal of Neurology, Neurosurgery, and Psychiatry, 64*(3), 325–330.

Herman, T., Giladi, N., Gruendlinger, L., & Hausdorff, J. M. (2007). Six weeks of intensive treadmill training improves gait and quality of life in patients with Parkinson's disease: A pilot study. *Archives of Physical Medicine and Rehabilitation, 88*(9), 1154–1158.

Herman, T., Giladi, N., Gurevich, T., & Hausdorff, J. M. (2005). Gait instability and fractal dynamics of older adults with a "cautious" gait: Why do certain older adults walk fearfully? *Gait & Posture, 21*(2), 178–185.

Herman, T., Giladi, N., & Hausdorff, J. M. (2009). Treadmill training for the treatment of gait disturbances in people with Parkinson's disease: A mini-review. *Journal of Neural Transmission, 116*(3), 307–318.

Herman, T., Mirelman, A., Giladi, N., Schweiger, A., & Hausdorff, J. M. (2010). Executive control deficits as a prodrome to falls in healthy older adults: A prospective study linking thinking, walking, and falling. *Journals of Gerontology. Series A, Biological Sciences and Medical Sciences, 65*(10), 1086–1092.

Holden, M. K. (2005). Virtual environments for motor rehabilitation: Review. *Cyberpsychology & Behavior, 8*(3), 187–211.

Jobges, M., Heuschkel, G., Pretzel, C., Illhardt, C., Renner, C., & Hummelsheim, H. (2004). Repetitive training of compensatory steps: A therapeutic approach for postural instability in Parkinson's disease. *Journal of Neurology, Neurosurgery, and Psychiatry, 75*(12), 1682–1687.

Jueptner, M., Frith, C. D., Brooks, D. J., Frackowiak, R. S., & Passingham, R. E. (1997). Anatomy of motor learning. II. Subcortical structures and learning by trial and error. *Journal of Neurophysiology, 77*(3), 1325–1337.

Kalron, A., Dvir, Z., & Achiron, A. (2010). Walking while talking—Difficulties incurred during the initial stages of multiple sclerosis disease process. *Gait & Posture, 32*(3), 332–335.

Kannus, P., Sievanen, H., Palvanen, M., Jarvinen, T., & Parkkari, J. (2005). Prevention of falls and consequent injuries in elderly people. *Lancet, 366*(9500), 1885–1893.

Keshner, E. A., & Weiss, P. T. (2007). Introduction to the special issue from the proceedings of the 2006 International Workshop on Virtual Reality in Rehabilitation. *Journal of Neuroengineering and Rehabilitation, 4*, 18.

Klinger, E., Chemin, I., Lebreton, S., & Marie, R. M. (2006). Virtual action planning in Parkinson's disease: A control study. *Cyberpsychology & Behavior, 9*(3), 342–347.

Kurtais, Y., Kutlay, S., Tur, B. S., Gok, H., & Akbostanci, C. (2008). Does treadmill training improve lower-extremity tasks in Parkinson disease? A randomized controlled trial. *Clinical Journal of Sport Medicine, 18*(3), 289–291.

Larocca, N. G. (2011). Impact of walking impairment in multiple sclerosis: Perspectives of patients and care partners. *Patient, 4*(3), 189–201.

Laufer, Y., Dickstein, R., Chefez, Y., & Marcovitz, E. (2001). The effect of treadmill training on the ambulation of stroke survivors in the early stages of rehabilitation: A randomized study. *Journal of Rehabilitation Research and Development, 38*(1), 69–78.

Legters, K. (2002). Fear of falling. *Physical Therapy, 82*(3), 264–272.

Lezak, M. D. (1995). *Neuropsychological assessment*. New York, NY: Oxford University Press.

Li, F., Harmer, P., Fitzgerald, K., Eckstrom, E., Stock, R., Galver, J., et al. (2012). Tai chi and postural stability in patients with Parkinson's disease. *The New England Journal of Medicine, 366*(6), 511–519.

Lin, M. T., & Beal, M. F. (2006). Mitochondrial dysfunction and oxidative stress in neurodegenerative diseases. *Nature, 443*(7113), 787–795.

Lord, S. R., Smith, S. T., & Menant, J. C. (2010). Vision and falls in older people: Risk factors and intervention strategies. *Clinics in Geriatric Medicine, 26*(4), 569–581.

Lowenthal, J., Gruedlinger, L., Baltadjieva, R., Herman, T., Hausdorff, J. M., & Giladi, N. (2004). Effects of rhythmic auditory stimulation on gait dynamics in Parkinson's disease. *Movement Disorders, 19*, S139.

Lowrey, C. R., Watson, A., & Vallis, L. A. (2007). Age-related changes in avoidance strategies when negotiating single and multiple obstacles. *Experimental Brain Research, 182*(3), 289–299.

Lundin-Olsson, L., Nyberg, L., & Gustafson, Y. (1997). "Stops walking when talking" as a predictor of falls in elderly people. *Lancet, 349*(9052), 617.

Lundin-Olsson, L., Nyberg, L., & Gustafson, Y. (1998). Attention, frailty, and falls: The effect of a manual task on basic mobility. *Journal of the American Geriatrics Society, 46*(6), 758–761.

Mahoney, J. E. (2010). Why multifactorial fall-prevention interventions may not work: Comment on "Multifactorial intervention to reduce falls in older people at high risk of recurrent falls". *Archives of Internal Medicine, 170*(13), 1117–1119.

Marchese, R., Diverio, M., Zucchi, F., Lentino, C., & Abbruzzese, G. (2000). The role of sensory cues in the rehabilitation of parkinsonian patients: A comparison of two physical therapy protocols. *Movement Disorders, 15*(5), 879–883.

Marsh, A. P., & Geel, S. E. (2000). The effect of age on the attentional demands of postural control. *Gait & Posture, 12*(2), 105–113.

Matar, E., Shine, J. M., Naismith, S. L., & Lewis, S. J. (2013). Using virtual reality to explore the role of conflict resolution and environmental salience in freezing of gait in Parkinson's disease. *Parkinsonism & Related Disorders, 19*(11), 937–942.

Mathiowetz, V., & Haugen, J. B. (1994). Motor behavior research: Implications for therapeutic approaches to central nervous system dysfunction. *The American Journal of Occupational Therapy, 48*(8), 733–745.

Menant, J. C., St George, R. J., Fitzpatrick, R. C., & Lord, S. R. (2010). Impaired depth perception and restricted pitch head movement increase obstacle contacts when dual-tasking in older people. *Journals of Gerontology. Series A, Biological Sciences and Medical Sciences, 65*(7), 751–757.

Messier, J., Adamovich, S., Jack, D., Hening, W., Sage, J., & Poizner, H. (2007). Visuomotor learning in immersive 3D virtual reality in Parkinson's disease and in aging. *Experimental Brain Research, 179*(3), 457–474.

Mirelman, A., Maidan, I., & Deutsch, J. E. (2013). Virtual reality and motor imagery: Promising tools for assessment and therapy in Parkinson's disease. *Movement Disorders, 28*(11), 1597–1608.

Mirelman, A., Maidan, I., Herman, T., Deutsch, J. E., Giladi, N., & Hausdorff, J. M. (2010). Virtual reality for gait training: Can it induce motor learning to enhance complex walking and reduce fall risk in patients with Parkinson's disease? *Journals of Gerontology. Series A, Biological Sciences and Medical Sciences, 66*(2), 234–240.

Mirelman A, Raphaeli Baer N, Dorfman M, Brozgol M, Giladi N, Hausdorff JM. (2011). Virtual Reality in Idiopathic fallers - A pilot study.: *IEEE*. doi: 10.1109/ICVR.2011.5971846.

Miyai, I., Fujimoto, Y., Ueda, Y., Yamamoto, H., Nozaki, S., Saito, T., et al. (2000). Treadmill training with body weight support: Its effect on Parkinson's disease. *Archives of Physical Medicine and Rehabilitation, 81*(7), 849–852.

Miyai, I., Fujimoto, Y., Yamamoto, H., Ueda, Y., Saito, T., Nozaki, S., et al. (2002). Long-term effect of body weight-supported treadmill training in Parkinson's disease: A randomized controlled trial. *Archives of Physical Medicine and Rehabilitation, 83*(10), 1370–1373.

Montero-Odasso, M., Bergman, H., Phillips, N. A., Wong, C. H., Sourial, N., & Chertkow, H. (2009). Dual-tasking and gait in people with mild cognitive impairment. The effect of working memory. *BMC Geriatrics, 9*, 41–42.

Morris, M. E., Huxham, F. E., McGinley, J., & Iansek, R. (2001). Gait disorders and gait rehabilitation in Parkinson's disease. *Advances in Neurology, 87*, 347–361.

Morris, M. E., Iansek, R., Matyas, T. A., & Summers, J. J. (1994). The pathogenesis of gait hypokinesia in Parkinson's disease. *Brain, 117*(Pt 5), 1169–1181.

Morris, M. E., Iansek, R., Matyas, T. A., & Summers, J. J. (1996). Stride length regulation in Parkinson's disease. Normalization strategies and underlying mechanisms. *Brain, 119*(Pt 2), 551–568.

Muir, G. D., & Steeves, J. D. (1997). Sensorimotor stimulation to improve locomotor recovery after spinal cord injury. *Trends in Neurosciences, 20*(2), 72–77.

Muslimovic, D., Post, B., Speelman, J. D., & Schmand, B. (2005). Cognitive profile of patients with newly diagnosed Parkinson disease. *Neurology, 65*(8), 1239–1245.

Nieuwboer, A., Kwakkel, G., Rochester, L., Jones, D., van Wegen, E., Willems, A. M., et al. (2007). Cueing training in the home improves gait-related mobility in Parkinson's disease: The RESCUE trial. *Journal of Neurology, Neurosurgery, and Psychiatry, 78*(2), 134–140.

Nutt, J. G., Bloem, B. R., Giladi, N., Hallett, M., Horak, F. B., & Nieuwboer, A. (2011). Freezing of gait: Moving forward on a mysterious clinical phenomenon. *Lancet Neurology, 10*(8), 734–744.

O'Sullivan, S. B. (1984). Perceived exertion. A review. *Physical Therapy, 64*(3), 343–346.

Overstall, P. W., Exton-Smith, A. N., Imms, F. J., & Johnson, A. L. (1977). Falls in the elderly related to postural imbalance. *British Medical Journal, 1*(6056), 261–264.

Pashler, H. (1994). Dual-task interference in simple tasks: Data and theory. *Psychological Bulletin, 116*(2), 220–244.

Passingham, R. E. (1996). Attention to action. *Philosophical Transactions of the Royal Society of London. Series B: Biological Sciences, 351*(1346), 1473–1479.

Peyser, J. M., Rao, S. M., LaRocca, N. G., & Kaplan, E. (1990). Guidelines for neuropsychological research in multiple sclerosis. *Archives of Neurology, 47*(1), 94–97.

Pichierri, G., Wolf, P., Murer, K., & de Bruin, E. D. (2011). Cognitive and cognitive-motor interventions affecting physical functioning: A systematic review. *BMC Geriatrics, 11*, 29.

Pilutti, L. A., Lelli, D. A., Paulseth, J. E., Crome, M., Jiang, S., Rathbone, M. P., et al. (2011). Effects of 12 weeks of supported treadmill training on functional ability and quality of life in progressive multiple sclerosis: A pilot study. *Archives of Physical Medicine and Rehabilitation, 92*(1), 31–36.

Plotnik, M., Giladi, N., & Hausdorff, J. M. (2009). Bilateral coordination of gait and Parkinson's disease: The effects of dual tasking. *Journal of Neurology, Neurosurgery, and Psychiatry, 80*(3), 347–350.

Plotnik, M., & Hausdorff, J. M. (2008). The role of gait rhythmicity and bilateral coordination of stepping in the pathophysiology of freezing of gait in Parkinson's disease. *Movement Disorders, 23*(Suppl. 2), S444–S450.

Radford, K., Lincoln, N., & Lennox, G. (2004). The effects of cognitive abilities on driving in people with Parkinson's disease. *Disability and Rehabilitation, 26*(2), 65–70.

Rao, S. M., Leo, G. J., Ellington, L., Nauertz, T., Bernardin, L., & Unverzagt, F. (1991). Cognitive dysfunction in multiple sclerosis. II. Impact on employment and social functioning. *Neurology, 41*(5), 692–696.

Robinson, K., Dennison, A., Roalf, D., Noorigian, J., Cianci, H., Bunting-Perry, L., et al. (2005). Falling risk factors in Parkinson's disease. *NeuroRehabilitation, 20*(3), 169–182.

Rochester, L., Baker, K., Hetherington, V., Jones, D., Willems, A. M., Kwakkel, G., et al. (2010). Evidence for motor learning in Parkinson's disease: Acquisition, automaticity and retention of cued gait performance after training with external rhythmical cues. *Brain Research, 1319*, 103–111.

Rowe, J., Stephan, K. E., Friston, K., Frackowiak, R., Lees, A., & Passingham, R. (2002). Attention to action in Parkinson's disease: Impaired effective connectivity among frontal cortical regions. *Brain, 125*(Pt 2), 276–289.

Rubenstein, T. C., Giladi, N., & Hausdorff, J. M. (2002). The power of cueing to circumvent dopamine deficits: A review of physical therapy treatment of gait disturbances in Parkinson's disease. *Movement Disorders, 17*(6), 1148–1160.

Rubenstein, L. Z., & Josephson, K. R. (2006). Falls and their prevention in elderly people: What does the evidence show? *The Medical Clinics of North America, 90*(5), 807–824.

Rubinsztein, D. C. (2006). The roles of intracellular protein-degradation pathways in neurodegeneration. *Nature, 443*(7113), 780–786.

Schaafsma, J. D., Giladi, N., Balash, Y., Bartels, A. L., Gurevich, T., & Hausdorff, J. M. (2003). Gait dynamics in Parkinson's disease: Relationship to Parkinsonian features, falls and response to levodopa. *Journal of the Neurological Sciences, 212*(1–2), 47–53.

Schenkman, M., & Butler, R. B. (1989). A model for multisystem evaluation treatment of individuals with Parkinson's disease. *Physical Therapy, 69*(11), 932–943.

Schwenk, M., Zieschang, T., Oster, P., & Hauer, K. (2010). Dual-task performances can be improved in patients with dementia: A randomized controlled trial. *Neurology, 74*(24), 1961–1968.

Sheridan, P. L., Solomont, J., Kowall, N., & Hausdorff, J. M. (2003). Influence of executive function on locomotor function: Divided attention increases gait variability in Alzheimer's disease. *Journal of American Geriatrics Society, 51*(11), 1633–1637.

Shine, J. M., Matar, E., Bolitho, S. J., Dilda, V., Morris, T. R., Naismith, S. L., et al. (2012). Modeling freezing of gait in Parkinson's disease with a virtual reality paradigm. *Gait Posture, 38*(1), 104–108.

Shine, J. M., Matar, E., Ward, P. B., Bolitho, S. J., Gilat, M., Pearson, M., et al. (2013). Exploring the cortical and subcortical functional magnetic resonance imaging changes associated with freezing in Parkinson's disease. *Brain, 136*(Pt 4), 1204–1215.

Shine, J. M., Naismith, S. L., Palavra, N. C., Lewis, S. J., Moore, S. T., Dilda, V., et al. (2013). Attentional set-shifting deficits correlate with the severity of freezing of gait in Parkinson's disease. *Parkinsonism & Related Disorders, 19*(3), 388–390.

Shine, J. M., Ward, P. B., Naismith, S. L., Pearson, M., & Lewis, S. J. (2011). Utilising functional MRI (fMRI) to explore the freezing phenomenon in Parkinson's disease. *Journal of Clinical Neuroscience, 18*(6), 807–810.

Shumway-Cook, A., Woollacott, M., Kerns, K. A., & Baldwin, M. (1997). The effects of two types of cognitive tasks on postural stability in older adults with and without a history of falls. *Journals of Gerontology. Series A, Biological Sciences and Medical Sciences, 52*(4), M232–M240.

Stuss, D. T., & Alexander, M. P. (2000). Executive functions and the frontal lobes: A conceptual view. *Psychological Research, 63*(3–4), 289–298.

Thaut, M. H., McIntosh, G. C., Rice, R. R., Miller, R. A., Rathbun, J., & Brault, J. M. (1996). Rhythmic auditory stimulation in gait training for Parkinson's disease patients. *Movement Disorders, 11*(2), 193–200.

The Panel on Prevention of Falls in Older Persons American Geriatrics Society and British Geriatrics Society. (2011). Summary of the Updated American Geriatrics Society/British Geriatrics Society clinical practice guideline for prevention of falls in older persons. *Journal of the American Geriatrics Society, 59*(1), 148–157.

Tinetti, M. E., Speechley, M., & Ginter, S. F. (1988). Risk factors for falls among elderly persons living in the community. *The New England Journal of Medicine, 319*(26), 1701–1707.

Tomassini, V., Johansen-Berg, H., Jbabdi, S., Wise, R. G., Pozzilli, C., Palace, J., et al. (2012). Relating brain damage to brain plasticity in patients with multiple sclerosis. *Neurorehabilitation and Neural Repair, 26*(6), 581–593.

Toole, T., Maitland, C. G., Warren, E., Hubmann, M. F., & Panton, L. (2005). The effects of loading and unloading treadmill walking on balance, gait, fall risk, and daily function in Parkinsonism. *NeuroRehabilitation, 20*(4), 307–322.

van Iersel, M. B., Kessels, R. P., Bloem, B. R., Verbeek, A. L., & Olde Rikkert, M. G. (2008). Executive functions are associated with gait and balance in community-living elderly people. *Journals of Gerontology. Series A, Biological Sciences and Medical Sciences, 63*(12), 1344–1349.

Van Wegen, E., Lim, I., de Goede, C., Nieuwboer, A., Willems, A., Jones, D., et al. (2006). The effects of visual rhythms and optic flow on stride patterns of patients with Parkinson's disease. *Parkinsonism & Related Disorders, 12*(1), 21–27.

Verghese, J., Buschke, H., Viola, L., Katz, M., Hall, C., Kuslansky, G., et al. (2002). Validity of divided attention tasks in predicting falls in older individuals: A preliminary study. *Journal of the American Geriatrics Society, 50*(9), 1572–1576.

Vitorio, R., Pieruccini-Faria, F., Stella, F., Gobbi, S., & Gobbi, L. T. (2010). Effects of obstacle height on obstacle crossing in mild Parkinson's disease. *Gait & Posture, 31*(1), 143–146.

Weerdesteyn, V., Rijken, H., Geurts, A. C., Smits-Engelsman, B. C., Mulder, T., & Duysens, J. (2006). A five-week exercise program can reduce falls and improve obstacle avoidance in the elderly. *Gerontology, 52*(3), 131–141.

Weinshenker, B. G. (1994). Natural history of multiple sclerosis. *Annals of Neurology, 36*(Suppl.), S6–S11.

Winstein, C. J. (1990). *Designing practice for motor learning: Clinical implications*. Paper presented at II STEP Conference, 1990.

Wood, B. H., Bilclough, J. A., Bowron, A., & Walker, R. W. (2002). Incidence and prediction of falls in Parkinson's disease: A prospective multidisciplinary study. *Journal of Neurology, Neurosurgery, and Psychiatry, 72*(6), 721–725.

Woollacott, M., & Shumway-Cook, A. (2002). Attention and the control of posture and gait: A review of an emerging area of research. *Gait & Posture, 16*(1), 1–14.

Wu, T., & Hallett, M. (2005). A functional MRI study of automatic movements in patients with Parkinson's disease. *Brain, 128*(Pt 10), 2250–2259.

Yogev, G., Giladi, N., Peretz, C., Springer, S., Simon, E. S., & Hausdorff, J. M. (2005). Dual tasking, gait rhythmicity, and Parkinson's disease: Which aspects of gait are attention demanding? *The European Journal of Neuroscience, 22*(5), 1248–1256.

Yogev, G., Plotnik, M., Peretz, C., Giladi, N., & Hausdorff, J. M. (2006). Gait asymmetry in patients with Parkinson's disease and elderly fallers: When does the bilateral coordination of gait require attention? *Experimental Brain Research, 177*(3), 336–346.

Yogev-Seligmann, G., Giladi, N., Brozgol, M., & Hausdorff, J. M. (2012). A training program to improve gait while dual tasking in patients with Parkinson's disease: A pilot study. *Archives of Physical Medicine and Rehabilitation, 93*(1), 176–181.

Yogev-Seligmann, G., Hausdorff, J. M., & Giladi, N. (2008). The role of executive function and attention in gait. *Movement Disorders, 23*(3), 329–342.

Chapter 9
Virtual Reality Reveals Mechanisms of Balance and Locomotor Impairments

Anouk Lamontagne, Emily A. Keshner, Nicoleta Bugnariu, and Joyce Fung

Objective To review how VR can be used to investigate normal and disturbed mechanisms of balance and locomotor control.

9.1 Multimodal Influences on Balance and Locomotor Control

Postural control requires integration of sensory information to assess the position of body in space and the ability to generate forces for controlling body position. The maintenance of upright equilibrium is essentially a sensorimotor integration task. The central nervous system (CNS) has to generate task-specific and goal-directed

A. Lamontagne (✉) • J. Fung
School of Physical and Occupational Therapy, McGill University,
3654 prom Sir-William-Osler, Montréal, QC, Canada, H3G 1Y5
e-mail: anouk.lamontagne@mcgill.ca; joyce.fung@mcgill.ca

E.A. Keshner
Department of Physical Therapy and Department of Electrical and Computer Engineering,
Temple University, 3307 N. Broad ST, Philadelphia, PA 19140, USA
e-mail: ekeshner@temple.edu

N. Bugnariu
Physical Therapy Program, University of North Texas Health Science Center,
3500 Camp Bowie Blvd., MET 531, Fort Worth, TX 76107, USA
e-mail: nicoleta.bugnariu@unthsc.edu

P.L. (Tamar) Weiss et al. (eds.), *Virtual Reality for Physical and Motor Rehabilitation*, Virtual Reality Technologies for Health and Clinical Applications,
DOI 10.1007/978-1-4939-0968-1_9,

complex motor responses based on the selective and rapid integration of sensory information from multiple sources. Since each sensory system has its own coordinate framework, specific time delay, and reliability, sensory conflicts may arise and requires the CNS to recalibrate the weight attributed to each particular sensory input. Adaptive or reactive postural control involves modifying sensory and motor systems in response to changing tasks and environmental demands. Humans can tread on changing and uneven terrains without falling because the intact CNS can make ongoing corrections.

Effective postural control requires more than the ability to generate and apply forces for controlling the body's position in space. In order to know when and how to apply restoring forces, the CNS must have accurate information of where the body is in space and whether it is stationary or in motion. Somatosensory afferents provide information regarding the body's position and motion in space with respect to the support surface. Visual inputs provide information concerning the position and motion of the head with respect to the surrounding environment. With the semicircular canals sensing angular accelerations of the head in different planes and the otoliths signaling linear position and acceleration of the head with respect to gravity and inertial forces, the vestibular system provides a gravito-inertial frame of reference for postural control (Chap. 5).

9.1.1 Visual Influences on Postural and Locomotor Control

It was once thought that visual inputs were too slow to have any effect on the rapid response due to sudden perturbations of stance, since the sensation of motion induced by moving visual fields has a relatively long latency (–1 s), and the influence on body sway is too slow (Nasher and Berthoz, 1978). Subsequent experiments have shown that visual information that conflicts with those arising from other sensory channels can have a rapid and profound effect on postural responses (Keshner, Kenyon, Dhaher, & Streepey, 2004; Vidal et al., 1982). For instance, when visual inputs are stabilized with respect to the head during the time of the perturbation only, the initial triceps surae burst can be significantly attenuated and forward sway increases. In contrast, merely closing the eyes during a postural perturbation has no effect on early evoked responses or on the performance, suggesting that sensory context is an important factor in shaping the strategy for postural responses (Vidal et al., 1982). Absence of vision under these conditions does not compromise postural performance since other sensory channels provide sufficient information. In contrast, visual information that conflicts with those from other sensory channels can have a rapid and profound effect on postural responses. The influence of moving visual fields on postural stability depends on the characteristics not only of the visual environment but also of the support surface, including the size of the base of support and its rigidity or compliance (Keshner & Kenyon, 2000; Streepey et al., 2007)

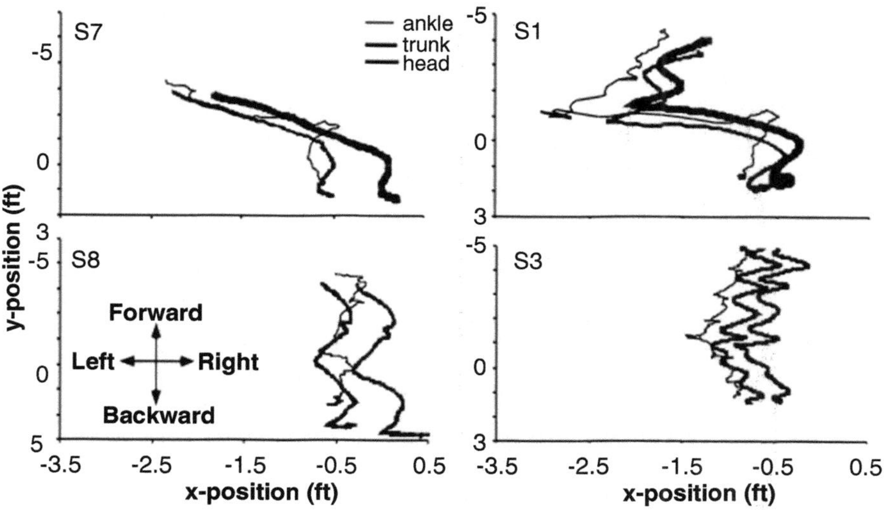

Fig. 9.1 Natural locomotion was combined with visual field motion in the roll plane with two different virtual environments (*left* and *right*). Each plot is of a different subject exhibiting one of the two response strategies in the (*top and bottom*) traces

The strong influence of a moving visual field observed on the kinematic parameters of posture and gait suggests that optic flow is an important component of the motor program when somatosensory feedback is fluctuating (Varraine, Bonnard, & Pailhous, 2002). For example, when natural locomotion was combined with visual field motion (Keshner & Kenyon, 2000; Varraine et al., 2002), kinematic parameters of gait were strongly influenced by the moving visual field (Fig. 9.1). Standing subjects viewing a wide-screen visual scene exhibited little sway when the scene was stationary, but large center of pressure (COP) changes when the scene was moving at 25°/s (Ferman, Collewijn, Jansen, & Van den Berg, 1987; Previc, 1992). Responses to visual field motion were even more strongly potentiated when body motion was added to visual field motion even though the visual inputs were incongruent with the somatosensory inputs. With only support surface translation (Keshner, Kenyon, Dhaher, et al., 2004; Keshner, Kenyon, & Langston, 2004) or tilt (Wang, Kenyon, & Keshner, 2009), segmental responses were small and mostly countering the direction of the perturbation. When the base of support and visual field disturbances were presented concurrently, however, response amplitudes became large for all subjects (Fig. 9.2). Average root mean square (RMS) values across subjects were significantly greater with combined stimuli than for either stimulus presented alone, and areas under the power curve across subjects were significantly increased at the frequency of the visual input when both inputs were presented. Kinematic changes were directly related to the velocity of the visual field (Wang et al., 2009). Therefore, virtual reality environments that manipulate the optic flow field present a compelling tool for the rehabilitation of sensorimotor disorders (Chaps. 4 and 6).

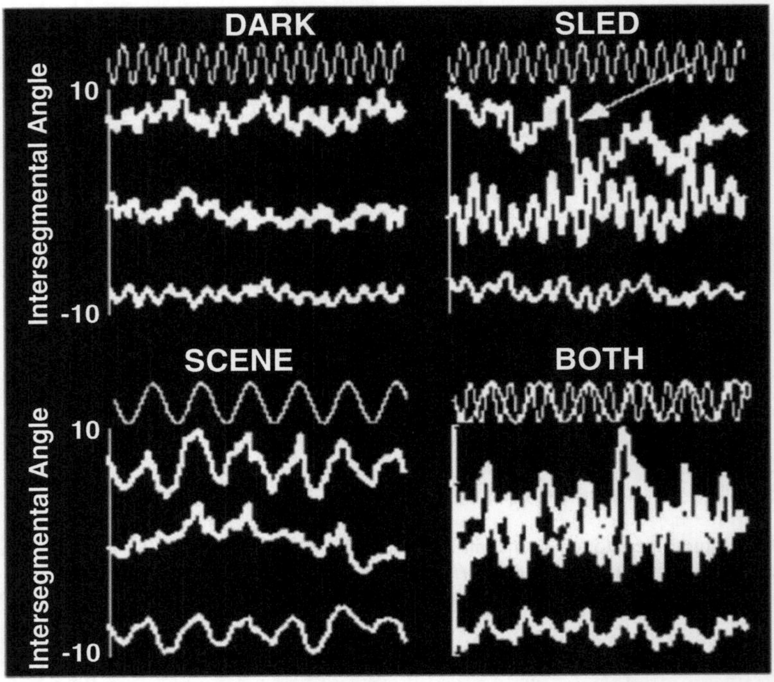

Fig. 9.2 Base of support and visual field disturbances presented concurrently (BOTH) produce more complex response behaviors than either one (SCENE or SLED) alone across 60 s of each trial. Trace above each plot is the stimulus waveform. In each plot, *top trace* is head re trunk; *middle trace* is trunk re shank; *bottom trace* is shank re platform

9.1.2 Sensory Preferences and Sensory Conflict

All of the sensory modalities are guided by, and provide updates to, a shared world model (Masumoto, Yamakawa, Kimoto, & Nagata, 1994). Conflicts between these channels have been observed through motor behaviors exhibited in the virtual world. Large movements of the visual field induce postural instability even when our bodies are not capable of performing equivalent magnitudes of motion (Dokka, Kenyon, Keshner, 2009). Both visual field velocity and direction have significant effects on the magnitude of the trunk and lower limb responses in healthy individuals (Dokka et al., 2009; Keshner & Dhaher, 2008; Keshner & Kenyon, 2000; Keshner, Kenyon, & Langston, 2004; Wang et al., 2009). Visual field motion influenced orientation of the head even when there was no physical disturbance to the position of the body suggesting a predominant impact on motion of the upper body. When conflicting self-motion from disturbances at the base of support was added to the visual field motion, kinematics of the whole body became more complex so that frequency parameters from both the visual field and the base of support motion were incorporated into the responses (Keshner, Kenyon, & Langston, 2004). Once destabilization resulting from platform motion had subsided, however, orientation of the body again became biased toward the direction of visual field motion and magnitude of joint motion increased as the visual velocity increased (Dokka et al., 2009). However, if we have prior knowledge of the characteristics of the upcoming visual motion, we are often able to reduce the size of these physical responses (Amblard, Cremieux, Marchand, & Carblanc, 1985; Day & Guerraz, 2007; Guerraz et al., 2001) from which we can infer that there is cortical control of these behaviors.

Intersensory dependencies apparent through the increased responses to the visual inputs when there were two simultaneous inputs (Keshner, Kenyon, Dhaher, & Streepey, 2005; Keshner, Kenyon, & Langston, 2004) indicate that the conflict between visual and vestibular pathways does not produce a simple switch from one modality to another. Resolving ambiguity between motion of objects in the world and motion of oneself is likely a combination of multisensorial feedback and perceptual choice and not just the identification of sensory relevance which, in the real world, may not be easily apparent (Lambrey & Berthoz, 2003). In fact, there is evidence that healthy individuals demonstrate preferences for particular sensory channels (Dumontheil, Panagiotaki, & Berthoz, 2006; Lambrey & Berthoz, 2003). When standing subjects viewed a virtual corridor in which forward movements were simulated at a constant linear velocity, and rotations were actually performed. When subjects were asked to learn the trajectory and then reproduce it from memory, half of the subjects placed more weight on visual than on non-visual information. The other subjects placed more weight on non-visual than on visual information. The difference between "visual" and "non-visual" subjects in their use of conflicting information was their own awareness of the sensory conflict. The conflicting sensory inputs were combined linearly in order to estimate the angular displacements until subjects became aware of the conflict and then produced nonlinear behaviors.

Multisensory calibration is fundamental for proficient interaction within a changing environment, but studies suggest a visual-dominant mechanism (Chap. 5). A study of both humans and monkeys performing a heading-discrimination task with either visual (optic-flow) or vestibular (motion-platform) or combined (visual–vestibular) stimuli revealed that directional adaptation of both visual and vestibular cues was required to reduce cue conflict. However, cue calibration did not depend on the reliability of the cue. Vestibular adaptation was greater than visual adaptation regardless of reliability suggesting that calibration is based on cue accuracy and that visual cue accuracy is greater than the vestibular cue accuracy (Zaidel, Turner, & Angelaki, 2011).

Visual preference, or dependence, has been measured through the "Rod and Frame" test (Asch & Witkin, 1992; Witkin & Asch, 1948). Based on performance on this test, perceptual style is classified as either field-independent or field-dependent. Field-independent individuals rely on gravitational and egocentric cues. Such individuals are able to adjust the rod to its true vertical and horizontal orientations with a high level of accuracy of about 1–2° although there is some variation in the degree to which people are influenced by the surrounding frame. Field-dependent individuals use mainly visual cues for estimating subjective vertical and body orientation.

These individuals are unable to accurately adjust the rod to its true vertical and horizontal orientations due to the influence of the surrounding tilted frame. Visual field dependence was found to be a good predictor of an individual's reliance on visual reafference to stabilize posture during Romberg stance in front of tilted visual field (Amblard et al., 1985; Isableu, Ohlmann, Cremieux, & Amblard, 1997).

9.1.3 Impact of Visual–Vestibular Conflict on Balance and Locomotion

A characteristic unique to the virtual reality environment is that it can become the observer's visual reality. This effect is more convincing when there are no cues to the physical environment, such as occurs in a CAVE or with head mounted displays (HMD). Even brief exposures to motion of a wide field of view visual environment can produce illusions of self-motion and create instability or reshape a planned movement (Dvorkin, Kenyon, & Keshner, 2009). If the environment around us is stationary, it is relatively easy to identify our physical motion. But when the world is moving, we have to determine whether it is the environment or oneself that is moving, and then shape our movements to accurately match the demands of the environment. To do this we must use the sensory information linked to the movement and identify any mismatch that may exist between the visual motion and our own sensory feedback (Dokka, Kenyon, Keshner, & Kording, 2010; Keshner & Kenyon, 2009). The perception of self-motion and orientation in space is derived from a convergence of vestibular, proprioceptive, and visual signals. Even in the physical environment, we rely on both visual and vestibular signals to define our spatial orientation and our self-motion. But when an immersive virtual environment presents no external cues to vertical, being able to distinguish between the body motion induced by visual field motion and that which is self-generated becomes a computational problem for the central nervous system (CNS) (Reymond, Droulez, & Kemeny, 2002).

This computational problem is not always accurately resolved because the perception of verticality is greatly influenced by the current optic flow field (Varraine et al., 2002; Warren, Kay, Zosh, Duchon, & Sahuc, 2001). For example, consider the feeling of self-motion when seeing movement of a train out of the corner of your eye even though you are standing still (Previc, 1992; Previc & Donnelly, 1993; Previc, Kenyon, Boer, & Johnson, 1993; Wang et al., 2009). This illusion of self-motion generated by motion of the visual surround is called vection. An extensive literature, ranging from behavioral studies (Dichgans, Brandt, & Held, 1975; Slobounov, Tutwiler, Sebastianelli, & Slobounov, 2006; Tanahashi, Ujike, Kozawa, & Ukai, 2007; Thurrell & Bronstein, 2002) to neuroimaging studies (Brandt et al., 2002; Kleinschmidt et al., 2002; Wiest et al., 2001), has demonstrated that both vestibular and visual inputs interact at the brainstem and cortical levels during vection and that both of these sensory inputs are likely to participate in the perception of self-motion. Major characteristics of vection such as the shape of the perceived path of self-motion (e.g., linear, curvilinear, circular) and its direction are defined with respect to visual input only, as if they are independent from vestibular input. However, when visual perspective is coupled to head position, a direct linkage between the perception of vection and postural orientation is demonstrated (Keshner, Dokka, & Kenyon, 2006) suggesting a strong vestibular contribution to the perception of self-motion. In fact, onset of vection has been shown to occur more readily in subjects that do not perceive conflict between visual and vestibular afferent inputs (Lepecq, Giannopulu, Mertz, & Baudonniere, 1999), suggesting that information from the vestibular system is dominating the inappropriate visual inputs (Black, Wall, & Nashner, 1983; Keshner, Kenyon, & Langston, 2004).

Conflicting results are seen in attempts to determine whether the impact of visual information on postural reactions is due to the same perceptual mechanisms that also produce the sway resulting from the illusion of self-motion produced by an optic flow field (vection) (Clement, Gurfinkel, Lestienne, Lipshits, & Popov, 1984; Previc, 1992; Previc & Donnelly, 1993). Studies that examined body sway on a stable surface while in the Rhomberg position (Kuno, Kawakita, Kawakami, Miyake, & Watanabe, 1999; Tanahashi et al., 2007) concluded that postural sway and sway elicited by vection relied upon a shared central mechanism. When standing on an unstable support surface such as foam (Guerraz & Bronstein, 2008) or a sinusoidally moving platform (Keshner, Kenyon, & Langston, 2004) so that the direction of the two sway responses could be differentiated, postural instability occurred earlier and in the opposite direction from the later vection response.

The different time course and mismatch between the direction of postural responses and the direction of vection support a conclusion that the perceptual and postural sway responses were not generated from a single visual control mechanism (Previc & Donnelly, 1993). When subjects experienced concomitant disturbances of the visual and proprioceptive/vestibular systems, the initial recovery of vertical orientation in space was very sensitive to the dynamics of the visual field (Wang et al., 2009). Such adaptations to an active visual environment, particularly when combined with an unstable base of support, will have significant impact on the ability to maintain upright stance when negotiating challenging environmental demands, and the absence of this rapid response to visual information may contribute to postural instability in elderly individuals.

The contribution of vestibular inputs to the perception of the direction of self-motion was investigated with galvanic vestibular stimulation (GVS) on visually induced self-motion (i.e., vection) in healthy subjects (Lepecq et al., 2006). Seated subjects were submitted to optokinetic stimulation inducing either forward or upward linear vection. Subjects indicated the shape and direction of their perceived self-motion path throughout the experiment with a joystick. Results indicated that GVS induced alterations in the path of vection. GVS acts through both otolith and canal afferents (Fitzpatrick, Marsden, Lord, & Day, 2002), and thus, the linear upward or forward self-motion perception, induced by combining vection and GVS, suggests a fusion of the vestibular and visual pathways. The impact of individual sensory preferences on postural behavior are being examined in the Keshner laboratory (Keshner, Slaboda, Buddharaju, Lanaria, & Norman, 2011) by combining mismatched visual and vestibular signals by combining galvanic vestibular stimulation

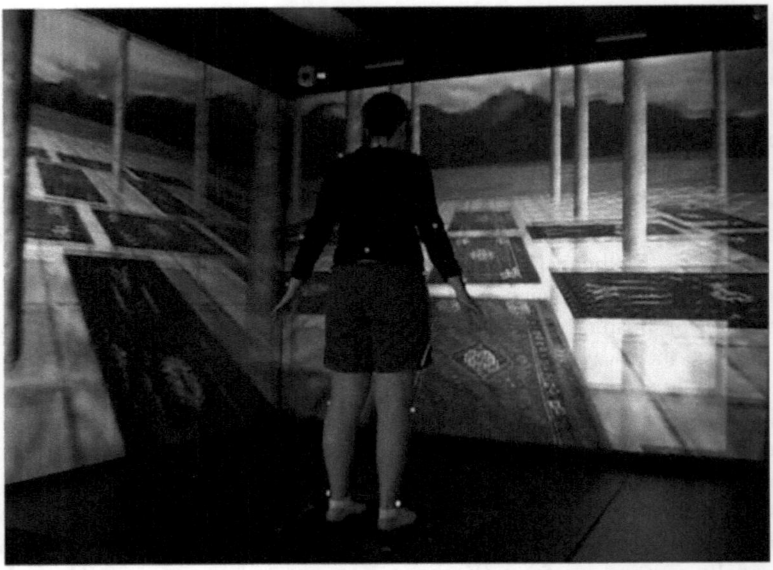

Fig. 9.3 A virtual room with carpets and columns and a distant horizon and a subject standing on the dual forceplates

(GVS) with rotations of the visual field. Healthy young adults stood quietly in a 3-wall immersive stereo virtual environment (Fig. 9.3). When exposed to a moving visual field, both prior to and after application of GVS, responses at the head and COP were significantly correlated with the frequency of the visual field oscillation (Fig. 9.4, left and right). When visual motion was combined with GVS, the FFT of head angular displacement revealed responses at both the GVS and visual scene frequencies (Fig. 9.4, center). The previous 0.25 Hz response of the COP was shifted down towards 0.2 Hz suggesting that performers adapted their postural behaviors to whatever confluence of sensory information was available.

9.1.4 *Effects of Visual–Vestibular Conflict with Aging and Neuromuscular Disorders*

The ability to manipulate sensory conflict is particularly important when dealing with older adults and those with neurological impairment such as stroke or Parkinson's disease. With the loss of vestibular information, as occurs with destruction of the labyrinths through disease, trauma, or chemical intervention, vertigo, dizziness, and instability often result. In labyrinthine deficient patients, when visual (Bles, Vianney de Jong, & de Wit, 1983) or somatosensory (Black et al., 1983; Horak, Nashner, & Diener, 1990) information becomes unreliable, postural

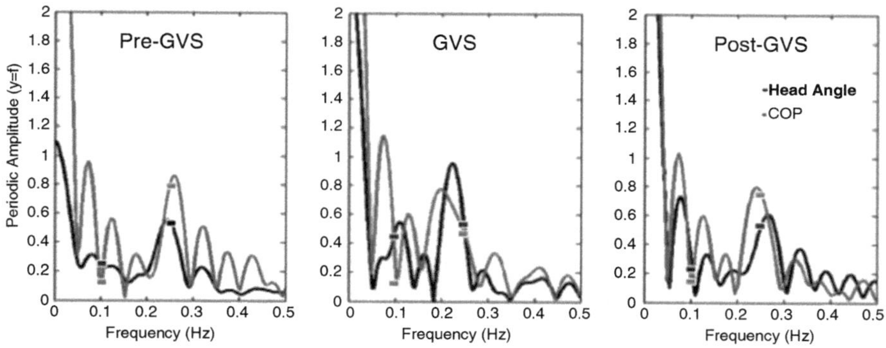

Fig. 9.4 Frequency responses of head angular displacement (*black*) and COP (*gray*) during 20 s of 0.25 Hz scene rotation (*left*), 20 s of 0.1 Hz galvanic vestibular stimulation (GVS) and 0.25 Hz scene rotation (*center*), and 20 s following GVS with 0.25 Hz scene rotation (*right*) show that GVS produced responses at the head and in the COP that were significantly correlated with the frequency of the visual field

disorientation can be explained by the fact that neither signal can adequately specify the orientation of the body in all situations.

It is not clear whether increased body sway with visual–vestibular conflict is due to optic flow streaming along the peripheral visual field, or the oculomotor motion generated by scanning the moving visual field. Studies of locomotion with combined central and peripheral radial flow have demonstrated that both central and peripheral regions of the visual field are sensitive to optic flow and will differentially influence postural stability in both healthy subjects and patients with vestibular disorders (Bardy, Warren, & Kay, 1999; Redfern & Furman, 1994; Straube, Krafczyk, Paulus, & Brandt, 1994). When elderly subjects tracked a focal object while the visual background and support surface were moving either congruently or incongruently, inappropriate peripheral visual inputs increased the amplitude of postural sway whereas appropriate peripheral visual inputs decreased postural sway (Keshner, Kenyon et al., 2004). The stabilizing effect of an object in the central visual field was altered depending upon the presence of a conflict in the peripheral visual region.

There is also evidence that the effect of visual motion on posture is modified by perceptual preference. Elderly individuals with a history of falling were significantly more visually field-dependent than those without (Lord & Webster, 1990; Slaboda, Lauer, & Keshner, 2011). Patients having cortical or sub-cortical stroke exhibited significantly larger absolute angular deviations than both healthy young and older adults for vertical and horizontal alignment of the rod even though their absolute angular deviations were highly variable between trials and within the group. Absolute angular deviations were also significantly different between older and young adults. Increased visual dependence was significantly correlated with increased postural sway when standing quietly in front of a moving visual field. Therefore, elderly adults and those with neurological impairment are more visually dependent than young adults and less responsive to somatosensory feedback, which could promote instability when vision conflicts with physical motion.

Older women in particular have been shown to be more visually sensitive than younger adults (Bugnariu & Fung, 2007; Guerraz & Bronstein, 2008; Slaboda et al., 2011). Older women exhibited significantly larger body's center of mass (COM) and COP responses in the direction of visual field motion and less muscle modulation as the platform returned to neutral than younger women. It appears that a stiffer body combined with heightened visual sensitivity in older women critically interferes with their ability to counteract postural destabilizing environments. Postural responses that are more closely matched to the visual environment but not temporally matched to the immediate demands of the postural disturbance (Dokka et al., 2010; Wright, DiZio, & Lackner, 2005) produce a greater mismatch between the visual motion feedback and somatosensory feedback and rapidly elicit spatial disorientation (Previc, 1992; Previc et al., 1993; Previc & Donnelly, 1993). In addition, postural reactions slow with aging (Gill et al., 2001; Keshner et al., 1993; Keshner, Allum, & Pfaltz, 1987; Woollacott, 1993), thereby creating even more of a window for slowly processed visual inputs to modify postural behavior.

The heightened impact of visual field motion with aging could be a significant factor in the increased occurrence of falls (Isableu et al., 2010). In addition, the changes in postural behavior in older adults as a result of visual and vestibular conflict are consistent with physiological changes of diminished vestibular sensitivity and visual acuity as we age (Allum, Carpenter, Honegger, Adkin, & Bloem, 2002; Bergstrom, 1973; Peterka, Black, & Schoenhoff, 1990a, 1990b; Rosenhall, 1973). A large body of evidence also proposes that postural instability in elderly individuals is caused by their inability to process multiple simultaneous demands on attention (Shumway-Cook & Woollacott, 2000; Silsupadol, Lugade et al., 2009; Silsupadol, Shumway-Cook et al., 2009; Siu, Chou, Mayr, Donkelaar, & Woollacott, 2008; Siu, Chou, Mayr, van Donkelaar, & Woollacott, 2009; Stelmach, Zelaznik, & Lowe, 1990; Verhoeff, Horlings, Janssen, Bridenbaugh, & Allum, 2009). When faced with multiple postural demands, such as a surface that changes in gradient and frictional characteristics in a busy visual environment, compensation for one disturbance will impinge on how our responses are organized to meet successive disturbances, and this influence becomes more overpowering with aging (Slaboda et al., 2011).

9.2 Visuomotor Control of Locomotion in Virtual Reality

Virtual reality (VR) can be used to investigate normal and disturbed mechanisms of visuo-locomotor control (Chap. 8). We explain how this technology provides opportunities to manipulate visual information pertaining to self-motion and environmental characteristics as a means to investigate and shape locomotor features such as speed, trajectory, and obstacle circumvention behaviors.

9.2.1 Changing Speed Using Visual Motion Paradigms

While comfortable walking speed is determined by biomechanical, physiological, and energetic factors (Bohannon, 1997; Saibene & Minetti, 2003; Taylor, Heglund, & Maloiy, 1982), it is also influenced and monitored by the perception of self-motion of the observer with respect to its surrounding, also referred to as optic flow (Warren, 1998). Investigations on the role of optic flow in the control of walking speed were initiated in the 1990s with projections of basic luminous patterns such as spots or diamond shapes on the floor, walls, or half-spherical screens (Chou et al., 2009; Konczak, 1994; Pailhous, Ferrandez, Fluckiger, & Baumberger, 1990; Prokop, Schubert, & Berger, 1997; Schubert, Prokop, Brocke, & Berger, 2005). Experiments were repeated in rich-textured and meaningful environments, with similar results (Lamontagne, Fung, McFadyen, & Faubert, 2007; Mohler, Thompson, Creem-Regehr, Pick, & Warren, 2007). Two main paradigms with distinct purposes emerge from the literature: a first paradigm that is designed to investigate *unintentional* modulations of walking speed and a second paradigm that requires the participants to *volitionally* alter walking speed based on visual perception.

9.2.2 Unintentional Modulations

Unintentional changes in walking speed is obtained by instructing participants to maintain their comfortable walking speed while having them exposed to continuous (Konczak, 1994; Pailhous et al., 1990; Prokop et al., 1997; Schubert et al., 2005) or discrete "steady-state" variations in optic flow speed (Chou et al., 2009; Francois, Morice, Bootsma, & Montagne, 2011; Lamontagne et al., 2007; Mohler et al., 2007). In most instances, the experiment takes place on a self-paced treadmill that allows the participants to change their walking speed at will. A common observation across studies is that faster optic flow causes a reduction in walking speed while slower optic flow yields a faster walking speed. Optic flow speed manipulations also shift walk-to-run and run-to-walk transitions, with faster optic flow rates eliciting lower transition speeds (Mohler et al., 2007). The proposed explanation for optic flow-induced unintentional speed modulations is that participants attempt to recalibrate the mismatch induced by the experimental manipulation between visual and body-based cues (Mohler et al., 2007; Prokop et al., 1997). Hence, a fast optic flow indicating a larger walking speed compared to that specified by body-based cues causes participants to slow down whereas a slower optic flow would do just the opposite.

Altering the speed of a visual display also modifies two features of optic flow that contribute to the perception of the speed of self-motion: global optic flow rate, referred to as the angular velocity of texture elements in a given visual direction, and edge rate, which is the number of texture elements per unit of time that pass by a reference point in a given visual direction (Francois, Morice, & Bootsma, et al., 2011; Larish & Flach, 1990). In a recent study, Francois and collaborators used a clever design based on manipulations of the participants' perceived height and density of texture elements on the floor (tiles) to dissociate the contribution of these two optic features. Both were found to contribute to walking speed modulations, with larger modifications of walking velocity being observed with the manipulations of global optic flow rate compared to edge rate. This observation indicates that both elements can potentially be manipulated in a virtual environment in order to maximize walking speed adaptations (Chap. 5).

In the context of locomotor rehabilitation, the choice of a training paradigm is guided by the nature and magnitude of the desired changes. A review of the different studies on unintentional speed modulations mediated by changing optic flows reveals that changes remain relatively modest in magnitude, that is, in the order of 10–20 % (Lamontagne et al., 2007; Pailhous et al., 1990; Prokop et al., 1997; Schubert et al., 2005). Speed adaptations are mediated through changes in both spatial and temporal dimensions, as reflected by concomitant modifications in stride length and frequency (Francois, Morice, & Bootsma, et al., 2011; Konczak, 1994; Pailhous et al., 1990; Prokop et al., 1997). Unlike normal walking with absent or congruent optic flow, however, the ratio of stride length over frequency is modified as optic flow-driven speed adaptations are predominantly induced by changes in stride length (Prokop et al., 1997; Schubert et al., 2005). In addition, modulation effects on speed were shown to diminish by 45 % over a walking distance of 800 m, indicating a habituation or, as proposed by Prokop and colleagues, a reweighting towards a more proprioceptive (spinal) control of locomotion (Prokop et al., 1997). Altogether, these observations suggest that while optic flow-based unintentional speed modulation paradigms can be useful to address matters of sensory reweighting, the modest magnitude of the speed adaptations, the altered temporal-distance relationship in stride adaptations, and attenuation of the modulation effects over time make this approach less relevant as a training paradigm to favor gait speed adaptations

9.2.3 Volitional Modulations

Lamontagne and colleagues have developed a paradigm in which participants are required to use optic flow to modulate walking speed (Lamontagne et al., 2007). It consists of having the participants walking in a short virtual corridor while presenting them with pairs of visual stimuli: a control stimulus which display an optic flow speed corresponding to the participants' comfortable walking speed followed by a test stimulus in which a steady state optic flow speed is set to a ratio (e.g., 0.25 to 2 times) of the control comfortable speed. Participants walk at comfortable speed in the control trials and are instructed, in the test trials, to walk the corridor distance within the same time as the preceding control trial. While using this gaming paradigm, an inverse linear relationship was demonstrated between optic flow and walking speed (Lamontagne et al., 2007), similar to the unintentional paradigm. As further detailed in the next section, this paradigm was proposed as a means to train walking speed adaptations in older adults, as well as in subjects with stroke.

9.3 Changing Locomotor Heading Using Visual Motion Paradigms

Heading can be broadly defined as the angular orientation, in the horizontal plane, of a motion trajectory. This section is concerned with manipulations of visual motion direction as a strategy to alter heading direction while walking. The optic flow manipulations are achieved by exposing the individuals to translating or rotating virtual environments, usually in the horizontal plane but also in the frontal plane, or by inducing a lateral asymmetry in the speed of the optic flow.

9.3.1 Manipulating Optic Flows in the Horizontal Plane

The optic flow theory stipulates that, as one moves in the environment, the flow field that is generated has a radial structure with a focus of expansion (FOE) located in the direction of self-motion which can be used to guide heading (Gibson, 1994; Warren, 1998). Warren and his colleagues were the first to demonstrate that optic flow direction information is used to guide heading during locomotion on foot (Warren et al., 2001). To do so, they offset the FOE to the side while instructing young participants to steer toward a goal and showed that the resulting trajectory in the physical world coordinates described a more or less linear path that veered away from the FOE. They also demonstrated that the reliance on the optic flow, as opposed to the visual direction of a goal (e.g., egomotion theory (Rushton, Harris, Lloyd, & Wann, 1998)), increased with greater flow and motion parallax. The latter finding suggests that providing richly textured environment to participants is ideal for enhancing or training optic flow induced steering behaviors.

In addition to the richness of the flow, its characteristics also contribute to shape steering behaviors. For instance, the larger the shift in the FOE, the larger the walking trajectory deviation in the physical walking world (Berard, Fung, McFadyen, & Lamontagne, 2009; Sarre, Berard, Fung, & Lamontagne, 2008). The structure of the flow, that is whether it is manipulated along the rotational or translational dimension, also has a profound influence on the steering behavior (Sarre et al., 2008). A translational flow that describes a lateral shift of the virtual environment lead to a steering behavior characterized by a change of locomotor trajectory that is accompanied by little reorientation of the head, thorax, pelvis, and feet, also referred to as a "crab walk" pattern (Fig. 9.5). When exposed to rotational flows, changes in the walking trajectory are accompanied by a horizontal reorientation of the head and other axial body segments in the direction of veering (Sarre et al., 2008), as observed when steering in the physical world (Grasso, Glasauer, Takei, & Berthoz, 1996; Patla, Adkin, & Ballard, 1999). These findings have a few implications that can be of interest for rehabilitation. First, by selectively shifting the FOE to one side or another, it is possible to promote veering toward a desired direction. Second, changing the magnitude of the FOE shift allows changing the extent of veering, from a

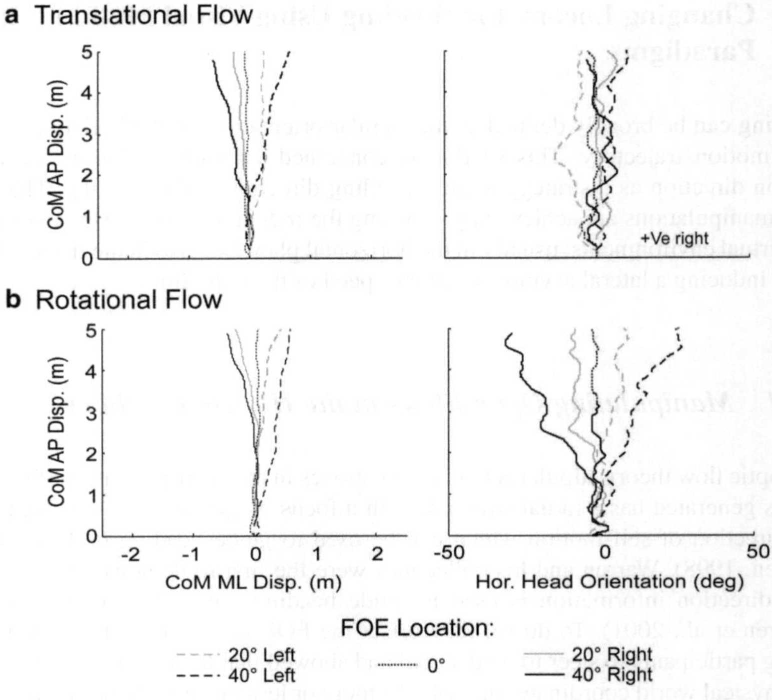

Fig. 9.5 Mediolateral displacement (*left panel*) and horizontal head reorientation (*right panel*) as a function of center of mass (COM) forward displacement in the physical world coordinates while walking in a virtual room describing optic flows having different focus of expansion (FOE) locations. The two optic flow conditions illustrated are (**a**) translational flows, where the scene was horizontally shifted to the side as the participant progressed forward, and (**b**) rotational flows, where the scene appeared as rotating around a vertical axis located at the center of the head. The participant was instructed to walk straight in the virtual world as viewed in the helmet mounted display. Note that both translational and rotational flows induced a walking deviation in the direction opposite to the FOE. This change in trajectory was accompanied by a horizontal head reorientation for the rotational flow (**b**) but not for the translational flow (**a**). This figure was modified from (Sarre et al., 2008)

small to a larger deviation. Finally, while the rotational vs. translational dimensions of the flow allows for selective steering behaviors in terms of body segment coordination, rotational flows appear to describe more ecological and commonly encountered visual stimuli, as when walking along a curved path, which in turn induces a more natural steering behavior.

9.3.2 *Optic Flow Speed Asymmetry and Visual Roll*

Other visual motion stimuli that were used to manipulate locomotor heading include lateral asymmetries in optic flow speed as well as visual roll stimulation. In the optic flow speed asymmetry paradigm, individuals exposed to different speeds of optic flow projected onto a right vs. left wall veer or drift away from the faster moving wall, with larger speed differences leading to larger lateral drifts (Chou et al., 2009; Duchon & Warren, 2002). A roll of the virtual environment at constant speeds ranging from 5°/s to 15°/s also lead to a lateral deviation of the walking trajectory (Keshner & Kenyon, 2000; Schneider, Jahn, Dieterich, Brandt, & Strupp, 2008). This walking deviation, which is towards the left in presence of a counter-clockwise rotation and towards the right for a clockwise rotation, could be mediated by an altered perception of verticality, as well as the sense of vection provided by the stimulus (Keshner & Kenyon, 2000; Schneider et al., 2008). The effects of a visual roll stimulation on the walking deviation can be overridden by some individuals (Keshner & Kenyon, 2000) and disappears after a walking distance beyond 2 m (Schneider et al., 2008), which suggests the presence of a sensory reweighting toward non-visual sources of information. It should be noted, however, that no such observations were reported in studies where participants were clearly instructed to control their heading within the *virtual world* coordinates (Berard et al., 2009; Warren et al., 2001). The instructions provided to participants, especially in a context where the sensory information specified in the virtual vs. physical world is incongruent, can be a key factor that contributes to shape the steering responses.

9.3.3 Adaptations to Repeated Exposure

Another issue that is of interest to rehabilitation concerns the effects of a prolonged exposure to a stimulus, as in the context of a training session (Chap. 3). When aiming at a virtual target while exposed to a rotating (yaw) optic flow over repeated walking trials, heading errors with respect to the target decrease, especially within the first 10 trials, provided that the adaptation is done overground to allow the participants to adjust their walking trajectory (Bruggeman, Zosh, & Warren, 2007; Saunders & Durgin, 2011). These results suggest the presence of a learning effect with repeated exposure. Full-field or richer optic flow conditions allow for faster and larger heading adaptations (Bruggeman et al., 2007; Saunders & Durgin, 2011), further supporting the idea that rich visual environments may be optimal for rehabilitation. A prolonged (20 min) or repeated (20 trials) exposure to a horizontal rotational flow while walking either overground or on a treadmill were reported to be sufficient to yield after-effects that are characterized by a change in torso orientation and heading direction (Mulavara et al., 2005; Nomura, Mulavara, Richards, Brady, & Bloomberg, 2005; Saunders & Durgin, 2011). Whether this after-effect persists over time and could thus be used for therapeutic purposes remains unknown.

9.4 Obstacle Avoidance Paradigms

When walking, individuals also need to adapt their locomotor behavior to environmental constraints that can present in the form of changing terrains, luminosity as well as presence of static and dynamic bodies. Obstacle circumvention abilities can be altered by various conditions such as post-stroke visuospatial neglect (Punt, Kitadono, Hulleman, Humphreys, & Riddoch, 2008; Webster, Rapport, Godlewski, & Abadee, 1994), traumatic brain injury (Fait, McFadyen, Swaine, & Cantin, 2009), or simply older age (Gerin-Lajoie, Richards, & McFadyen, 2006; Paquette & Vallis, 2010), leading to an increased risk of collisions and limited mobility in the community. The VR technology, because of its configurability, reproducibility, and safety, is an ideal tool to investigate and train complex visuo-locomotor tasks, especially when using a moving obstacle paradigm that would otherwise be challenging to design and control in a physical environment. Yet very few VR studies in this area are so far available, especially in individuals with disabilities. The section below highlights the salient findings from these few studies and introduces new perceptuo-motor paradigms developed in our laboratory which could help provide insights into the altered obstacle circumvention abilities presented by individuals with perceptual or motor problems.

The first studies that used the VR technology to investigate locomotor adaptations to virtual objects emerged from the field of psychology and have proposed different mathematical models to capture behaviors during interceptive, steering, and obstacle circumvention tasks (Chardenon, Montagne, Laurent, & Bootsma, 2004; Cutting & Vishton, 1995; Fajen & Warren, 2003). When both the participant and virtual object of interest are moving, as when intercepting a moving ball while walking, the locomotor adaptations depend on multiple sources of optical information, including the global optic flow perceived at the eye of the moving participants, the local optic flow due to the ball movement and the egocentric position (non-flow information) of the ball (Chardenon et al., 2004; Cutting & Vishton, 1995; Fajen & Warren, 2003). It is proposed that interceptive, steering, and obstacle circumvention tasks would rely on similar optical information and share a similar architecture of control law (Chardenon et al., 2004; Fajen & Warren, 2003; Fink, Foo, & Warren, 2007).

A first question of interest to the field of rehabilitation concerning obstacle circumvention in virtual environments is whether it resembles that observed in the physical world. Features that are peculiar to the VR technology and that may influence obstacle circumvention include, but are not limited to, a lack of physical consequence in presence of a collision, a greater uncertainty about the position of virtual objects and that of the participant, as well as a perceived distance compression (Chap. 4, Fink et al., 2007). In two studies that compared circumvention strategies of young adults in response to real vs. virtual static obstacles, it was found that the curvature and shape of the participants' trajectory was the same but that subjects maintained slightly larger distances from the obstacles in the virtual world compared to the physical world (Fink et al., 2007; Gerin-Lajoie, Richards, Fung, & McFadyen, 2008). This similarity in terms of strategy, at least for young adults walking in the presence of static obstacles, suggests that obstacle circumvention paradigms in virtual environments can be used for evaluation and training purposes and may translate into improvements in the physical world.

By varying the characteristics of the obstacles, it was also shown that the perception of a potential collision and the actual avoidance strategies can be modified. For instance, changing the proximity at which a virtual pedestrian will pass with respect to the participant impacts on the ability to detect a potential collision (Ouellette, Chagnon, & Faubert, 2009). Indeed, while predictions are highly accurate for "head-on" approaches and reasonably good when the virtual pedestrian passes at ±10° on either side of the participants' shoulders, there is much more uncertainty, hence larger errors, when the pedestrian passes close (±5°) to the participants. The side of approach also makes a difference with larger errors in collision prediction being reported for moving obstacles passing to the right (Ouellette et al., 2009) and larger clearances when circumventing a static obstacle towards the left (obstacle on the right) (Gerin-Lajoie et al., 2008). The latter observations indicate the presence of asymmetries in terms of perceptual and motor responses to right vs. left obstacles, which have to be taken into consideration when dealing with populations with unilateral sensory and/or motor disorders such as a stroke. Finally, although this is yet to be confirmed in virtual environments, circumvention strategies remain the same for static vs. dynamic obstacle but are characterized by later onsets in terms of step pattern modulation and smaller clearances with dynamic obstacles (Gerin-Lajoie, Richards, & McFadyen, 2005, 2006). The number of obstacles can also add to the complexity of the locomotor adjustments (Berard & Vallis, 2006) and the addition of distractors that challenge attentional resources can impact on the task performance (Gerin-Lajoie et al., 2006). A VR training paradigm for obstacle circumvention can thus be graded in complexity, starting with environments where obstacles have an easily identifiable risk of collision and where the presence of distractors and locomotor adjustments are minimized, and progressing to scenarios where perceptual, attentional, and motor demands become increasingly challenging.

9.4.1 Investigating Perceptuo-motor Strategies with Visuospatial Neglect

The ability to perform a circumvention task depends on the integrity of the perceptual, motor, and cognitive systems. We have recently developed a series of experiments that allow investigating the perceptual and motor strategies used by healthy individuals (Darekar, Lamontagne, & Fung submitted) and subjects with post-stroke visuospatial neglect (Aravind & Lamontagne, 2012). These experiments probe questions such as: How early is an obstacle movement perceived in the virtual environment? Are perceptual abilities related the persons' ability to avoid an obstacle while walking?

We have recently tested 12 subjects in a virtual environment consisting of a room with 3 obstacles, one of which randomly approached from head-on or 30° to the left or right (Aravind & Lamontagne, 2012). Subjects pressed a joystick button on perception of a moving obstacle in the perceptuo-motor task and walked toward a target while avoiding a collision with the moving obstacle in the walking task. Detection times in the perceptuo-motor task and minimum distances maintained from the obstacles in the walking task were examined. Results indicate that more than half ($n=7$) of the participants with neglect showed longer detection times (28 %) in the perceptuo-motor task as well as smaller minimal distances (−35 %) and higher collision rates (140 %) in the walking task when the obstacles approaching from the contralesional side compared to the ipsilesional side. These participants also avoided steering toward the contralesional side in 90 % of the walking trials, irrespective of the obstacle approach. Other participants with neglect showed less severe alterations and asymmetries in their performance for the ipsilesional and contralesional obstacles. More recent analyses revealed that the total number of collisions while walking was moderately associated with the ability to detect the obstacles on the contralesional side (Pearson's $r = 0.64$, $p < 0.05$), but not with the number of omissions on the Bell's test, a clinical test for visuospatial neglect. These results indicate that obstacle circumvention abilities are affected by visuospatial neglect, thereby confirming several anecdotal reports of an increased risk of collisions with objects in this population. With virtual reality, it was possible to establish a relationship between the participants' perceptuo-motor and locomotor performances in a similar, controlled environment. The lack of relationship between the walking performance and the clinical "pencil and pencil" test for neglect further emphasizes the utility of virtual reality which can provide task-specific and functionally relevant environments in which perceptual and motor strategies can be assessed, and eventually trained.

9.5 Effects of Optic Flow and on Elderly and Neurologically Impaired Individuals

9.5.1 Modifying the Speed of Optic Flow

A few research groups have examined the effects of aging and CNS lesions on optic flow-driven speed modulation patterns. A common observation is that unintentional speed modulations are preserved in older adults (Chou et al., 2009; Konczak, 1994; Schubert et al., 2005). With the occurrence of a stroke, however, unintentional speed modulations are attenuated compared to healthy controls (Lamontagne et al., 2007). Changes are not attributable to the patients' functional gait capacity (Lamontagne et al., 2007) but may be explained by an altered perception of speed of visual motion information (Vaina et al., 2010) or defective sensorimotor integration (Lamontagne, Paquet, & Fung, 2003). At variance, individuals with Parkinson's disease show exaggerated responses to changing optic flow speeds (Schubert et al., 2005). Furthermore, they do not present with the attenuation over time of the speed responses that is normally observed in healthy adults. According to Shubert and collaborators, the abnormal speed responses observed in Parkinson's disease could be explained by the presence of deficits in proprioception that were likely compensated by a reweighting of visual kinesthesia (Schubert et al., 2005).

When engaged in volitionally using optic flow speed information to adapt their walking speed, young individuals do very well, as illustrated by a strong inverse relationship between optic flow speed and gait speed with a slope that approaches −1

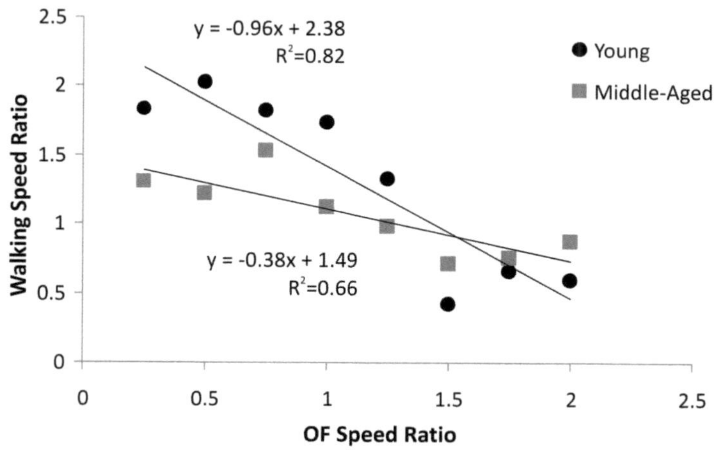

Fig. 9.6 Changes in walking speed in one young (27 YO) and one middle-aged individual (53 YO) walking on a self-pace treadmill while watching a virtual corridor of changing optic flow speed in a helmet mounted display. Values are expressed as ratios of the speed measured during comfortable walking. Linear regression equations and corresponding coefficients of determination (R^2) are illustrated for each participant. Note the attenuated slope in the middle-aged individual compared to the young adult

(Fig. 9.6). Older individuals that can be qualified as "young-old" (mean age 67 ± 4 years), however, already show attenuated speed responses compared to their younger counterpart (Lamontagne, Fung, Paquette, Faubert, & McFadyen, 2005).

Similarly, in a study that also involved controlling speed of self-motion but during a joystick driven locomotor interceptive task, middle-aged individuals (mean age 58 ± 2 years) displayed abnormally large errors compared to younger adults (Francois, Morice, Blouin, & Montagne, 2011). Performance at visuo-locomotor tasks that require the processing of visual motion speed can thus start deteriorating early in the process of aging. Potential explanatory factors include an altered perception of visual motion (Norman, Ross, Hawkes, & Long, 2003; Snowden & Kavanagh, 2006), slower information processing (Salthouse, 2000; Welford, 1988), and an altered sensorimotor integration. Interestingly, it is worth mentioning that while older adults were consistently reported to show exaggerated postural responses to moving visual surrounds (Bugnariu & Fung, 2007; Simoneau et al., 1999; Slaboda et al., 2011), they can at the same time experience a reduced sense of vection (Haibach, Slobounov, & Newell, 2009), suggesting that an enhanced susceptibility to visual motion information can coexist with an altered perception or utilization of visual motion during postural or locomotor tasks.

Individuals with stroke display volitional gait speed modulations that are within the range of age-matched control values, even when presenting with severely reduced gait capacities (Lamontagne et al., 2007), which suggest that the volitional paradigm has potential for training speed adaptations in this population. In fact, this paradigm was recently integrated in a VR training regimen to promote balance and faster walking speeds in subjects with chronic stroke (Kang, Kim, Chung, & Hwang, 2012).

9.5.2 *Modifying the Direction of Optic Flow*

Similar to optic flow speed, changing optic flow direction elicit changes in locomotor behaviors, which can be altered by aging and the occurrence of central nervous system pathologies. Berard and collaborators demonstrated that young-old adults (mean age 66 ± 4 years) failed to modify their walking trajectory in response to translational optic flows of changing direction, indicating a pronounced effect of aging, even at its very early stage (Berard et al., 2009). While this information is consistent with the altered discrimination abilities of older adults for the direction of radial or translational visual motion (Ball & Sekuler, 1986; Warren, Blackwell, & Morris, 1989), evidence of a relationship between visual motion perception and heading adaptations to visual motion while walking is still lacking.

At variance with translational optic flows, rotational flow stimuli do yield some degree of heading modulation in older adults, possibly due to the more "ecological" nature of the rotational flow stimuli for which the processing may be partially preserved with older age (Berard, Fung, & Lamontagne, 2011). In individuals with stroke, patterns of steering behaviors in response to both rotational and translational flows are altered and include reduced, absent, as well as asymmetrical patterns of responses that are biased either towards the paretic or non-paretic side (Berard, Fung, & Lamontagne, 2012; Lamontagne, Fung, McFadyen, Faubert, & Paquette, 2010). A history of visuospatial neglect, where symptoms are apparently resolved based on standard neurophysiological assessments, would be a common hallmark of stroke participants displaying either reduced or asymmetrical steering responses (Berard et al., 2012). This suggests that persistent visuospatial neglect, especially for far space and/or dynamic visual cues, may not be detected through conventional static pen and paper tests and should be addressed using ecological virtual environments where dynamic visual information about near and far space is integrated.

9.6 Sensorimotor Conflicts Support Virtual Reality as a Rehabilitation Tool

VR can be a valuable tool for therapeutic interventions that require adaptation to complex, multimodal environments (Chaps. 3 and 6). When designing VR protocols involving multisensory modalities, one should be aware of the potential of sensory conflicts and their effects. Conflicting visual and somatosensory stimuli can modulate automatic postural responses in both healthy young and old adults (Bugnariu & Fung, 2007). Aging affects the interaction of the somatosensory and visual systems on the ability of the CNS to resolve sensory conflicts and to maintain upright stance equilibrium.

Visual dependence may be a compensatory strategy for coping with poor balance post stroke. Compounding effects of age and neurological injury can skew the sensory recalibration processes required for resolution of sensory conflicts toward an excessive reliance on visual inputs. In addition to motor impairment, postural imbalance in patients with hemiparesis may be caused not only by elementary sensory impairment (visual, somatosensory, vestibular) but also by the inability to resolve sensory conflicts and to select pertinent sensory information. Thus, excessive reliance on vision may become problematic when the visual information is not reliable.

In a study that investigated the effects of aging and stroke on the capability of the CNS to select appropriate sensorimotor strategies and regulate balance while under conditions of sensory conflict created by VR, both young and older adults were tested during quiet stance while wearing a helmet-mounted display (HMD, Kaiser Optics ProView™ XL50). Subjects were exposed to random visual and/or surface perturbations consisting of ramp-and-hold tilts under four conditions: (1) visual-only; (2) surface-only; (3) discordant where visual perturbation was combined with synchronized surface perturbation in the same direction, and (4) concordant where visual perturbation was combined with synchronized surface perturbation in the opposite direction.

During visual-only perturbations, minimal displacements of COP and COM were observed in both subject groups (Figs. 9.7 and 9.8). The presence of sensory conflicts in surface-only and discordant perturbations induced significantly larger COM excursions than concordant perturbations in both young and old adults. However, the presence of sensory conflicts required a larger correction in older adults.

Average EMG latencies of ventral muscles during surface-only, discordant, and concordant perturbations in young and old adults are shown in Fig. 9.9. In young adults, muscle recruitment generally followed a distal-to-proximal sequence, regardless of perturbation direction or sensory conflicts. In older adults, the distal-to-proximal sequence of EMG activation was less consistent, especially under sensory conflict, during surface-only and discordant perturbations where a reverse sequence was observed (Fig. 9.9). Generally, the EMG onset latencies of older adults, which were already delayed as compared to young adults, were further prolonged in conditions of sensory conflict. Thus, the presence of sensory conflict had a larger impact on the selection of appropriate strategies for balance control in older adults.

Similar age-related postural instability was reported by Mahboobin, Loughlin, Redfern, & Sparto (2005) who showed that optic flow induced larger postural responses in older subjects than in subjects who had adapted from unilateral loss of vestibular function. It is plausible that delayed or diminished vestibular and somatosensory inputs in older adults increases their sensory thresholds to complex multimodal stimuli, thereby inducing a greater reliance on visual inputs and making it more difficult for them to respond selectively to visual and physical destabilization. However, we must consider that the use of a HMD to deliver the visual perturbation might have also limited the influence of visual inputs. Postural responses coupled with optic flow are less frequent when the optic flow is delivered in a central field of view, like the HMD, as compared to large field of view display (Sparto et al., 2006; Whitney et al., 2002).

The effects of aging and sensory motor deficits following stroke on the capability of CNS to select pertinent sensory information and resolve sensory conflict created by virtual reality were also examined in subjects with chronic stroke and age-matched healthy old adults (Fig. 9.10). With repeated exposure to VR-induced sensory conflict,

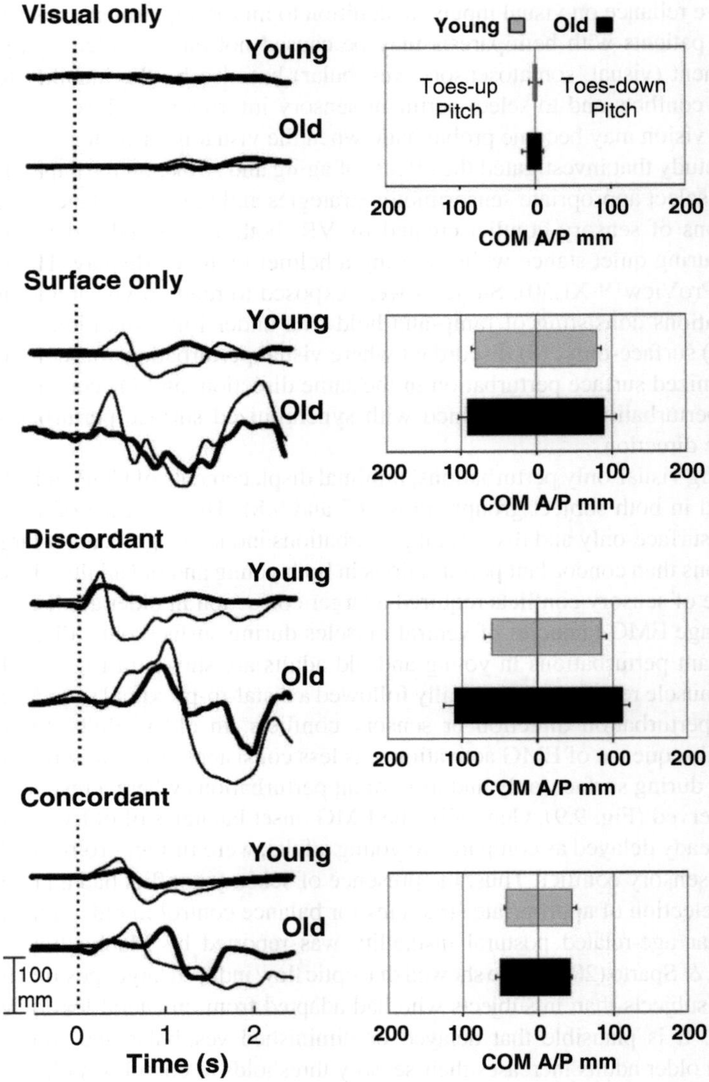

Fig. 9.7 Representative example of individual traces of COP (*thin lines*) and COM (*thick lines*) from one young and one old subject (*left panel*) exposed to toes-up tilt of the surface. Bar graphs on the *right panel* show COM peak-to-peak excursions (mean ± SD) averaged across 10 young subjects (*gray bars*) and 10 older subjects (*black bars*) in both toes-up (*left column*) and toes-down (*right column*) directions

a general training effect associated with fewer stepping responses and improved ability to maintain balance was observed in older adults but was less evident in stroke subjects. Stroke subjects exhibited under-activated responses in the paretic leg and

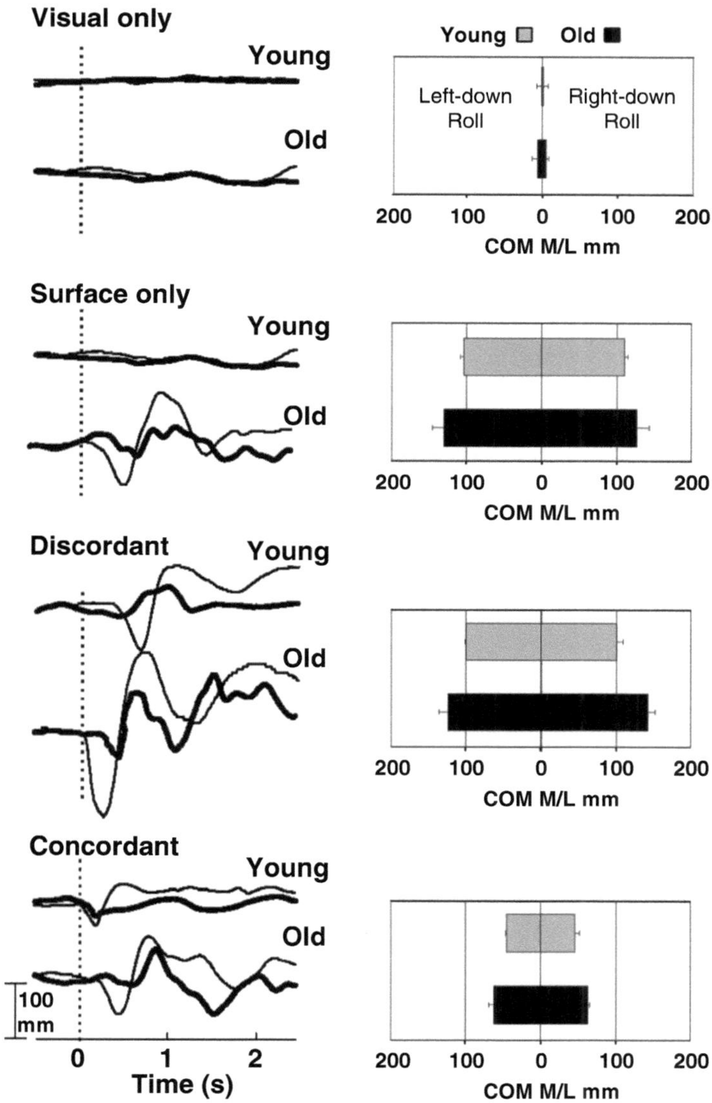

Fig. 9.8 Representative example of individual traces of COP (*thin lines*) and COM (*thick lines*) from one young and one old subject (*left panel*) exposed to right-down roll of the surface. Bar graphs on the *right panel* show COM peak-to-peak excursions (mean ± SD) averaged across 10 young subjects (*gray bars*) and 10 older subjects (*black bars*) in both left-down (*left column*) and right-down roll (*right column*) directions

exaggerated responses in the non-paretic limb (Fig. 9.11). In general, aging disrupted the distal-to-proximal muscle recruitment sequence and the presence of sensory conflict and stroke exacerbated the inconsistencies.

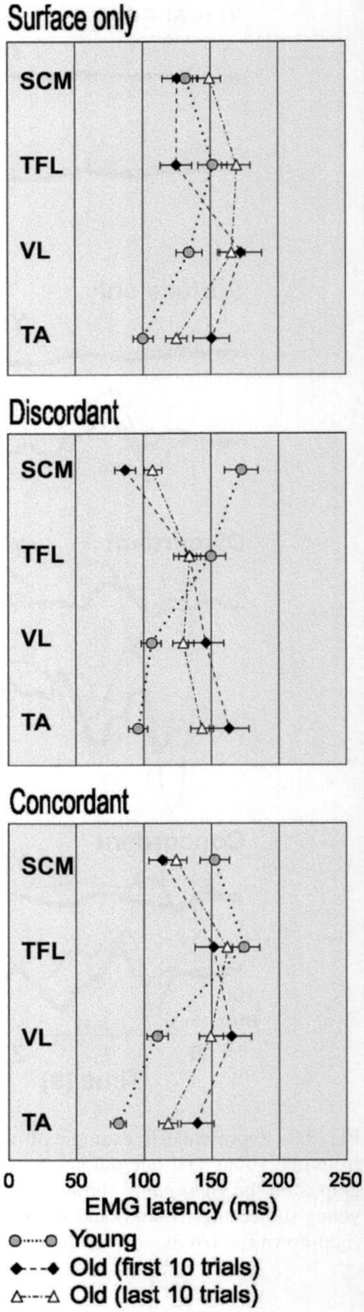

Fig. 9.9 EMG latencies (mean ± SD) of ventral muscles responding to toes-up pitch surface perturbations across young (*gray circles*) and old subjects. Note the decrease in the latencies in old subjects from the first 10 (*black diamonds*) to the last 10 (*open triangles*) trials

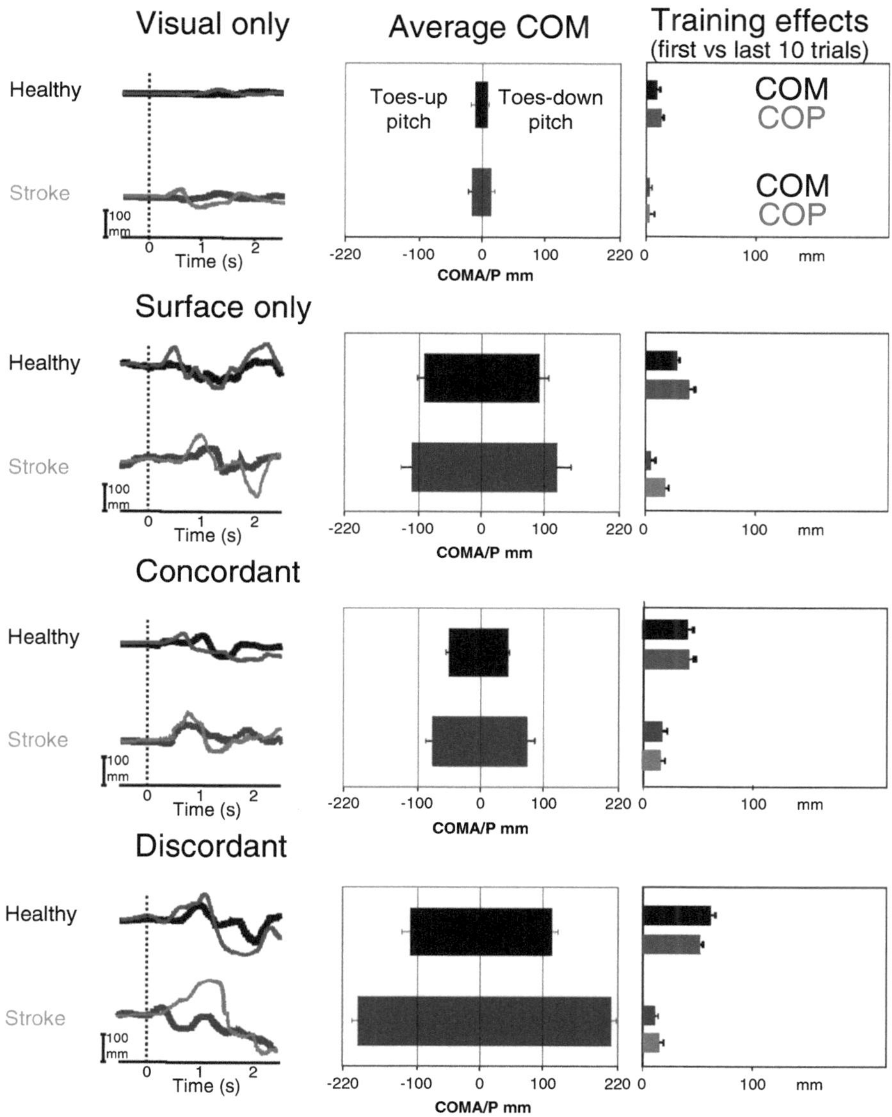

Fig. 9.10 Representative example of individual traces of COP (*thin lines*) and COM (*thick lines*) from one control healthy and one stroke subject (*left panels*) exposed to pitch plane tilt (toes-up). Bar graphs on the *middle panels* show COM peak-to-peak excursions (mean ± SD) averaged across groups of subjects in both directions of perturbations. Bar graphs on the right panels show data differences between first and last 10 trials

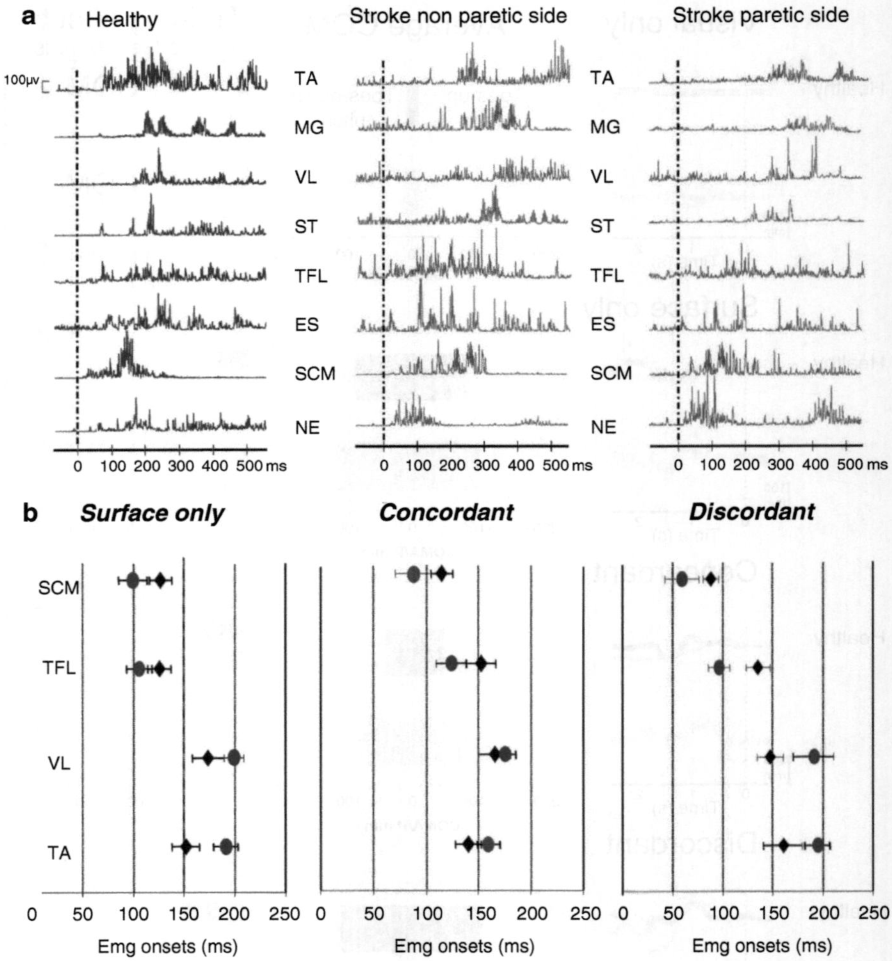

Fig. 9.11 (**a**) Example of muscle activation sequence following toes up rotation in a healthy control subject (*left panel*) and in stroke patient non paretic side (*middle panel*) and paretic side (*right panel*). (**b**) Group Mean ± SD for muscles onset latencies following pitch rotations (toes-up) for healthy control subjects (*black diamonds*) and stroke subjects (*gray circles*) in different sensory conditions: surface only, concordant and discordant in *left*, *middle* and *right panels*, respectively

The frequency-response function of each one of the four sensory conditions (Fig. 9.12) showed that young adults displayed low visual gains and high values of surface gains. In conditions of visual–somatosensory conflict, they increased surface gain and decreased visual gain, suggesting that young adults deal with the sensory conflict by either attempting to suppress visual information or attributing more weight and increased reliance on somatosensory feedback. Healthy older subjects and stroke patients displayed higher visual gains than young adults regardless of the sensory conditions. Moreover, in conditions of sensory conflict, they adopted

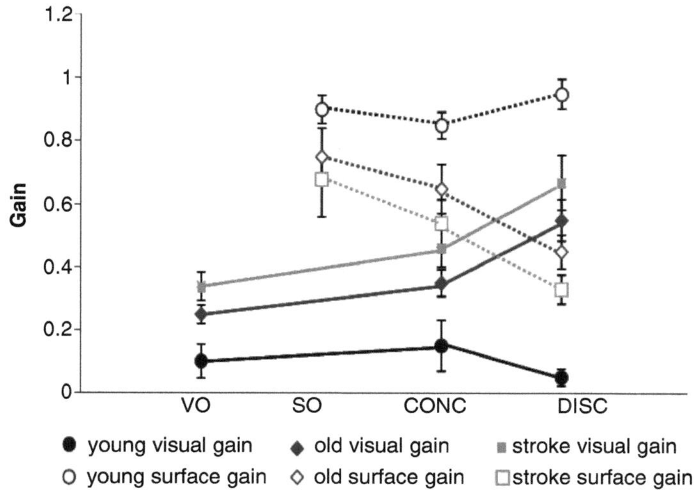

Fig. 9.12 Group Mean ± SD for COM gain relative to visual (*filled symbols*) and surface stimulus (*open symbols*) in four different sensory conditions, for healthy young (*circles*), old subjects (*diamonds*) and stroke patients (*squares*)

an opposite strategy increasing the visual gain and lowering the surface gain. This demonstrates an excessive reliance on visual inputs or a need to first stabilize their head, a common strategy adopted by people with balance impairments.

The resolution of sensory conflict is affected by aging and stroke but can be enhanced by training. Repeated exposure to VR-induced sensory conflict improved balance performance in all healthy older subjects and to some extent in stroke subjects (note differences between the first 10 trials and last 10 trials out of a total of 72 perturbation trails in Figs. 9.9 and 9.10). Even with a 1-h immersion in virtual environments and exposure to sensory conflict, it is possible for the CNS to recalibrate and adapt to the changes. A training program of longer durations is needed to confirm sustainable long-term effects.

9.7 Conclusions

Rehabilitation of postural control and balance has included practice of specific, well-defined automatic postural reactions (Horak, 2006; O'Neill, Gill-Body, & Krebs, 1998; Wrisley et al., 2007). But if relearning of postural control is to have any functional carryover, it needs to be incorporated into more complex motor behaviors (Keshner, Kenyon, & Langston, 2004; McCollum, 1999; Varraine et al., 2002). Adaptation of motor commands to functional circumstances are driven by error signals (Shadmehr, Smith, & Krakauer, 2010), and thus, the impact of rehabilitation interventions might increase if the sensory feedback can be manipulated so that it does not precisely match the expected afference.

Virtual reality is an excellent tool for presenting environments that contain controlled sensory incongruities thereby requiring constant correction to the sensory reafference (Chap. 2). The most recognized sensory characteristics of virtual reality are the absence of haptic and force feedback. But VR also creates a strong conflict between visual and vestibular senses (Lepecq et al., 2006). By adding tools such as robots (Adamovich, Fluet, Merians, Mathai, & Qiu, 2009; Qiu et al., 2010), treadmills (Kizony, Levin, Hughey, Perez, & Fung, 2010), and dynamic platforms (Keshner & Kenyon, 2004; Keshner, Kenyon et al., 2004) into the virtual environment, we can further manipulate the demands during motor tasks. Preventive and rehabilitation programs should take into account the possible impairment of sensory organization or sensorimotor integration and include VR training under conditions of sensory conflict.

Acknowledgements This work was supported in part by NIH-NIA grants AG16359 and AG26470 to E.A. Keshner and the Canadian Institutes of Health Research (CIHR, RMF-111622) and the Jewish Rehabilitation Hospital Foundation to J. Fung. A. Lamontagne was supported by CIHR (MOP- 77548) and the Canada Foundation for Innovation. A.L. and J.F. are researchers of the Multidisciplinary SensoriMotor Rehabilitation Research Team [http://www.errsm.ca/], an emerging research team in Regenerative Medicine and Nanomedicine funded by the CIHR. N. Bugariu was funded by a Tomlinson postdoctoral research fellowship award at McGill University.

References

Adamovich, S. V., Fluet, G. G., Merians, A. S., Mathai, A., & Qiu, Q. (2009). Incorporating haptic effects into three-dimensional virtual environments to train the hemiparetic upper extremity. *IEEE Transactions on Neural Systems and Rehabilitation Engineering, 17*, 512–520.

Allum, J. H., Carpenter, M. G., Honegger, F., Adkin, A. L., & Bloem, B. R. (2002). Age-dependent variations in the directional sensitivity of balance corrections and compensatory arm movements in man. *Journal of Physiology, 542*, 643–663.

Amblard, B., Cremieux, J., Marchand, A. R., & Carblanc, A. (1985). Lateral orientation and stabilization of human stance: static versus dynamic visual cues. *Experimental Brain Research, 61*, 21–37.

Aravind, G., & Lamontagne, A. (2012). *Ability of subjects with post—stroke visuospatial neglect to avoid dynamic obstacles while walking in a virtual environment.* In: 13th Research Colloquium in Rehabilitation, pp 5–6 Montreal.

Asch, S. E., & Witkin, H. A. (1992). Studies in space orientation. II. Perception of the upright with displaced visual fields and with body tilted. *Journal of Experimental Psychology: General, 121*, 407–418. discussion 404–406.

Ball, K., & Sekuler, R. (1986). Improving visual perception in older observers. *Journal of Gerontology, 41*, 176–182.

Bardy, B. G., Warren, W. H., Jr., & Kay, B. A. (1999). The role of central and peripheral vision in postural control during walking. *Perception & Psychophysics, 61*, 1356–1368.

Berard, J. R., Fung, J., & Lamontagne, A. (2011). Evidence for the use of rotational optic flow cues for locomotor steering in healthy older adults. *Journal of Neurophysiology, 106*, 1089–1096.

Berard, J., Fung, J., & Lamontagne, A. (2012). Visuomotor control post stroke can be affected by a history of visuospatial neglect. *Journal of Neurology & Neurophysiology, S8*, 1–8.

Berard, J. R., Fung, J., McFadyen, B. J., & Lamontagne, A. (2009). Aging affects the ability to use optic flow in the control of heading during locomotion. *Experimental Brain Research Experimentelle Hirnforschung Experimentation Cerebrale, 194*, 183–190.

Berard, J. R., & Vallis, L. A. (2006). Characteristics of single and double obstacle avoidance strategies: a comparison between adults and children. *Experimental Brain Research Experimentelle Hirnforschung Experimentation Cerebrale, 175*, 21–31.

Bergstrom, B. (1973). Morphology of the vestibular nerve. II. The number of myelinated vestibular nerve fibers in man at various ages. *Acta Oto-Laryngologica, 76*, 173–179.

Black, F. O., Wall, C., 3rd, & Nashner, L. M. (1983). Effects of visual and support surface orientation references upon postural control in vestibular deficient subjects. *Acta Oto-Laryngologica, 95*, 199–201.

Bles, W., Vianney de Jong, J. M., & de Wit, G. (1983). Compensation for labyrinthine defects examined by use of a tilting room. *Acta Oto-Laryngologica, 95*, 576–579.

Bohannon, R. W. (1997). Comfortable and maximum walking speed of adults aged 20-79 years: reference values and determinants. *Age and Ageing, 26*, 15–19.

Brandt, T., Glasauer, S., Stephan, T., Bense, S., Yousry, T. A., Deutschlander, A., et al. (2002). Visual-vestibular and visuovisual cortical interaction: new insights from fMRI and pet. *Annals of the New York Academy of Sciences, 956*, 230–241.

Bruggeman, H., Zosh, W., & Warren, W. H. (2007). Optic flow drives human visuo-locomotor adaptation. *Current Biology, 17*, 2035–2040.

Bugnariu, N., & Fung, J. (2007). Aging and selective sensorimotor strategies in the regulation of upright balance. *Journal of Neuroengineering and Rehabilitation, 4*, 19.

Chardenon, A., Montagne, G., Laurent, M., & Bootsma, R. J. (2004). The perceptual control of goal-directed locomotion: a common control architecture for interception and navigation? *Experimental Brain Research Experimentelle Hirnforschung Experimentation Cerebrale, 158*, 100–108.

Chou, Y. H., Wagenaar, R. C., Saltzman, E., Giphart, J. E., Young, D., Davidsdottir, R., et al. (2009). Effects of optic flow speed and lateral flow asymmetry on locomotion in younger and older adults: a virtual reality study. *The Journals of Gerontology. Series B, Psychological Sciences and Social Sciences, 64*, 222–231.

Clement, G., Gurfinkel, V. S., Lestienne, F., Lipshits, M. I., & Popov, K. E. (1984). Adaptation of postural control to weightlessness. *Experimental Brain Research, 57*, 61–72.

Cutting, J. E., & Vishton, P. M. (1995). How we avoid collisions with stationary and moving objects. *Psychological Review, 102*, 627–651.

Darekar, A., Goussev, V., McFadyen, B. J., Lamontagne, A., & Fung, J. (2013). Spatial navigation in the presence of dynamic obstacles in a virtual environment: A preliminary study. *International Conference on Virtual Rehabilitation, IEEE Conference Proceedings*, 2 pages.

Day, B. L., & Guerraz, M. (2007). Feedforward versus feedback modulation of human vestibular-evoked balance responses by visual self-motion information. *Journal of Physiology, 582*, 153–161.

Dichgans, J., Brandt, T., & Held, R. (1975). The role of vision in gravitational orientation. *Fortschritte der Zoologie, 23*, 255–263.

Dokka, K., Kenyon, R. V., & Keshner, E. A. (2009). Influence of visual scene velocity on segmental kinematics during stance. *Gait & Posture, 30*, 211–216.

Dokka, K., Kenyon, R. V., Keshner, E. A., & Kording, K. P. (2010). Self versus environment motion in postural control. *PLoS Computational Biology, 6*, e1000680.

Duchon, A. P., & Warren, W. H., Jr. (2002). A visual equalization strategy for locomotor control: of honeybees, robots, and humans. *Psychological Science, 13*, 272–278.

Dumontheil, I., Panagiotaki, P., & Berthoz, A. (2006). Dual adaptation to sensory conflicts during whole-body rotations. *Brain Research, 1072*, 119–132.

Dvorkin, A. Y., Kenyon, R. V., & Keshner, E. A. (2009). Effects of roll visual motion on online control of arm movement: reaching within a dynamic virtual environment. *Experimental Brain Research, 193*(1), 95–107.

Fait, P., McFadyen, B. J., Swaine, B., & Cantin, J. F. (2009). Alterations to locomotor navigation in a complex environment at 7 and 30 days following a concussion in an elite athlete. *Brain Injury, 23*, 362–369.

Fajen, B. R., & Warren, W. H. (2003). Behavioral dynamics of steering, obstacle avoidance, and route selection. *Journal of Experimental Psychology. Human Perception and Performance, 29*, 343–362.

Ferman, L., Collewijn, H., Jansen, T. C., & Van den Berg, A. V. (1987). Human gaze stability in the horizontal, vertical and torsional direction during voluntary head movements, evaluated with a three-dimensional scleral induction coil technique. *Vision Research, 27*, 811–828.

Fink, P. W., Foo, P. S., & Warren, W. H. (2007). Obstacle avoidance during walking in real and virtual environments. *ACM Transactions on Applied Perception, 4*, 18.

Fitzpatrick, R. C., Marsden, J., Lord, S. R., & Day, B. L. (2002). Galvanic vestibular stimulation evokes sensations of body rotation. *Neuroreport, 13*, 2379–2383.

Francois, M., Morice, A. H., Blouin, J., & Montagne, G. (2011). Age-related decline in sensory processing for locomotion and interception. *Neuroscience, 172*, 366–378.

Francois, M., Morice, A. H., Bootsma, R. J., & Montagne, G. (2011). Visual control of walking velocity. *Neuroscience Research, 70*, 214–219.

Gerin-Lajoie, M., Richards, C. L., Fung, J., & McFadyen, B. J. (2008). Characteristics of personal space during obstacle circumvention in physical and virtual environments. *Gait & Posture, 27*, 239–247.

Gerin-Lajoie, M., Richards, C. L., & McFadyen, B. J. (2005). The negotiation of stationary and moving obstructions during walking: anticipatory locomotor adaptations and preservation of personal space. *Motor Control, 9*, 242–269.

Gerin-Lajoie, M., Richards, C. L., & McFadyen, B. J. (2006). The circumvention of obstacles during walking in different environmental contexts: a comparison between older and younger adults. *Gait & Posture, 24*, 364–369.

Gibson, J. J. (1994). The visual perception of objective motion and subjective movement. 1954. *Psychological Review, 101*, 318–323.

Gill, J., Allum, J. H., Carpenter, M. G., Held-Ziolkowska, M., Adkin, A. L., Honegger, F., et al. (2001). Trunk sway measures of postural stability during clinical balance tests: effects of age. *Journals of Gerontology. Series A, Biological Sciences and Medical Sciences, 56*, M438–M447.

Grasso, R., Glasauer, S., Takei, Y., & Berthoz, A. (1996). The predictive brain: anticipatory control of head direction for the steering of locomotion. *Neuroreport, 7*, 1170–1174.

Guerraz, M., & Bronstein, A. M. (2008). Mechanisms underlying visually induced body sway. *Neuroscience Letters, 443*, 12–16.

Guerraz, M., Gianna, C. C., Burchill, P. M., Gresty, M. A., & Bronstein, A. M. (2001). Effect of visual surrounding motion on body sway in a three-dimensional environment. *Perception & Psychophysics, 63*, 47–58.

Haibach, P., Slobounov, S., & Newell, K. (2009). Egomotion and vection in young and elderly adults. *Gerontology, 55*, 637–643.

Horak, F. B. (2006). Postural orientation and equilibrium: what do we need to know about neural control of balance to prevent falls? *Age and Ageing, 35*(Suppl 2), ii7–ii11.

Horak, F. B., Nashner, L. M., & Diener, H. C. (1990). Postural strategies associated with somatosensory and vestibular loss. *Experimental Brain Research, 82*, 167–177.

Isableu, B., Ohlmann, T., Cremieux, J., & Amblard, B. (1997). Selection of spatial frame of reference and postural control variability. *Experimental Brain Research, 114*, 584–589.

Isableu, B., Ohlmann, T., Cremieux, J., Vuillerme, N., Amblard, B., & Gresty, M. A. (2010). Individual differences in the ability to identify, select and use appropriate frames of reference for perceptuo-motor control. *Neuroscience, 169*, 1199–1215.

Kang, H. K., Kim, Y., Chung, Y., & Hwang, S. (2012). Effects of treadmill training with optic flow on balance and gait in individuals following stroke: randomized controlled trials. *Clinical Rehabilitation, 26*, 246–255.

Keshner, E. A., Allum, J. H., & Honegger, F. (1993). Predictors of less stable postural responses to support surface rotations in healthy human elderly. *Journal of Vestibular Research, 3*, 419–429.

Keshner, E. A., Allum, J. H., & Pfaltz, C. R. (1987). Postural coactivation and adaptation in the sway stabilizing responses of normals and patients with bilateral vestibular deficit. *Experimental Brain Research, 69*, 77–92.

Keshner, E. A., & Dhaher, Y. (2008). Characterizing head motion in three planes during combined visual and base of support disturbances in healthy and visually sensitive subjects. *Gait Posture, 28*(1), 127–134.

Keshner, E. A., Dokka, K., & Kenyon, R. V. (2006). Influences of the perception of self-motion on postural parameters. *Cyberpsychology & Behavior, 9*, 163–166.
Keshner, E. A., & Kenyon, R. V. (2000). The influence of an immersive virtual environment on the segmental organization of postural stabilizing responses. *Journal of Vestibular Research, 10*, 207–219.
Keshner, E. A., & Kenyon, R. V. (2004). Using immersive technology for postural research and rehabilitation. *Assistive Technology, 16*, 54–62.
Keshner, E. A., & Kenyon, R. V. (2009). Postural and spatial orientation driven by virtual reality. *Studies in Health Technology and Informatics, 145*, 209–228.
Keshner, E., Kenyon, R.V., Dhaher, Y.Y., & Streepey, J.W. (2004a). *Employing a virtual environment in postural research and rehabilitation to reveal the impact of visual information*. Internation conference on disability, Virtual reality, and Associated Technologies New College, Oxford, UK.
Keshner, E. A., Kenyon, R. V., Dhaher, Y., & Streepey, J. (2005). Employing a virtual environment in postural research and rehabilitation to reveal the impact of visual information. *International Journal on Disability and Human Development, 4*, 177–182.
Keshner, E. A., Kenyon, R. V., & Langston, J. (2004). Postural responses exhibit multisensory dependencies with discordant visual and support surface motion. *Journal of Vestibular Research, 14*, 307–319.
Keshner, E. A., Slaboda, J. C., Buddharaju, R., Lanaria, L., & Norman, J. (2011). Augmenting sensory-motor conflict promotes adaptation of postural behaviors in a virtual environment. *IEEE Engineering in Medicine & Biology Society, 2011*, 1379–1382.
Kizony, R., Levin, M. F., Hughey, L., Perez, C., & Fung, J. (2010). Cognitive load and dual-task performance during locomotion poststroke: a feasibility study using a functional virtual environment. *Physical Therapy, 90*, 252–260.
Kleinschmidt, A., Thilo, K. V., Buchel, C., Gresty, M. A., Bronstein, A. M., & Frackowiak, R. S. (2002). Neural correlates of visual-motion perception as object- or self-motion. *NeuroImage, 16*, 873–882.
Konczak, J. (1994). Effects of optic flow on the kinematics of human gait: a comparison of young and older adults. *Journal of Motor Behavior, 26*, 225–236.
Kuno, S., Kawakita, T., Kawakami, O., Miyake, Y., & Watanabe, S. (1999). Postural adjustment response to depth direction moving patterns produced by virtual reality graphics. *Japanese Journal of Physiology, 49*, 417–424.
Lambrey, S., & Berthoz, A. (2003). Combination of conflicting visual and non-visual information for estimating actively performed body turns in virtual reality. *International Journal of Psychophysiology, 50*, 101–115.
Lamontagne, A., Fung, J., McFadyen, B. J., & Faubert, J. (2007). Modulation of walking speed by changing optic flow in persons with stroke. *Journal of Neuroengineering and Rehabilitation, 4*, 22.
Lamontagne, A., Fung, J., McFadyen, B., Faubert, J., & Paquette, C. (2010). Stroke affects locomotor steering responses to changing optic flow directions. *Neurorehabilitation and Neural Repair, 24*, 457–468.
Lamontagne, A., Fung, J., Paquette, C., Faubert, J., & McFadyen, B. J. (2005). Influence of optic flow on speed and heading control of locomotion due to ageing. *Gait & Posture, 21*(1), S18, 4.7.
Lamontagne, A., Paquet, N., & Fung, J. (2003). Postural adjustments to voluntary head motions during standing are modified following stroke. *Clinical Biomechanics (Bristol, Avon), 18*, 832–842.
Larish, J. F., & Flach, J. M. (1990). Sources of optical information useful for perception of speed of rectilinear self-motion. *Journal of Experimental Psychology. Human Perception and Performance, 16*, 295–302.
Lepecq, J. C., De Waele, C., Mertz-Josse, S., Teyssedre, C., Huy, P. T., Baudonniere, P. M., et al. (2006). Galvanic vestibular stimulation modifies vection paths in healthy subjects. *Journal of Neurophysiology, 95*, 3199–3207.
Lepecq, J. C., Giannopulu, I., Mertz, S., & Baudonniere, P. M. (1999). Vestibular sensitivity and vection chronometry along the spinal axis in erect man. *Perception, 28*, 63–72.
Lord, S. R., & Webster, I. W. (1990). Visual field dependence in elderly fallers and non-fallers. *International Journal of Aging and Human Development, 31*, 267–277.

Mahboobin, A., Loughlin, P. J., Redfern, M. S., & Sparto, P. J. (2005). Sensory re-weighting in human postural control during moving-scene perturbations. *Experimental Brain Research, 167*(2), 260–267.

Masumoto, D., Yamakawa, E., Kimoto, T., Nagata, S. (1994). *Hierarchical sensory-motor fusion model with neural networks.* In: Multisensor Fusion and Integration for Intelligent Systems, 1994 IEEE International Conference on MFI '94, pp 630–638 Las Vegas, NV, USA.

McCollum, G. (1999). Sensory and motor interdependence in postural adjustments. *Journal of Vestibular Research, 9*, 303–325.

Mohler, B. J., Thompson, W. B., Creem-Regehr, S. H., Pick, H. L., Jr., & Warren, W. H., Jr. (2007). Visual flow influences gait transition speed and preferred walking speed. *Experimental Brain Research Experimentelle Hirnforschung Experimentation Cerebrale, 181*, 221–228.

Mulavara, A. P., Richards, J. T., Ruttley, T., Marshburn, A., Nomura, Y., & Bloomberg, J. J. (2005). Exposure to a rotating virtual environment during treadmill locomotion causes adaptation in heading direction. *Experimental Brain Research Experimentelle Hirnforschung Experimentation Cerebrale, 166*, 210–219.

Nashner, L., & Berthoz, A. (1978). Visual contribution to rapid motor responses during postural control. *Brain Research, 150*(2), 403–407.

Nomura, Y., Mulavara, A. P., Richards, J. T., Brady, R., & Bloomberg, J. J. (2005). Optic flow dominates visual scene polarity in causing adaptive modification of locomotor trajectory. *Brain Research. Cognitive Brain Research, 25*, 624–631.

Norman, J. F., Ross, H. E., Hawkes, L. M., & Long, J. R. (2003). Aging and the perception of speed. *Perception, 32*, 85–96.

O'Neill, D. E., Gill-Body, K. M., & Krebs, D. E. (1998). Posturography changes do not predict functional performance changes. *American Journal of Otology, 19*, 797–803.

Ouellette, M., Chagnon, M., & Faubert, J. (2009). Evaluation of human behavior in collision avoidance: A study inside immersive virtual reality. *Cyberpsychology & Behavior : The Impact of the Internet, Multimedia and Virtual Reality on Behavior and Society, 12*, 215–218.

Pailhous, J., Ferrandez, A. M., Fluckiger, M., & Baumberger, B. (1990). Unintentional modulations of human gait by optical flow. *Behavioural Brain Research, 38*, 275–281.

Paquette, M. R., & Vallis, L. A. (2010). Age-related kinematic changes in late visual-cueing during obstacle circumvention. *Experimental Brain Research Experimentelle Hirnforschung Experimentation Cerebrale, 203*, 563–574.

Patla, A. E., Adkin, A., & Ballard, T. (1999). Online steering: coordination and control of body center of mass, head and body reorientation. *Experimental Brain Research Experimentelle Hirnforschung Experimentation Cerebrale, 129*, 629–634.

Peterka, R. J., Black, F. O., & Schoenhoff, M. B. (1990a). Age-related changes in human vestibulo-ocular and optokinetic reflexes: pseudorandom rotation tests. *Journal of Vestibular Research, 1*, 61–71.

Peterka, R. J., Black, F. O., & Schoenhoff, M. B. (1990b). Age-related changes in human vestibulo-ocular reflexes: sinusoidal rotation and caloric tests. *Journal of Vestibular Research, 1*, 49–59.

Previc, F. H. (1992). The effects of dynamic visual stimulation on perception and motor control. *Journal of Vestibular Research, 2*, 285–295.

Previc, F. H., & Donnelly, M. (1993). The effects of visual depth and eccentricity on manual bias, induced motion, and vection. *Perception, 22*, 929–945.

Previc, F. H., Kenyon, R. V., Boer, E. R., & Johnson, B. H. (1993). The effects of background visual roll stimulation on postural and manual control and self-motion perception. *Perception & Psychophysics, 54*, 93–107.

Prokop, T., Schubert, M., & Berger, W. (1997). Visual influence on human locomotion. Modulation to changes in optic flow. *Experimental Brain Research, 114*, 63–70.

Punt, T. D., Kitadono, K., Hulleman, J., Humphreys, G. W., & Riddoch, M. J. (2008). From both sides now: crossover effects influence navigation in patients with unilateral neglect. *Journal of Neurology, Neurosurgery and Psychiatry, 79*, 464–466.

Qiu, Q., Fluet, G. G., Saleh, S., Lafond, I., Merians, A. S., & Adamovich, S. V. (2010). Integrated versus isolated training of the hemiparetic upper extremity in haptically rendered virtual environments. *Conference proceedings IEEE Engineering in Medicine & Biology Society, 2010*, 2255–2258.

Redfern, M. S., & Furman, J. M. (1994). Postural sway of patients with vestibular disorders during optic flow. *Journal of Vestibular Research, 4*, 221–230.

Reymond, G., Droulez, J., & Kemeny, A. (2002). Visuovestibular perception of self-motion modeled as a dynamic optimization process. *Biological Cybernetics, 87*, 301–314.

Rosenhall, U. (1973). Degenerative patterns in the aging human vestibular neuro-epithelia. *Acta Oto-Laryngologica, 76*, 208–220.

Rushton, S. K., Harris, J. M., Lloyd, M. R., & Wann, J. P. (1998). Guidance of locomotion on foot uses perceived target location rather than optic flow. *Current Biology, 8*, 1191–1194.

Saibene, F., & Minetti, A. E. (2003). Biomechanical and physiological aspects of legged locomotion in humans. *European Journal of Applied Physiology, 88*, 297–316.

Salthouse, T. A. (2000). Aging and measures of processing speed. *Biological Psychology, 54*(1–3), 35–54.

Sarre, G., Berard, J., Fung, J., & Lamontagne, A. (2008). Steering behaviour can be modulated by different optic flows during walking. *Neuroscience Letters, 436*, 96–101.

Saunders, J. A., & Durgin, F. H. (2011). Adaptation to conflicting visual and physical heading directions during walking. *Journal of Vision, 11*.

Schneider, E., Jahn, K., Dieterich, M., Brandt, T., & Strupp, M. (2008). Gait deviations induced by visual stimulation in roll. *Experimental brain research Experimentelle Hirnforschung Experimentation Cerebrale, 185*, 21–26.

Schubert, M., Prokop, T., Brocke, F., & Berger, W. (2005). Visual kinesthesia and locomotion in Parkinson's disease. *Movement Disorders: Official Journal of the Movement Disorder Society, 20*, 141–150.

Shadmehr, R., Smith, M. A., & Krakauer, J. W. (2010). Error correction, sensory prediction, and adaptation in motor control. *Annual Review of Neuroscience, 33*, 89–108.

Shumway-Cook, A., & Woollacott, M. (2000). Attentional demands and postural control: the effect of sensory context. *Journals of Gerontology. Series A, Biological Sciences and Medical Sciences, 55*, M10–M16.

Silsupadol, P., Lugade, V., Shumway-Cook, A., van Donkelaar, P., Chou, L. S., Mayr, U., et al. (2009). Training-related changes in dual-task walking performance of elderly persons with balance impairment: a double-blind, randomized controlled trial. *Gait & Posture, 29*, 634–639.

Silsupadol, P., Shumway-Cook, A., Lugade, V., van Donkelaar, P., Chou, L. S., Mayr, U., et al. (2009). Effects of single-task versus dual-task training on balance performance in older adults: a double-blind, randomized controlled trial. *Archives of Physical Medicine and Rehabilitation, 90*, 381–387.

Simoneau, M., Teasdale, N., Bourdin, C., Bard, C., Fleury, M., & Nougier, V. (1999). Aging and postural control: postural perturbations caused by changing the visual anchor. *Journal of American Geriatrics Society, 47*, 235–240.

Siu, K. C., Chou, L. S., Mayr, U., Donkelaar, P., & Woollacott, M. H. (2008). Does inability to allocate attention contribute to balance constraints during gait in older adults? *Journals of Gerontology. Series A, Biological Sciences and Medical Sciences, 63*, 1364–1369.

Siu, K. C., Chou, L. S., Mayr, U., van Donkelaar, P., & Woollacott, M. H. (2009). Attentional mechanisms contributing to balance constraints during gait: the effects of balance impairments. *Brain Research, 1248*, 59–67.

Slaboda, J. C., Lauer, R. T., & Keshner, E. A. (2011). Continuous visual field motion impacts the postural responses of older and younger women during and after support surface tilt. *Experimental Brain Research, 211*(1), 87–96.

Slobounov, S., Tutwiler, R., Sebastianelli, W., & Slobounov, E. (2006). Alteration of postural responses to visual field motion in mild traumatic brain injury. *Neurosurgery, 59*, 134–139. discussion 134-139.

Snowden, R. J., & Kavanagh, E. (2006). Motion perception in the ageing visual system: minimum motion, motion coherence, and speed discrimination thresholds. *Perception, 35*, 9–24.

Sparto, P. J., Redfern, M. S., Jasko, J. G., Casselbrant, M. L., Mandel, E. M., & Furman, J. M. (2006). The influence of dynamic visual cues for postural control in children aged 7-12 years. *Experimental Brain Research, 168*(4), 505–516. PMID: 16151780.

Stelmach, G. E., Zelaznik, H. N., & Lowe, D. (1990). The influence of aging and attentional demands on recovery from postural instability. *Aging (Milano), 2*, 155–161.
Straube, A., Krafczyk, S., Paulus, W., & Brandt, T. (1994). Dependence of visual stabilization of postural sway on the cortical magnification factor of restricted visual fields. *Experimental Brain Research, 99*, 501–506.
Streepey, J. W., Kenyon, R. V., & Keshner, E. A. (2007). Field of view and base of support width influence postural responses to visual stimuli during quiet stance. *Gait & Posture, 25*(1), 49–55.
Tanahashi, S., Ujike, H., Kozawa, R., & Ukai, K. (2007). Effects of visually simulated roll motion on vection and postural stabilization. *Journal of Neuroengineering and Rehabilitation, 4*, 39.
Taylor, C. R., Heglund, N. C., & Maloiy, G. M. (1982). Energetics and mechanics of terrestrial locomotion. I. Metabolic energy consumption as a function of speed and body size in birds and mammals. *The Journal of Experimental Biology, 97*, 1–21.
Thurrell, A. E., & Bronstein, A. M. (2002). Vection increases the magnitude and accuracy of visually evoked postural responses. *Experimental Brain Research, 147*, 558–560.
Vaina, L. M., Sikoglu, E. M., Soloviev, S., LeMay, M., Squatrito, S., Pandiani, G., et al. (2010). Functional and anatomical profile of visual motion impairments in stroke patients correlate with fMRI in normal subjects. *Journal of Neuropsychology, 4*, 121–145.
Varraine, E., Bonnard, M., & Pailhous, J. (2002). Interaction between different sensory cues in the control of human gait. *Experimental Brain Research, 142*, 374–384.
Verhoeff, L. L., Horlings, C. G., Janssen, L. J., Bridenbaugh, S. A., & Allum, J. H. (2009). Effects of biofeedback on trunk sway during dual tasking in the healthy young and elderly. *Gait & Posture, 30*, 76–81.
Vidal, P. P., Berthoz, A., & Millanvoye, M. (1982). Difference between eye closure and visual stabilization in the control of posture in man. *Aviation, Space, and Environmental Medicine, 53*(2), 166–170.
Wang, Y., Kenyon, R. V., & Keshner, E. A. (2009). Identifying the control of physically and perceptually evoked sway responses with coincident visual scene velocities and tilt of the base of support. *Experimental Brain Research, 201*(4), 663–672.
Warren, B. R. (1998). Visually Controlled Locomotion: 40 years Later. *Ecological Psychology, 10*, 177.
Warren, W. H., Jr., Blackwell, A. W., & Morris, M. W. (1989). Age differences in perceiving the direction of self-motion from optical flow. *Journal of Gerontology, 44*, P147–P153.
Warren, W. H., Jr., Kay, B. A., Zosh, W. D., Duchon, A. P., & Sahuc, S. (2001). Optic flow is used to control human walking. *Nature Neuroscience, 4*, 213–216.
Webster, J. S., Rapport, L. J., Godlewski, M. C., & Abadee, P. S. (1994). Effect of attentional bias to right space on wheelchair mobility. *Journal of Clinical and Experimental Neuropsychology, 16*, 129–137.
Welford, A. T. (1988). Reaction time, speed of performance, and age. *Annals of the New York Academy of Sciences, 515*, 1–17.
Whitney, S. L., Sparto, P. J., Brown, K., Furman, J. M., Jacobson, J. L., & Redfern, M. S. (2002). The potential use of virtual reality in vestibular rehabilitation: Preliminary findings with the BNAVE. *Neurology Report, 26*(2), 72–78.
Wiest, G., Amorim, M. A., Mayer, D., Schick, S., Deecke, L., & Lang, W. (2001). Cortical responses to object-motion and visually-induced self-motion perception. *Brain Research. Cognitive Brain Research, 12*, 167–170.
Witkin, H. A., & Asch, S. E. (1948). Studies in space orientation; further experiments on perception of the upright with displaced visual fields. *Journal of Experimental Psychology, 38*, 762–782.
Woollacott, M. H. (1993). Age-related changes in posture and movement. *Journal of Gerontology, 48*, 56–60.
Wright, W. G., DiZio, P., & Lackner, J. R. (2005). Vertical linear self-motion perception during visual and inertial motion: more than weighted summation of sensory inputs. *Journal of Vestibular Research, 15*, 185–195.
Wrisley, D. M., Stephens, M. J., Mosley, S., Wojnowski, A., Duffy, J., & Burkard, R. (2007). Learning effects of repetitive administrations of the sensory organization test in healthy young adults. *Archives of Physical Medicine and Rehabilitation, 88*, 1049–1054.
Zaidel, A., Turner, A. H., & Angelaki, D. E. (2011). Multisensory calibration is independent of cue reliability. *Journal of Neuroscience, 31*, 13949–13962.

Chapter 10
Applications of VR Technologies for Childhood Disability

Dido Green and Peter Wilson

Objective To provide an overview of the evolution of VR technologies across domains of childhood disability that focuses on the evidence base for applications in research, clinical and community settings in order to optimise outcomes for the child and family.

10.1 Introduction

10.1.1 Theoretical Models of Rehabilitation: Where Does VR Fit In?

The ICF-CY represents a seismic shift away from the notion of disability as a purely medical construct in which the disability or impairment resides entirely with the child. Rather, there has been a move to a more ecological approach which considers the physical and psychological as well as the political *and* societal experiences of the child who has the "impairment" that then gives rise to disability and potential discrimination. An ecological approach to rehabilitation considers the impact of childhood disability on both the child and their family. Interventions therefore need to address the interaction between factors that lie within the child, the task and/or

D. Green (✉)
Centre for Rehabilitation, Faculty of Health and Life Sciences, Oxford Brookes University, Marston Road Campus, Jack Straw's Lane, Oxford, OX3 0FL, UK
e-mail: dido.green@brookes.ac.uk

P. Wilson
School of Psychology, Australian Catholic University, 115 Victoria Pde., Melbourne, VIC 3450, Australia
e-mail: peterh.wilson@acu.edu.au

P.L. (Tamar) Weiss et al. (eds.), *Virtual Reality for Physical and Motor Rehabilitation*, Virtual Reality Technologies for Health and Clinical Applications,
DOI 10.1007/978-1-4939-0968-1_10, © Springer Science+Business Media New York 2014

the environment in order to maximise participation across contexts. The downside of adopting an ecological approach to intervention is the breadth of areas that may need to be addressed when taking into consideration individual experiences and perspectives. Such a model presents a number of practical and financial barriers in health care delivery.

10.1.2 Child Motor and Cognitive Development: Implications for VR-Based Applications

Object knowledge is available to young infants in the form of perceptual primitives, as well as information conveyed by physical interaction with objects in space. Put another way, the rudiments of veridical object concepts are evident in the first 6 months after birth (Johnson, 2005) but more sophisticated object concept knowledge requires volitional interactions. Exploratory actions in both peripersonal and extrapersonal space, particularly those directed at objects, occur readily in infants and promote learning of the systematic co-variation between visual and somatic information (Bremner, Holmes, & Spence, 2008). The plasticity of the neural system enables this active learning by allowing the reinforcement of neural networks that support replication of successful (goal-directed) interactions (Cheung, in press). Ultimately, the child generates a sense of body schema that is attuned to their external world, and that can better anticipate the outcomes of their own actions.

The perception of self in relation to the environment develops from active movements in peri-personal space, extending to interactions in extra-personal space, and gradually to actions which may have an impact on imaginary environments or those extended in both time and space. The extension of action planning (anticipatory planning) for potential outcomes of behaviour requires knowledge of alternative or occluded perspectives and is related to the complex interactions underpinning social cognition (Green, 1997). Intriguing is the fact that perception of three dimensional depth cues are not necessary for the perception of occluded objects but rather that this spatial knowledge can arise from motion information (Baillargeon, Spekle, & Wasserman, 1985; Shuwairi, Tran, DeLoache, & Johnson, 2010; Slater, Johnson, & Kellman, 1994). Moreover, projected two-dimensional (2D) images of impossible objects have also been shown to encourage manual exploration, socialisation and vocalisation in infants, reflecting the interrelationship between perceptual and motor mechanisms in development (Shuwairi et al., 2010). Taken together, while infants have a primitive system for spatial (object) perception, they need to interact dynamically with the object in space in order to learn higher-order object concepts and to build knowledge of the dynamics of their own motor system and its potentialities (i.e. the force–time relationships that are needed to impact the physical world and achieve action goals). In short, in order to develop advanced perceptual understanding, the infant needs to interact with objects and interaction of the objects in space in order to understand the dynamics of their own system.

The opportunity to present learning environments that provide affordances for interaction can be achieved in both 2D and three-dimensional (3D) projection, provided that the display makes use of kinematic cues. While a 2-D display allows us to derive spatial and perceptual information, manipulation of real objects in 3D space provides a stronger basis for the development of spatial knowledge (Bertenthal, 1996). VR systems that employ tangible interfaces can enhance perceptual experiences for children with disabilities, affording opportunities for manual interactions and exploration they might not otherwise have access to. This can assist children in mapping the relationship between their own actions and object and environment interactions.

10.1.3 Patterns of Neural Development Supporting Goal Directed Actions: Trends in Typical and Atypical Development

The recent concept of *interactive specialisation* suggests that the emergence of a new behaviour is the result of weighted activity from several brain regions whose modular architecture and rate of maturation may vary (Johnson, 2005). Functional circuits within the central nervous system (CNS) are initially ill-defined and may be activated in response to a broad range of stimuli. With the advent of time and experience, these circuits or networks become more specialised. For a given band of stimuli, there develops a shift in activation from diffuse to more focal regions (Durston et al., 2006).

The overarching hypothesis is that the functional output of a given cortical region is dependent on the nature of its reciprocal couplings to other regions. As such, new behaviours are seen to emerge as a result of changes to multiple regions rather than particular sites within the CNS.

Frontal systems play a particularly important role in the control of goal-directed movement throughout development, enabling more flexible behaviour in the face of changing or more complex environmental constraints (Brocki & Bohlin, 2004). For example, high task complexity and variable constraints during reaching place significant demands on limited capacity working memory systems which are supported by the dorsolateral prefrontal cortex and parietal cortex (Suchy, 2009). Furthermore, differential neural activation of the medial prefrontal cortex versus left premotor cortex has been shown during imitation, depending on knowledge of the intention (or goal) underlying the observed action (Chaminade, Meltzoff, & Decety, 2002). It is a rule of thumb that the amount of top-down (or front to back) control increases substantially over childhood to enable more complex actions (Sommerville, Hare, & Casey, 2011).

One important implication of these developmental changes is that younger children and those with motor difficulties show limitations in the ability to enlist online control under complex task constraints (i.e. when demand on executive function is high). We see greater reliance on pure feedback systems under these conditions (e.g. Chicoine, Lassonde, & Proteau, 1992; Wilson, Ruddock, Smits-Engelsman, Polatajko, & Blank, 2013). Indeed, given the strong evidence for executive function deficits in Developmental Coordination Disorders (DCD), we may see a double disadvantage in the control of action: poor predictive control coupled with deficits of executive function, resulting in significant delays in skill acquisition and perhaps self-regulation. There is strong evidence of a link between executive control and the development of movement skill, more generally. Levels of inhibitory control, for example, are correlated with movement skill in both younger (Livesey, Keen, Rouse, & White, 2006) and older (Mandich, Buckolz, & Polatajko, 2003; Piek, Dyck, Francis, & Conwell, 2007; Wilmot, Brown, & Wann, 2007) children.

10.1.4 Atypical Development/Neurodevelopmental Disorders

In cases of neural damage or problems of functional connectivity, reorganisation of the developing system has been shown to be influenced by activity. Eyre and colleagues (2001) have shown activity dependent withdrawal of ipsilateral corticospinal neural connections during the first 2 years of life which are retained in some children with hemiplegic cerebral palsy with a functional cost (Eyre et al., 2001). Accumulating evidence shows the importance of task specific intense and repetitive training for motor skill acquisition and neural plasticity for improved functional ability (French et al., 2010; Kuhnke et al., 2008; Sutcliffe, Logan, & Fehlings, 2009). However, less evidence is present for the translation of specific gains shown in the clinical setting to longer-term functional benefits. Furthermore, engaging children in such repetitive exercise is challenging and the potential benefits of these therapy programmes can be compromised by frustration and poor compliance (Campbell, 2002; Gilmore, Ziviani, Sakzewski, Shields, & Boyd, 2010).

10.2 Evolution of Technology-Mediated Rehabilitation in Childhood Disability

VR technologies offer solutions that can be relatively easily engineered to accommodate to the reduced capabilities of children with varying disabilities. In addition, these may offer ecologically valid interventions, that are also acceptable from a psychosocial perspective, provide motivating and engaging exercise environments that can be scaled to individual needs and encourage repeated practice of functional actions under different task constraints (Bryanton et al., 2006; Snider, Majnemer, & Darsaklis, 2010).

Early approaches using VR systems in rehabilitation in childhood disability reported use of video capture technology for children with cerebral palsy (CP) or acquired brain injury (ABI) initially used systems such as the GestureTek Interactive Rehabilitation Exercise virtual reality system (http://www.gesturetekhealth.com/) to target specific areas of motor or cognitive impairment (see Laufer & Weiss, 2011 for review of use of VR systems in both assessment and treatment of children with motor impairments). As there have been only a few randomised controlled trials (RCT) of VR systems which have included children with specific types of CP and as performance profiles differ significantly between groups (and individuals), it is difficult to generalise results; changes in skill and participation have not been demonstrated across settings. While one RCT did not yield significant evidence of a positive treatment effect ($n=31$; Reid & Cabell, 2006), a smaller RCT ($n=10$, Jannink et al., 2008) using the Eye-Toy system (http://us.playstation.com/ps2/) showed treatment effects only at the body function level without reports of functional activity benefit for children with mixed types of CP. These mixed results are consistent with those summarised in a recent review by Laufer and Weiss (2011) and a study by Jelsma and colleagues (2013). For children with spastic hemiplegic CP, Jelsma et al. (2013) showed benefits from training on the Nintendo Wii Fit (http://wiifit.com/) on clinical measures of balance control; however, these effects did not translate into function.

Recommendations for the use of VR for children with CP are thus inconclusive and clinical guidelines emphasise the need for intensive motor based and task specific therapies such as Constraint Induced Movement therapy (Anttila, Autti-Rämö, Suoranta, Mäkelä, & Malmivaara, 2008; NICE guidelines UK, 2012; Sakzewski, Ziviani, & Boyd, 2009).

Research using 2D video capture systems (GestureTek IREX) has been undertaken with children with Traumatic Brain Injury (Galvin & Levac, 2011); a glove is used to identify the body part and indirectly embed the "child" into the environment. However, the temporal and sensory experiences are offset by the nature of the interface design such that the sensory feedback is not correlated in a way that reinforces the natural spatiotemporal relationship between modalities, nor reinforces the pragmatics of the task/game at hand (Golomb et al., 2009). By comparison, the use of objects known as tangible-user interfaces (TUIs), which enlist more intuitive forms of workspace interaction and real-time decision making, may provide opportunities to effect higher levels of presence and more natural movement kinematics and have shown stronger treatment effects and greater generalisation, in the main (e.g. Mumford et al., 2010; Subramanian, Massie, Malcolm, & Levin, 2010).

Akhutina et al. (2003) successfully recruited an avatar based VE with additional desktop tasks for children with cerebral palsy. However, children with lower levels of cognitive performance did not show benefit from the additional training, indicative of the difficulties of scaling some systems sufficiently at lower levels of ability (Chen et al., 2007). The use of virtual tutors has been exploited within education environments. Of note, is the potential for the use of VR technologies with children with intellectual impairment. Protocols combining a software tutor and human tutor suggest that computer-aided learning may be helpful in assisting people with intellectual disabilities in learning that transfers to the real-life situation (Standen, Brown, & Cromby, 2001). However, the variability within and between subjects and wide range of user requirements restrict interpretation.

Interesting extensions of VR technologies in paediatric rehabilitation have recently emerged. Bart and colleagues (2008) successfully used VR training to improve confidence in street crossing abilities in children aged 7–12 years and also used the IREX system to distinguish between attentional and behaviour factors of children with and without ABI (Bart, Agam, Weiss, & Kizony, 2011), but less is known about the potential of such systems to improve real "street crossing". The latter study attempts to address the elements of activity performance and participation in its research design however focusses on the measurement of specific levels of impairment as primary outcomes with as yet, little evidence showing change in specific functions transferring to real-time changes in activity performance or participation. A promising development, extending the role of VR to activity performance is evidenced by Kirshner, Weiss, and Tirosh (2011) in considering a virtual meal preparation environment for children with cerebral palsy. While research has tended to focus on the assessment role of the system, opportunities exist to extend these principles for the training of skills required for successful improvements in skills and participation in an important practical and social activity.

Mixed reality environments may offer more opportunities to bridge the virtual to real task divide. Pridmore and colleagues (2007) have focused on developing mixed-reality environments to "soften" the real–virtual divide with the aim of improved transfer of rehabilitation activities into everyday life. By placing the markers on objects, the interaction with a virtual world can be bridged by a tangible—or real—interface. The use of TUIs can enable a direct mode of wireless interaction within a visual display unit that has the advantage of overcoming the delay inherent in more "traditional" VR systems. Mixed-reality systems permit real-time tracking of an individual's movements relative to events presented in a virtual workspace/environment along with more direct feedback of sensory perceptual characteristics of object/action environmental interactions. The Elements system, used in (Mumford & Wilson, 2009), adapted for paediatric use as the Reaction system (Green & Wilson, 2012), shows promise in promoting real-time responses for improved reaching and targeting for adults with acquired brain injury and children with cerebral palsy, respectively. The latter study also showed transfer to improvements in skills affecting performance in daily activities such as ability to open a (real) door. Interaction with multimodal interfaces may support the acquisition of intuitive movements, based on individual and subjective experience (and hence accommodating naturally to constraints of the specific impairments), as well as support the perception–action experiences required for performance of useful actions (Morganti, Goulene, Gaggioli, Stramba-Badiale, & Riva, 2006). Further research is required to see if these early results extend to larger and/or different paediatric populations.

Another use of mixed environments has been explored by embedded groups of children (young adults) in real time, within play/games, designed to promote socio-cognitive understanding of social engagement to facilitate actual social engagement behaviours in children with Autism (Bauminger-Zviely, Eden, Zancanaro, Weiss, &

Gal, 2013; Gal et al., 2009; Kandalaft, Didehbani, Krawczyk, Allen, & Chapman, 2013). This methodology shows potential in harnessing children's interest in a mutual goal to promote implicit social learning for participation in interactive play activities with further research required to determine whether the impressive gains evidenced transfer beyond the research diads to novel and unexperienced social situations. The use of these technologies by Kandalaft et al. (2013) in young adults with high functioning autism show promise in transfer of skills to real-life social and occupational functioning (Gal, in press).

The entertainment field has generated a number of readily available and increasingly more affordable technologies enhancing at one end leisure opportunities for children with disabilities as well as rehabilitation at the impairment level. Figure 9.1 illustrates the areas in which evidence or potential exists for the use of VR technologies across ICF levels. Commercially available gaming consoles using motion sensors such as the Nintendo Wii offer low cost virtual reality therapy options (www.nintendo.co.uk). The motion sensors use differences in the applied forces and movements to change the amount of visual and audio feedback provided. Case-study reports, as well as randomised trials, have suggested the Nintendo Wii Fit to be useful in enhancing motor proficiency in stroke patients (Mouawad, Doust, Max, & McNulty, 2011; Saposnik et al., 2010) and a child with diplegic cerebral palsy (Deutsch, Borbely, Filler et al., 2008) 'and also 18 children with Developmental Coordination Disorder (Hammond, Jones, Hill, Green, & Male, 2013); however robust empirical data remain limited in childhood disability (Laver, George, Ratcliffe, & Crotty, 2011). Deutsch et al. (2008) demonstrated the effective use of the Wii gaming console, of a minimum of 7 h, in improving postural and functional mobility (distance walked with forearm crutches). The Wii fit programme has recently been used to promote motor and psychosocial skills of children with Developmental Coordination Disorder (DCD) in a programme run during school lunch break (Hammond et al., 2013). This latter study, while measuring the effects on balance and motor coordination, engaged children in a daily activity considered desirable to their non-DCD peers during recess. The use of Sony's PlayStation2® EyeToy was equally effective as conventional physiotherapy for young children with DCD on balance and functional mobility tasks (Ashkenazi, Orian, Weiss, & Laufer, 2013).

The extent to which such systems not only promote specific motor or social skills but act as a mechanism for engagement and enjoyment in meaningful social and leisure activities has yet to be explored. Children without disabilities are reporting an increased amount of time using computers and computer based technologies for both educational as well as leisure tasks (Rideout, Vandewater, & Wartella, 2003; Roberts, Foehr, & Rideout, 2005). Increasing evidence shows many children, with and without disabilities, to be using and engaging with computer and electronic games technologies in both play and educational activities (Green, Meroz, Margalit, & Ratson, 2012; Laufer & Weiss, 2011; Reid, 2002, 2004). While the targeted area of practice effects of research of different VR and mixed reality systems may focus on the impairment level, the outcomes of rehabilitation programmes should be targeted towards developing activity skills for enhanced participation across meaningful areas of performance.

While research to date has continued to focus on outcomes related to body function levels, the participation in computer/VR games in and of themselves corresponds with participation in activities that are meaningful to children at various levels across educational, leisure and social contexts. Bauminger-Zviely and colleagues (2013) begin to address this question through their studies exploring the use of the Diamond Touch system in developing social cognition for enhanced interactive play. The capacity to adapt and scale access to VR technologies may permit children with motor, social and cognitive deficits to participate in activities not only with matched disability peer groups but also with contemporaries without disabilities. As children with physical disabilities rarely have the opportunity to "compete" in physical activities on an equal playing field with their "non-disabled" peers, VR technologies have the potential to provide competitive/sporting opportunities for these children. Figure 9.1 illustrates the number of areas within the ICFDH-CY framework in which VR technologies have shown promise in promoting function and skills in young people.

10.3 Horses for Courses: Tailored Solutions for Specific Conditions Affecting Movement

Rehabilitation systems using new (interactive) technologies can be classified in a number of ways. First, a distinction can be drawn between game-like systems that use the logic of many off-the-shelf technologies, and those systems designed more specifically for learning and rehabilitation (i.e. Virtual tutor/animation and telerehabilitation, respectively). Second, systems can be divided according to the particular behavioural or psychological focus of therapy, e.g. upper- or lower-limb rehabilitation, physical fitness/balance, functional rehabilitation, participation and play, social interaction and self-esteem, and self-empowerment (For review see: Galvin & Levac, 2011). How these distinctions are drawn is often a reflection of the specific neurological condition or disability.

10.3.1 Evidence Across Varieties of Cerebral Palsy

Recent evaluations of off-the-shelf systems for children with ***hemiplegia*** are encouraging, albeit with small sample sizes. Applications vary across ICF domains targeting specific areas of impairment (upper limb control), activity performance (meal preparation, street crossing, etc.) and participation (notably in leisure activities). Golomb et al. (2010) showed improved manual ability (lifting objects with greater range of motion) in three adolescents with hemiplegic CP (HCP) using a 5DT 5 Ultra Glove and PlayStation3 game console; Chen et al. (2007) showed improved reaching (kinematics) translating to functional performance in three children with HCP using a series of reaching games programmed within the PlayStation2® EyeToy system;

and You et al. (2005) used the IREX VR system resulting in improved functional arm movements in a child with HCP with associated enhancement of cortical activation on functional magnetic resonance imaging. Use of these systems with their relatively low cost and fairly intuitive modes of interaction with children with HCP is promising, however it is not possible to separate out the specific benefits of the VR system from the intensity and duration of the protocols implemented in these studies (13–25 h over 36–67 days, 8 h over 4 weeks, 20 h over 4 weeks, respectively). Other intensive therapies such as constraint-induced movement therapy (CIMT) or hand–arm bimanual intensive therapy (HABIT), using protocols varying from 60 to 90 h across 2 weeks to 1 months, show evidence of positive motor skill translating to improved performance in activities of daily living (ADL) (Green et al., 2013).

Ready-made, off-the-shelf systems frequently necessitate a prerequisite level of skill and neuromotor integrity to interact effectively with the learning environments (Green & Wilson, 2012). Hence, it is more difficult to vary task constraints below a certain, minimum level to match the developmental and cognitive aspects of children with disabilities. This then restricts application to younger children with movement difficulties whose nervous system may well exhibit greater plasticity and be more responsive to intervention (Eyre, 2007). Recent definitions of CP have highlighted the individualised manner that motor deficits and the frequently accompanying sensory, perceptual, cognitive, psychological and communication deficits interact and contribute to the overall functional impairment and disability (Bax, Tydeman, & Flodmark, 2006; Goble, Hurvitz, & Brown, 2009; Guzzetta, Tinelli, & Cioni, 2008). With a shift in understanding of the importance of collaborative goal setting (Löwing et al., 2009), interventions systems need to provide intuitive interfaces for interaction for many children or young people with motor and intellectual disabilities which also enable identification of the goal of the activity to optimise appropriate responses (Akhutina et al., 2003; Chen et al., 2007; Weiss, Bialik, & Kizony, 2003).

Encouraging evidence of the potential of VR systems in rehabilitation of children with CP is provided by Akhutina et al. (2003). There was variation in severity of both motor and cognitive difficulties in their study, suggesting that progress in some aspects of the training was independent of initial severity. In contrast, the results of Jelsma et al. (2013) suggest a potential interaction effect between severity and the extent and nature of the therapeutic response. Consistent with the summary of Laufer and Weiss (2011), greater detail on individual variation and patterns of responses is required in reports of intervention effects, particularly in order to better understand *how* applications are working and to optimise programmes for individual children.

10.4 Future Directions

The capacity of VR technologies to support motor learning through manipulation of feedback is covered in Levac and Sveistrup (in press). Feedback on performance (explicit and implicit) and predictive control play important roles in the course of development (Hemayattalab & Rostami, 2009). Integrating technologies which manipulate/augment feedback has been shown to be effective in motor therapy for children with severe motor and cognitive disabilities (Green & Wilson, 2012). Critically, VR-based technologies afford many options for the provision of multisensory AF and avenues for future development in VR-assisted therapy. This form of therapy is an ideal solution for conditions that affect the predictive control of action, including CP and DCD.

A recent review of object affordance in therapy suggests that the incorporation of real objects within therapy interventions is more important than either the functionality or number of objects (Hetu & Mercier, 2012). However, definitions of "functionality" vary between studies and the extent to which "conflict/impossibility" may in fact provoke more spontaneous actions has also not been explored within VR environments (Shuwairi et al., 2010). The anticipatory nature of representation, essential for motor planning (Hyde & Wilson, 2011; Liu, Zaine, & Westcott, 2007; Pezzulo, 2008; Steenbergen & Gordon, 2006) may be exploited by VR technologies either in assessment, outcome measurements or in intervention itself. In view of the burgeoning evidence of the relationship of motor imitation and motor planning, an unexplored area for VR technologies could exploit participant generation of images that result in more/less successful outcomes at a motor, social or behavioural level. Contrasting embedded images of self-performing movements versus use of Avatars for replication via imitation or gesture generation may provide important information of the role of imagery in both social and motor development. With advancements in technology, programmes designed which incorporate motor imagery for developing predictive planning may not be too distant.

10.5 Conclusion

While little evidence is present for the translation of specific gains shown in the clinical setting to longer-term functional benefits, this may arguably be due to the different context of application across studies in which the variables of the person (motivation and capacity), task and the environment have been shifted in a nonlinear fashion, implicitly altering the nature of the task in both temporal and spatial spheres. Treatment targeting specific modalities such as reaching and grasping and spatial skills should not be considered in isolation from the motivational elements of the end-goal such as playfulness and functional everyday self-care and leisure activities (including ADL). Children need to be engaged in the therapeutic process for therapy to be effective (Löwing et al., 2009), supporting generalisation across specific skills to activity participation. Virtual Reality technologies have the potential to expand the opportunities available for engaging children in therapeutic activities across physical, social and cognitive domains. Indeed, past limitations that restricted access and extension into community and other settings, are being superseded by recent advances in portable, low-costs devices.

References

Akhutina, T., Foreman, N., Krichevets, A., Matikka, L., Narhi, V., Pylaeva, N., et al. (2003). Improving spatial functioning in children with cerebral palsy using computerized and traditional game tasks. *Disability and Rehabilitation, 25*, 1361–1371.

Anttila, H., Autti-Rämö, I., Suoranta, J., Mäkelä, M., & Malmivaara, A. (2008). Effectiveness of physical therapy interventions for children with cerebral palsy: A systematic review. *BMC Pediatrics*. doi:10.1186/1471-2431-8-14.

Ashkenazi, T., Orian, D., Weiss, PL., Laufer, Y. (2013). *Effect of training children with Developmental Coordination Disorders in a virtual environment compared with a conventional environment*. IEEE Intl. Conference Proceedings. Philadelphia, PA.

Baillargeon, R., Spekle, E. S., & Wasserman, S. (1985). Object permanence in five-month-old infants. *Cognition, 20*, 191–208.

Bart, O., Agam, T., Weiss, P. L., & Kizony, R. (2011). Using video capture virtual reality for children with acquired brain injury. *Disability and Rehabilitation, 33*, 1579–1586.

Bart, O., Katz, N., Weiss, P. L., & Josman, N. (2008). Street crossing by typically developed children in real and virtual environments. *OTJR: Occupation, Participation and Health, 28*, 89–97.

Bauminger-Zviely, N., Eden, S., Zancanaro, M., Weiss, P. L., & Gal, E. (2013). Increasing social engagement in high-functioning children with ASD using collaborative technologies in the school. *Autism: International Journal of Research and Practice, 17*, 317–339.

Bax, M., Tydeman, C., & Flodmark, O. (2006). Clinical and MRI correlates of cerebral palsy. *Journal of the American Medical Association, 296*, 1602–1608.

Bertenthal, B. I. (1996). Origins and early development of perception, action and representation. *American Review of Psychology, 47*, 431–459.

Bremner, A. J., Holmes, N. P., & Spence, C. (2008). Infants lost in (peripersonal) space? *Trends in Cognitive Science, 12*, 298–305.

Brocki, K. C., & Bohlin, B. (2004). Executive Functions in children aged 6 to 13: A dimensional and developmental study. *Developmental Neuropsychology, 26*, 571–593.

Bryanton, C., Bosse, J., Brien, M., Mclean, J., McCormick, A., & Sveistrup, H. (2006). Feasibility, Motivation and Selective Motor Control: Virtual Reality compared to conventional home exercise in children with cerebral palsy. *Cyberpsychology & Behavior, 9*, 123–128.

Campbell, M. (2002). The rehabilitation of brain injured children: The case for including physical exercise and virtual reality: A clinical perspective. *Developmental Neurorehabilitation, 5*, 43–45.

Chaminade, T., Meltzoff, A. N., & Decety, J. (2002). Does the End Justify the Means? A PET exploration of the mechanisms involved in human imitation. *NeuroImage, 15*, 318–328.

Chen, Y.-P., Kang, L.-J., Chuang, T.-Y., Doong, J.-L., Lee, S.-J., Tsai, M.-W., et al. (2007). Use of virtual reality to improve upper-extremity control in children with cerebral palsy: A single-subject design. *Physical Therapy, 87*, 1441–1457.

Cheung, K.L., Tunik, E., Adamovich, S. and Boyd, L.A. (in press) *Neuroplasticity and virtual reality*. Volume 1 of this book series.

Chicoine, A. J., Lassonde, M., & Proteau, L. (1992). Developmental aspects of sensorimotor integration. *Developmental Neuropsychology, 8*, 381–394.

Deutsch, J. E., Borbely, M., Filler, J., et al. (2008). Use of a low-cost, commercially available gaming console (Wii) for rehabilitation of an adolescent with cerebral palsy. *Physical Therapy, 88*, 196–1207.

Durston, S., Davidson, M. C., Tottenham, N., Galvan, A., Spicer, J., Fossella, J. A., et al. (2004). A shift from diffuse to focal cortical activity with development. *Developmental Science, 9*, 1–8.

Eyre, J. (2007). Corticospinal tract development and its plasticity after perinatal injury. *Neuroscience and Biobehavioral Review, 31*, 1136–1149.

French, B., Thomas, L., Leathley, M., Sutton, C., McAdam, J., Forster, A., et al. (2010). Does repetitive task training improve functional activity after stroke: A Cochrane systematic review and meta-analysis. *Journal of Rehabilitation Medicine, 42*(1), 9–14.

Gal, E., Zancanaro, M., Weiss, P.L. *Using innovative technologies as therapeutic and educational tools for children with Autism Spectrum Disorder*. [autism chapter in vol 2 of this book series].

Gal, E., Beuminger, N., Goren-Bar, D., Pianesi, F., Stock, O., Massimo, Z., et al. (2009). Enhancing social communication of children with high functioning autism through a co-located interface. *AI and Society, the Journal of Human-Centred Systems, 24*, 1–17.

Galvin, J., & Levac, D. (2011). Facilitating clinical decision-making about the use of virtual reality within paediatric motor rehabilitation: Describing and classifying virtual reality systems. *Developmental Neurorehabilitation, 14*, 112–122.

Gilmore, R., Ziviani, J., Sakzewski, L., Shields, N., & Boyd, R. (2010). A balancing act: Children's experience of modified constraint-induced movement therapy. *Developmental Medical and Child Neurology, 13*, 88–94.

Goble, D. J., Hurvitz, E. A., & Brown, S. H. (2009). Deficits in the ability to use proprioceptive feedback in children with hemiplegic cerebral palsy. *International Journal of Rehabilitation Research, 32*, 267–269.

Golomb, MR., Barkat-Masih, M., Rabin, B., Abdelbaky, M., Huber, M., Burdea, G. C. (2009). Eleven Months of Virtual Reality Telerehabilitation—Lessons Learned. Virtual Rehabilitation International Conference. doi: 10.1109/ICVR.2009.5174200.

Golomb, M. R., McDonald, B. L., Warden, S. J., Yonkman, J., Saykin, A. J., Shirley, B., et al. (2010). In-home VR videogame telerehabilitation in adolescents with hemiplegic cerebral palsy. *Archives Physical Medicine Rehabilitation, 91*, e1–e8.

Green, D. (1997). *Clumsiness in Asperger's syndrome*. Unpublished Master's Thesis: University of Surrey.

Green, D., Meroz, A., Margalit, A. E., & Ratson, N. Z. (2012). A validation study of the Keyboard Personal Computer Style instrument (K-PeCS) for use with children. *Applied Ergonomics, 43*(6), 985–992.

Green, D., Schertz, M., Gordon, A., Moore, A., Schejter-Margalit, T., Farquharson, Y., et al. (2013). A multi-site study of functional outcomes following a themed approach to hand-arm bimanual intensive therapy (HABIT) for children with hemiplegia. *Developmental Medicine and Child Neurology*. doi:10.1111/dmcn.12113.

Green, D., & Wilson, P. H. (2012). Use of virtual reality in rehabilitation of movement in children with hemiplegia—A multiple case study evaluation. *Disability Rehabilitation, 34*(7), 593–604.

Guzzetta, A., Tinelli, F., & Cioni, G. (2008). Alternative neural pathways for treatment of cerebral visual disorders. *Developmental Medicine and Child Neurology, 50*(S114), 5.

Hammond, J., Jones, V., Hill, E., Green, D., & Male, I. (2013). An investigation of the impact of regular use of the Wii Fit to improve motor and psychosocial outcomes in children with movement difficulties: A pilot study. *Child: Care, Health and Development*. doi:10.1111/cch.12029.

Hemayattalab, R., & Rostami, L. R. (2009). Effects of frequency of feedback on the learning of motor skill in individuals with cerebral palsy. *Research in Developmental Disabilities, 31*, 212–217.

Hetu, S., & Mercier, C. (2012). Using purposeful tasks to improve motor performance: Does object affordance matter? *British Journal of Occupational Therapy, 75*(8), 367–376.

Hyde, C., & Wilson, P. H. (2011). Online motor control in children with developmental coordination disorder: Chronometric analysis of double-step reaching performance. *Child: Care, Health and Development, 37*(1), 111–122.

Jannink, M. J. A., Van Der Wilden, G. J., Navis, D. W., Vsser, G., Gussinklo, J., & Ijzerman, M. (2008). A low-cost video game applied for training of upper extremity function in children with cerebral palsy: A pilot study. *CyberPsychology and Behavior, 11*, 27–32.

Jelsma, J., Pronk, M., Ferguson, G., & Jelsma-Smit, D. (2013). The effect of the Nintendo Wii Fit on balance control and gross motor function of children with spastic hemiplegic cerebral palsy. *Developmental Neurorehabilitation, 16*, 27–37.

Johnson, M. H. (2005). *Developmental cognitive neuroscience* (2nd ed.). Oxford: Blackwell.

Kandalaft, M. F., Didehbani, N., Krawczyk, D. C., Allen, T. T., & Chapman, S. B. (2013). Virtual Reality Social Cognition Training for young adults with high functioning autism. *Journal of Autism and Developmental Disorders, 43*, 34–44.

Kirshner, S., Weiss, P. L., & Tirosh, E. (2011). Meal-Maker: A virtual meal preparation environment for children with cerebral palsy. *European Journal of Special Needs Education, 26*, 323–336.
Kuhnke, N., Juenger, H., Walther, M., Berweck, S., Mall, V., & Staudt, M. (2008). Do patients with congenital hemiparesis and ipsilateral corticospinal projections respond differently to constraint-induced movement therapy? *Developmental Medicine and Child Neurolgy, 50*(12), 898–903.
Laufer, Y., & Weiss, P. L. (2011). Virtual reality in the assessment and treatment of children with motor impairment: A systematic review. *Journal of Physical Therapy Education, 25*, 59–71.
Laver, K., George, S., Ratcliffe, J., & Crotty, M. (2011). Virtual reality stroke rehabilitation—hype or hope? *Australian Occupational Therapy Journal, 58*, 215–219.
Levac, D.E., & Sveistrup, H. (in press). *Principles of motor learning in virtual environments* [this volume]
Liu, W.-Y., Zaine, C. A., & Westcott, S. (2007). Anticipatory postural adjustments in children with cerebral palsy and children with typical development. *Pediatric Physical Therapy, 19*, 88–195.
Livesey, D. J., Keen, J., Rouse, J., & White, F. (2006). The relationship between measures of executive function, motor performance and externalising behaviour in 5- and 6-year-old children. *Human Movement Science, 25*, 50–64.
Löwing, K., Bexelius, A., & Carlberg, E. B. (2009). Activity focused and goal directed therapy for children with cerebral palsy—Do goals make a difference? *Disability and Rehabilitation, 31*, 1808–1816.
Mandich, A., Buckolz, E., & Polatajko, H. (2003). Children with developmental coordination disorder (DCD) and their ability to disengage ongoing attentional focus: More on inhibitory function. *Brain Cognition, 51*, 346–366.
Morganti, F., Goulene, K., Gaggioli, A., Stramba-Badiale, M., & Riva, G. (2006). Grasping virtual objects: A feasibility study for an enactive interface application in stroke. *PsychNology, 4*, 181–197.
Mouawad, M. R., Doust, C. G., Max, M. D., & McNulty, P. A. (2011). Wii-based movement therapy to promote improved upper extremity function post-stroke: A pilot study. *Journal of Rehabilitation Medicine, 43*, 527–533.
Mumford, N., Duckworth, J., Thomas, P. R., Shum, D., Williams, G., & Wilson, P. H. (2010). Upper limb virtual rehabilitation for traumatic brain injury: Initial evaluation of the elements system. *Brain Injury, 24*, 780–791.
Mumford, N., & Wilson, P. H. (2009). Virtual reality in acquired brain injury upper limb rehabilitation: Evidence-based evaluation of clinical research. *Brain Injury, 179–91.*
NICE guidelines UK. (2012). *Spasticity in children and young people with non-progressive brain disorders: Management of spasticity and co-existing motor disorders and their early musculoskeletal complications.* NICE clinical guideline 145: http://www.nice.org.uk/CG145. Accessed 1 Aug 2012.
Pezzulo, G. (2008). Coordinating with the Future: The anticipatory nature of representation. *Minds and Machines, 18*, 179–225.
Piek, J. P., Dyck, M. J., Francis, M., & Conwell, A. (2007). Working memory, processing speed, and set-shifting in children with developmental coordination disorder and attention-deficit–hyperactivity disorder. *Developmental Medicine and Child Neurology, 49*, 678–683.
Pridmore, T., Cobb, S., Hilton, D., Green, J., & Eastgate, R. (2007). Mixed reality environments in stroke rehabilitation: Interfaces across the real/virtual divide. *International Journal of Disability and Human Development, 6*, 3–10.
Reid, D. (2002). Benefits of virtual play rehabilitation environment for children with cerebral palsy on perceptions of self-efficacy: A pilot study. *Pediatric Rehabilitation, 5*, 141–158.
Reid, D. (2004). The influence of virtual reality on playfulness in children with cerebral pasly: A pilot study. *Occupational Therapy International, 11*, 131–144.
Reid, D., & Cabell, K. (2006). The use of virtual reality with children with cerebral palsy: A pilot randomized trial. *Therapeutic Recreation Journal, 40*, 255–268.
Rideout, V. J., Vandewater, E. A., & Wartella, E. A. (2003). *Zero to six: Electronic media in the lives of infants, toddlers and preschoolers*. Menlo Park, CA: Kaiser Family Foundation.

Roberts, D. F., Foehr, U. G., & Rideout, V. J. (2005). *Generation M: Media in the lives of 8-18 year olds*. Menlo Park, CA: Kaiser Family Foundation.
Sakzewski, L., Ziviani, J., & Boyd, R. (2009). Systematic review and meta-analysis of therapeutic management of upper-limb dysfunction in children with congenital hemiplegia. *Pediatrics, 123*, e1111–e1122.
Saposnik, G., Mamdani, M., Bayley, M., Bayley, M., Thorpe, K. E., Hail, J., et al. (2010). Effectiveness of Virtual Reality Exercises in Stroke Rehabilitation (EVREST): Rationale, Design, and Protocol of a Pilot Randomized Clinical Trial Assessing the Wii Gaming System. *International Journal Stroke, 5*, 47–51.
Shuwairi, S. M., Tran, A., DeLoache, J. S., & Johnson, S. P. (2010). Infants' response to pictures of impossible objects. *Infancy, 15*, 636–649.
Slater, A., Johnson, S. P., & Kellman, P. J. (1994). The role of three-dimensional depth cues in infants' perception of occluded objects. *Early Development and Parenting, 3*, 187–191.
Snider, L., Majnemer, A., & Darsaklis, V. (2010). Virtual reality as a therapeutic modality for children with cerebral palsy. *Developmental Neurorehabilitation, 13*, 120–128.
Sommerville, L. H., Hare, T., & Casey, B. J. (2011). Frontostriatal maturation predicts cognitive control failure to appetitive cues in adolescents. *Journal Cognitive Neuroscience, 23*, 2123–2134.
Standen, P. J., Brown, D. J., & Cromby, J. J. (2001). The effective use of virtual environments in the education and rehabilitation of students with intellectual disabilities. *British Journal of Education and Technology, 32*, 289–299.
Steenbergen, B., & Gordon, A. M. (2006). Activity limitation in hemiplegic cerebral palsy: evidence for disorders in motor planning (review). *Developmental Medicine and Child Neurology, 48*, 780–783.
Subramanian, S. K., Massie, C. L., Malcolm, M. P., & Levin, M. F. (2010). Does provision of extrinsic feedback result in improved motor learning in the upper limb poststroke: A systematic review of the evidence. *Neurorehabilitation Neural Repair, 24*(2), 113–124.
Suchy, Y. (2009). Executive Functioning: Overview, assessment, and research issues for the non-neuropsychologist. *Annals of Behavioral Medicine, 37*, 106–116.
Sutcliffe, T. L., Logan, W. J., & Fehlings, D. L. (2009). Pediatric constraint-induced movement therapy is associated with increased contralateral cortical activity on functional magnetic resonance imaging. *Journal of Child Neurology, 24*(10), 1230–1235. doi:10.1177/0883073809341268. 24/10/1230 [pii].
Weiss, P. L., Bialik, P., & Kizony, R. (2003). Virtual reality provides leisure time opportunities for young adults with physical and intellectual disabilities. *CyberPsychology & Behavior, 6*, 335–342.
Wilmot, K., Brown, J. H., & Wann, J. P. (2007). Attention disengagement in children with Developmental Coordination Disorder. *Disability and Rehabilitation, 29*, 47–55.
Wilson, P. H., Ruddock, S., Smits-Engelsman, B., Polatajko, H., & Blank, R. (2013). Understanding performance deficits in developmental coordination disorder: A meta-analysis of recent research. *Developmental Medicine and Child Neurology, 55*(3), 217–228.
You, S. Y., Jan, S. H., Kim, Y.-H., Kwon, Y.-H., Barrow, I., & Gallett, M. (2005). Cortical reorganization induced by virtual reality therapy in a child with hemiparetic cerebral palsy. *Developmental Medicine and Child Neurology, 47*, 628–635.

Chapter 11
Current and Future Trends for VR and Motor Rehabilitation

Patrice L. (Tamar) Weiss, Emily A. Keshner, and Mindy F. Levin

Objective To summarize the current state of the art in applications of VR to motor rehabilitation and to set the stage for developments over the next 5–10 years.

11.1 Introduction

The faithful reader of this volume will have learned of some of the major issues that are important to consider when using virtual reality (VR) for motor rehabilitation. In this volume the neurophysiological principles underlying VR interventions for motor rehabilitation are discussed, including neuroplasticity, motor learning, sensorimotor integration, vision, and perception. In addition, the validity of virtual environments for motor rehabilitation is presented. This volume also summarizes the current state of knowledge regarding the effectiveness of VR interventions for improving rehabilitation outcomes for conditions such as stroke, degenerative diseases, vestibular pathology,

P.L. (Tamar) Weiss (✉)
Department of Occupational Therapy, Faculty of Social Welfare and Health Sciences, University of Haifa, Mount Carmel, Haifa 3498838, Israel
e-mail: tamar@research.haifa.ac.il

E.A. Keshner
Department of Physical Therapy and Department of Electrical and Computer Engineering, Temple University, 3307 N. Broad ST, Philadelphia, PA 19140, USA
e-mail: ekeshner@temple.edu

M.F. Levin
School of Physical and Occupational Therapy, McGill University, 3654 Promenade Sir William Osler, Montreal, QC, Canada, H3G 1Y5
e-mail: mindy.levin@mcgill.ca

P.L. (Tamar) Weiss et al. (eds.), *Virtual Reality for Physical and Motor Rehabilitation*, Virtual Reality Technologies for Health and Clinical Applications,
DOI 10.1007/978-1-4939-0968-1_11, © Springer Science+Business Media New York 2014

and cerebral palsy. The objective of this final chapter is to briefly summarize the current state of the art and to set the stage for future developments.

We begin with a review of the major technological "breakthroughs" (1986–1995; 1996–2005; 2006-present) that led to the use of VR for motor rehabilitation. We then present a summary overview of the evidence for the effectiveness of VR for motor rehabilitation. Finally, we present the results of a "Force Field" analysis to identify the major factors that "drive" or "restrain" the use of VR technologies in motor rehabilitation. This analysis facilitates a look into the future regarding developments that we anticipate will occur over the next 5–10 years.

11.2 Major Technological "Breakthroughs" that Led to the Use of VR for Motor Rehabilitation

Table 11.1 lists some of the key technological developments that influenced the use of VR technology for motor rehabilitation since its first adoption (1986–1995), through a period of development and initial implementation (1996–2005) and until the present stage of refinement and meaningful clinical research (2006–2013). The most characteristic features of the early technologies were their large size, high cost, and limited accuracy. These systems led to several pioneering motor rehabilitation applications (Deutsch et al., 2002; Holden, 2005; Jack et al., 2001; Krebs, Hogan, Aisen, & Volpe, 1998; Subramanian et al., 2007) while their clinical relevance was still uncertain due to very limited clinical access to either hardware or software. There was no real grass-roots clinical perception of the need for VR based interventions during this period.

The key changes that took place over the period between 1996 and 2005 include the emergence of platforms such as Superscape World Builder and OpenGL that supported easier development and distribution of desktop VR applications. VR began to be directed to specific rehabilitation applications although the focus was clearly research-oriented since only funded groups could support the creation of customized rehabilitation prototypes (e.g., Virtual Classroom, Virtual Office (Rizzo et al., 2002); Rutgers Arm (Burdea et al., 2010)). During this period, the first clinically oriented commercial VR systems emerged such as IREX (for motor rehabilitation) and Virtually Better (for treatment of phobias).

The period between 2006 and 2013 has seen development and commercialization of both high-end (e.g., CAREN) and low-cost VR systems. The latter were off-the-shelf (e.g., Nintendo Wii, Sony EyeToy) products that did not target rehabilitation but were nevertheless widely used by clinicians because of their accessibility and low cost. More recently, and in particular since 2010, a number of low-cost VR systems designed for and targeting rehabilitation (e.g., SeeMe, Timocco, Kinect) have become available. A variety of rehabilitation-oriented desktop gaming programs that implement VR properties (e.g., feedback, documentation, motivation) are also increasingly available. Still more recently, the increasing accessibility of embedded ambient technologies (e.g., inexpensive cameras, proximity sensors, wearable computing) that support the monitoring of motor and cognitive functioning under real-world conditions has extended VR-based interventions beyond the clinical setting.

Table 11.1 Key technological developments that influenced the use of VR technology in rehabilitation

Period	Key technology developments	Issues for rehabilitation
1986–1995	• Mainstream VR technologies (e.g., Head Mounted Displays); large installations (e.g., CAVE) • Initial development work in research labs that became the impetus for eventual rehabilitation prototypes (e.g., Myron Krueger's videoplace (Weiss, Sveistrup, Rand, & Kizony, 2009))	• Need for more precise, lower weight and lower cost hardware in order to ensure relevance and feasibility for rehabilitation (Rizzo, Buckwalter, & Neumann, 1997) • Need to bridge gaps in VR between goals of basic researchers, applied researchers, and developers
1996–2005	• Platforms such as Superscape World Builder and OpenGL support easier development and distribution of desktop VR applications • VR begins to be accessible for rehabilitation settings (e.g., GestureTek GX Software Developer's Kit) • Customized rehabilitation prototypes (e.g., Virtual Classroom, Virtual Office (Rizzo et al., 2000); Rutgers Arm (Burdea, Cioi, Martin, Fensterheim, & Holenski, 2010)) • Emergence of commercial clinically oriented VR systems (e.g., IREX, Virtually Better)	• System development more specific for rehabilitation (Keshner & Kenyon, 2004) • Proof of concept studies (Viau, Feldman, Mcfadyen, & Levin, 2004) • Reliability, validity, transfer of training studies • Literature reviews on specific rehabilitation applications (e.g., for VR-based motor rehabilitation by Sveistrup, 2004)
2006–2013	• Development of both high-end (e.g., CAREN; Knaut, Subramanian, McFadyen, Bourbonnais, & Levin, 2009; Subramanian et al., 2007) and low-end VR systems • Development and commercialization of numerous low-cost VR systems, some of which are off-the-shelf (e.g., Nintendo Wii, Sony EyeToy) for commercial use not targeting rehabilitation • Commercialization of numerous low-cost VR systems designed for and targeting rehabilitation (e.g., SeeMe, Timocco) • Increasing availability of embedded ambient VR technologies to monitor real-world activity	• Using VR as a paradigm for posing questions of relevance to motor control and motor learning (such as the effectiveness of feedback delivery for motor improvement (e.g., Keshner, Kenyon, Dhaher, & Streepey, 2005)) • Validation of movement kinematics (upper limb) used in VR (see Chap. 6) • Numerous studies showing how VR technology can address important rehabilitation questions about treatment effectiveness; these have been mostly small sample single-site clinical studies and very few Randomized Controlled Trials (e.g., Saposnik & Levin, 2011) • Exploration of novel clinical intervention paradigms feasible only with VR-supported technology (e.g., tele-rehabilitation applications) • Mixing of technologies to support augmented reality and "Living Lab" approaches
Future	• Proliferation of low-cost, turn-key VR systems with increasing clinical validity and reliability (e.g., more precise markerless non-encumbering motion tracking) • Increasing focus on VR applications supporting a personalized medicine approach	• Need for large, multi-center effectiveness studies that demonstrate capacity of VR to improve motor rehabilitation

11.3 Tools to Identify Technology Adoption

A number of different tools have been used to identify the readiness of a given technology for adoption. The most frequently used tool is the SWOT matrix, a method that was classically used to support strategic project planning, most often applied to business. Its origins are somewhat difficult to discern with attribution variously given to Harvard academics in the 1960s (King, 2004), Ansoff in 1987 (Turner, 2002) and contributions by Weihrich in 1982, Dealtry in 1992 and Wheelan and Hunger in 1998 (Koch, 2000). The initials stand for, respectively, *S*trengths, *W*eaknesses, *O*pportunities, and *T*hreats. A SWOT analysis is typically initiated by specifying the objective of a particular product or field of study and then identifying the internal and external factors that support or detract from its achievement. Rizzo and Kim (2005) carried out a SWOT analysis of the field of applications of VR to rehabilitation. They identified key factors that facilitated the initial growth of clinical and educational applications (strengths) and ensured continued development (opportunities). They further identified weaknesses that limited the field at that point in time as well as threats that warranted recognition in order to minimize their effect. The Rizzo and Kim (2005) SWOT matrix was based primarily on the literature and reflected input primarily from the research and clinical communities. Viewpoints of other stakeholders, in particular, direct users and funders were less well represented. Many of the opportunities (e.g., gaming industry development of special education-oriented applications) that were identified in this analysis have come to fruition, whereas some of the threats (e.g., unrealistic expectations of a given technology's capacity) continue to be of concern.

Gartner's "Hype Cycle" is another tool that has been used to identify the readiness of technologies for adoption (Rizzo & Kim, 2005; Weiss, 2005). The location of emerging technologies on the Hype Cycle helps a clinician assess its suitability for immediate adoption if it has reached a stable phase of development (i.e., a "plateau"). In contrast, in the case of less mature technologies, where performance expectations may be unrealistic (i.e., either too much or too little "hype"), a clinician may be advised that the usage of such technologies in clinical settings may require more financial and time resources than available. Most technologies require a 3–5 year cycle between their first emergence and their readiness for use in rehabilitation. One recent exception is the iPad that almost entirely skipped the stages from emergence to adoption.

11.4 Force Field Analysis

A Force-Field analysis is a less frequently considered tool for assessing the readiness of technology for adoption. As illustrated schematically in Fig. 11.1, a "Force Field" analysis provides a framework for examining the factors (forces) that influence the achievement of a designated objective. It was originally used in the fields of social science, psychology, and social psychology (Greer & Lei, 2012).

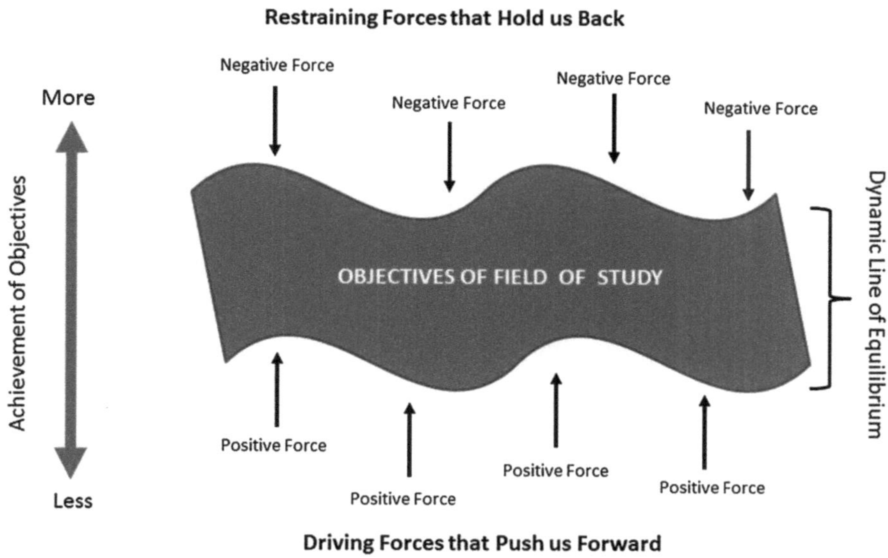

Fig. 11.1 Schema to illustrate the balance in a Force Field between the driving forces that push one forward towards the objectives of a given field of study and restraining forces that push one back from reaching these objectives

It identifies the forces that are causing a project to move towards achieving its goal (driving forces) or those that are causing it to become more distant from its goal (restraining forces). Developed by Lewin in 1943, it may be used to present the recommendations that we perceive as helping the field of virtual rehabilitation to move forward and to identify issues that need to be addressed in order to prevent the field from moving backwards.

A key advantage of a "Force Field" analysis is that it is dynamic with the location of the "push forward"/"hold-back" line susceptible to change as a project develops. This is shown in Fig. 11.1 as the thick, wavy grey band and referred to as the "Dynamic Line of Equilibrium". Thus, a given field may start to progress in accordance with objectives based on the identification of driving and restraining forces determined from reviews of the literature and meta-analyses. Changes in the location of the Line of Equilibrium may occur after reconsideration of the identity and potency of the driving forces and restraining forces on an ongoing basis.

Another advantage of a "Force Field" analysis is that it helps to distinguish among the sometimes overwhelming list of factors that are currently having the greatest influence on the achievement of objectives related to a given field of study, discipline, or project. Thus, the stakeholders[1] may use the results of this analysis as

[1] Stakeholders include all users of a given technology (both primary and secondary) as well as developers, distributors, funders, and researchers.

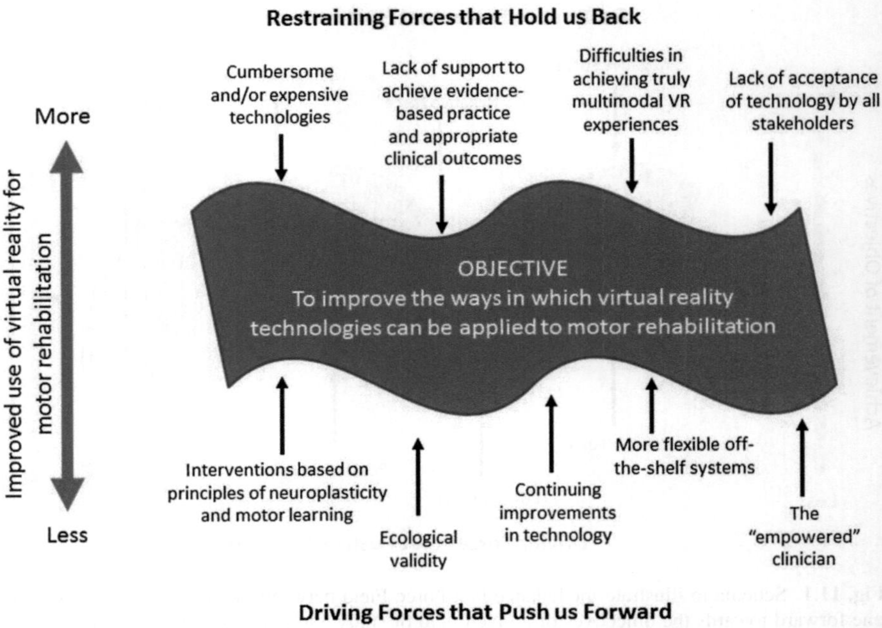

Fig. 11.2 Force Field analysis of the application of virtual reality technologies for motor rehabilitation

a tool to examine the major factors that affect performance, by developing a list of the primary driving forces that promote the achievement of goals and by identifying/resolving the key restraining forces that detract from these goals.

Figure 11.2 shows the Force Field analysis for the application of VR technologies for motor rehabilitation. Based on the reviews presented in the chapters in this volume, the key restraining forces that appear to "hold back" and the key driving forces that appear to "push forward" VR-base motor rehabilitation have been identified.

11.5 Key Driving Forces as Identified in this Volume

1. Improvements in *interventions based on principles of neuroplasticity and motor learning*. Examples include:
   - Chapter 2 (Cheung, Tunik, Adamovich, and Boyd) discusses how VR induces neuroplastic changes through repetitive practice and how this can be tracked by a variety of technologies during recovery from brain injury.
   - Chapter 3 (Levac and Sveistrup) reviews many VR applications that are constructed on the basis of the principles of neuroplasticity and motor learning.
   - Chapter 7 (Merians and Fluet) discusses how computer algorithms can use decision rules to progress the degree of difficulty of tasks in VR.

2. *Ecological validity*. Focus on new techniques for creating customized simulations based on specific needs of the client and interests that support functionality versus previous limited approaches (Riva et al., 2009). Examples of this include:
   - Chapter 4 (Kenyon and Ellis) discusses how the actual impact of the properties of a VR environment on visual-motor processing can be applied to future development of VR systems and environments.
   - Chapter 5 (Wright, Creem-Regehr, Warren, Anson, Jeka, and Keshner) discusses the selection of augmented rather than VR applications depending on the needs of the individual performer.
   - Chapter 6 (Levin, Deutsch, Kafri, and Liebermann) discusses how tasks in VR for the upper limb may be calibrated to the reaching space of the individual in order that they appear to be reachable. Another example is that exercise performed in VR creates the same stresses on the cardiovascular system as in real-world exercise environments.
   - Chapter 9 (Lamontagne, Keshner, Bugnariu, and Fung) discusses individual differences with aging and how optic flow and sensory conflict properties can be adjusted to elicit the desired behavior.

3. *Continuing improvements in technology* (e.g., more 3D systems are becoming available with improved resolution). Examples include:
   - Chapter 5 (Wright, Creem-Regehr, Warren, Anson, Jeka, and Keshner) discusses how advances in head mounted displays and more realistic computer generated images allow for the provision of augmented visual information to improve gait.
   - Chapter 6 (Levin, Deutsch, Kafri, and Liebermann) describes how reaching and grasping movements in VR can be improved by providing haptic feedback.
   - Chapters 5 (Wright, Creem-Regehr, Warren, Anson, Jeka, and Keshner) and Chap. 9 (Lamontagne, Keshner, Bugnariu, and Fung) discuss how we can capture and potentially modify cortical processing by presenting realistic, multisensory conflicts that engage the performer in both planning and performance of a motor task.

4. *More flexible off-the-shelf systems* (e.g., availability of Kinect Software Developer's Kit versus the previous non-accessibility to rehabilitation users).
   - Chapter 6 (Levin Deutsch, Kafri, and Liebermann) discusses the validity of the movements made by the user of commercially available systems compared to VR applications developed specifically for rehabilitation.
   - Chapter 10 (Green and Wilson) presents some of these systems for pediatric interventions.

5. *The "empowered" clinician*. Clinicians are more aware of the literature and more able to discern which technologies merit adoption and which have not yet reached the Hype cycle "plateau". All of the chapters in this volume provide considerable evidence about the clinical use of VR applications for motor rehabilitation. A recent review (e.g., Saposnik & Levin, 2011) summarizes the evidence.
   - Chapter 8 (Mirelman, Deutsch, and Hausdorff) and Chap. 9 (Green and Wilson) discuss the impact of VR tools on clinical practice.

11.6 Key Restraining Forces as Identified in this Volume

1. *Cumbersome and expensive equipment* (e.g., lack of fidelity). Examples include:

   - Chapter 6 (Levin, Deutsch, Kafri, and Liebermann) discusses several significant limitations that this technology has for rehabilitation. Discussed here are the weight and limited field of view available in HMDs, low-resolution motion tracking, size of devices that limit accurate hand and finger movement, and the lack of haptic feedback for collision detection and knowledge of results.
   - Chapters 4 (Kenyon and Ellis), Chap. 5 (Wright, Creem-Regehr, Warren, Anson, Jeka, and Keshner), and Chap. 9 (Lamontagne, Keshner, Bugnariu, and Fung) focus on the technological demands that require both engineering and computer skills and limit accessibility and maintenance by clinicians in the clinical environment.

2. *Lack of "strong" research design and rigorous measurement* and selection of *appropriate clinical outcomes* that can attest to the effectiveness of an intervention to evaluate clinical effectiveness of VR-based motor rehabilitation interventions. Although this may be related to the difficulty in obtaining funding, this issue limits the undertaking of large randomized controlled trials as well as the continuing development of technology (the system often changes before it has been fully evaluated). Examples include:

   - Chapter 2 (Cheung, Tunik, Adamovich, and Boyd) and Chap. 9 (Lamontagne, Keshner, Bugnariu, and Fung) discuss issues related to the specificity of the data collected, namely that it is dependent on additional technologies that are not always available or have not yet been correlated with the behaviors observed in the virtual environment. For example, measurement of changes in movement patterns requires access to high-resolution motion tracking technology.
   - Chapter 4 (Kenyon and Ellis) and Chap. 5 (Wright, Creem-Regehr, Warren, Anson, Jeka, and Keshner) discuss how VR impacts visual perception, which is inherently variable. Added to the variability found within clinical populations, this can weaken generalizations about the effectiveness of any intervention.

3. *Difficulties in achieving truly multimodal VR experiences*. Given the limitations of technology, it is not possible to provide clients with experiences in virtual rehabilitation that are truly reminiscent of the actual physical requirements e.g., true haptic feedback, realistic navigation while performing tasks. Examples include:

   - Chapter 6 (Levin, Deutsch, Kafri, and Liebermann) discusses applications aimed at upper limb rehabilitation that do not identify when motor compensations occur.
   - Chapter 3 (Levac and Sveistrup) discusses the lack of consistent and modifiable provision of feedback to the user in commercial applications.

4. *Lack of acceptance of technology* by some stakeholders due to insufficient familiarity with technology, cost, or technical barriers. Although not referred to directly in the chapters of this volume, Kizony, Weiss, and Rand provide related material about the acceptability of technology in their chapter in Volume 4 of this series.

11.7 Conclusion

There is a French expression "plus ça change, plus c'est la même chose" meaning the more things change, the more they remain the same. That is, many of the phenomena that we observe as new in our lives today have also been observed in the past. This expression is very applicable to many of the positive and negative "forces" that drive or constrain technology usage for motor rehabilitation. It is interesting to recall the following statement that was reported in the London Times in 1834 about the then new technology, the stethoscope:

> That it will ever come into general use, notwithstanding its value, is extremely doubtful; because its beneficial application requires much time and gives a good bit of trouble both to the patient and the practitioner; because its hue and character are foreign and opposed to all our habits and associations. Clinicians will not take kindly to accepting changes that are detrimental to existing working processes unless there are significant or proven benefits. (http://www.futurehealthit.com/2006/01/stethoscope.html).

A similar statement could have just as easily been made in more modern times about hundreds of invented technologies. Novel devices, techniques and programs will continue to challenge the abilities of both researchers to investigate them and clinicians to adopt them. Yet the example of the positive impact of the stethoscope on health care, as well as numerous other innovations, has been echoed throughout the chapters of this volume. Despite its acknowledged limitations, technology innovation in rehabilitation is clearly here to stay. Its success for rehabilitation will likely be the result of continuing careful analyses and reviews made by researchers and clinicians, notwithstanding a healthy dose of scepticism.

References

Burdea, G. C., Cioi, D., Martin, J., Fensterheim, D., & Holenski, M. (2010). The Rutgers Arm II Rehabilitation System—A Feasibility Study. *IEEE Transactions on Neural Systems and Rehabilitation Engineering, 18*(5), 505–514.

Deutsch, J. E., Merians, A. S., Burdea, G. C., Boian, R., Adamovich, S. V., & Poizner, H. (2002). Haptics and virtual reality used to increase strength and improve function in chronic individuals post-stroke: Two case reports. *Neurology Report, 26*, 79–86.

Greer, C. R., & Lei, D. (2012). Collaborative innovation with customers: A review of the literature and suggestions for future research. *International Journal of Management Reviews, 14*, 63–84.

Holden, M. K. (2005). Virtual environments for motor rehabilitation: Review. *CyberPsychology & Behavior, 8*(3), 187–211.

Jack, D., Boian, R., Merians, A. S., Tremaine, M., Burdea, G. C., Adamovich, S. V., et al. (2001). Virtual reality-enhanced stroke rehabilitation. *IEEE Transactions on Neural Systems and Rehabilitation Engineering, 9*(3), 308–318.

Keshner, E. A., & Kenyon, R. V. (2004). Using immersive technology for postural research and rehabilitation. *Assistive Technology, 16*, 54–62.

Keshner, E. A., Kenyon, R. V., Dhaher, Y. Y., & Streepey, J. W. (2005). Employing a virtual environment in postural research and rehabilitation to reveal the impact of visual information. *International Journal on Disability and Human Development, 4*, 177–182.

King, R. K. (2004). *Enhancing SWOT analysis using TRIZ and the bipolar conflict graph: A case study on the Microsoft Corporation, Proceedings of TRIZCON2004, 6th Annual Altshuller Institute*.

Knaut, L. A., Subramanian, S., McFadyen, B. J., Bourbonnais, D., & Levin, M. F. (2009). Kinematics of pointing movements made in a virtual versus a physical 3D environment in stroke. *Archives of Physical Medicine and Rehabilitation, 90*(5), 793–802.

Koch, A. J. (2000). *SWOT does not need to be recalled: It needs to be enhanced*. Retrieved from http://www.westga.edu/~bquest/2001/swot2.htm. Accessed 16 Sept 2013

Krebs, H. I., Hogan, N., Aisen, M. L., & Volpe, B. T. (1998). Robot-aided neurorehabilitation. *IEEE Transactions on Rehabilitation Engineering, 6*(1), 75–87.

Lewin, K. (1943; 1997). Defining the field at a given time. *Psychological Review, 50*, 292–310. Republished in *Resolving Social Conflicts & Field Theory in Social Science*, Washington, DC: American Psychological Association, 1997.

Riva, G., Carelli, L., Gaggioli, A., Gorini, A., Vigna, C., Corsi, R., et al. (2009). NeuroVR 1.5 - a free virtual reality platform for the assessment and treatment in clinical psychology and neuroscience. *Studies in Health Technology and Informatics, 142*, 268–270.

Rizzo, A. A., Buckwalter, J. G., Bowerly, T., van der Zaag, C., Humphrey, L., Neumann, U., et al. (2000). The virtual classroom: A virtual environment for the assessment and rehabilitation of attention deficits. *CyberPsychology & Behavior, 3*, 483–500.

Rizzo, A. A., Buckwalter, J. G., & Neumann, U. (1997). Virtual reality and cognitive rehabilitation: A brief review of the future. *Journal of Head Trauma and Rehabilitation, 12*, 1–15.

Rizzo, A. A., & Kim, G. (2005). A SWOT analysis of the field of Virtual Rehabilitation and Therapy. *Presence: Teleoperators and Virtual Environments, 14*, 1–28.

Rizzo, A. A., Buckwalter, J. G., & van der Zaag, C. (2002). Virtual environment applications for neuropsychological assessment and rehabilitation. In K. Stanney (Ed.), *Handbook of virtual environments* (pp. 1,027–1,064). New York: Erlbaum.

Saposnik, G., & Levin, M. F. (2011). Virtual reality in stroke rehabilitation: A metanalysis and implications for clinicians. *Stroke, 42*(5), 1380–1386.

Subramanian, S., Knaut, L. A., Beaudoin, B., McFadyen, B. J., Feldman, A. G., & Levin, M. F. (2007). Virtual reality environments for post-stroke arm rehabilitation. *Journal of NeuroEngineering and Rehabilitation, 4*, 20.

Sveistrup, H. (2004). Motor rehabilitation using virtual reality. *Journal of Neuroengineering and Rehabilitation, 1*, 10.

Turner, S. (2002). *Tools for success: A manager's guide*. London: McGraw-Hill.

Viau, A., Feldman, A. G., Mcfadyen, B. J., & Levin, M. F. (2004). Reaching in reality and virtual reality: A comparison of movement kinematics in healthy subjects and in adults with hemiparesis. *Journal of NeuroEngineering and Rehabilitation, 1*, 11.

Weiss, P. L. (2005). The future is already here: Aiming for excellence. *Israel Journal of Occupational Therapy, 14*, E59–E71.

Weiss, P. L., Sveistrup, H., Rand, D., & Kizony, R. (2009). Video capture virtual reality: A decade of rehabilitation assessment and intervention. *Physical Therapy Reviews, 14*, 307–321.

Index

P.L. (Tamar) Weiss et al. (eds.), *Virtual Reality for Physical and Motor Rehabilitation*, Virtual Reality Technologies for Health and Clinical Applications, DOI 10.1007/978-1-4939-0968-1, © Springer Science+Business Media New York 2014

MIX
Papier aus verantwortungsvollen Quellen
Paper from responsible sources
FSC® C105338

If you have any concerns about our products,
you can contact us on
ProductSafety@springernature.com

In case Publisher is established outside the EU,
the EU authorized representative is:
Springer Nature Customer Service Center GmbH
Europaplatz 3, 69115 Heidelberg, Germany

Printed by Libri Plureos GmbH
in Hamburg, Germany